EQUINE
MEDICINE
SECRETS

EQUINE MEDICINE SECRETS

CATHERINE J. SAVAGE, BVSc, MS, PhD, Dip ACVIM
Assistant Professor
Equine Internal Medicine
College of Veterinary Medicine and Biomedical Sciences
Veterinary Teaching Hospital
Colorado State University
Fort Collins, Colorado

HANLEY & BELFUS, INC./ Philadelphia

Publisher: HANLEY & BELFUS, INC.
              Medical Publishers
              210 South 13th Street
              Philadelphia, PA 19107
              (215) 546-7293; 800-962-1892
              FAX (215) 790-9330
              Web site: http://www.hanleyandbelfus.com

Note to the reader: Although the information in this book has been carefully reviewed for correctness of dosage and indications, neither the authors nor the editor nor the publisher can accept any legal responsibility for any errors or omissions that may be made. Neither the publisher nor the editor makes any warranty, expressed or implied, with respect to the material contained herein. Before prescribing any drug, the reader must review the manufacturer's current product information (package inserts) for accepted indications, absolute dosage recommendations, and other information pertinent to the safe and effective use of the product described.

Library of Congress Cataloging-in-Publication Data

Equine medicine secrets / edited by Catherine J. Savage.
        p.   cm. — (The Secrets Series®)
      Includes bibliographical references and index.
      ISBN 1-56053-263-7 (alk. paper)
        1. Horses—Diseases—Examinations, questions, etc.   2. Horses—
      Health—Examinations, questions, etc..   I. Savage, Catherine J.,
      1965–   . II. Series.
      SF951.E574   1998
      636.1'089—dc21
      DNLM/DLC
      for Library of Congress   98-40692
                                                                CIP

EQUINE MEDICINE SECRETS   ISBN 1-56053-263-7

Last digit is the print number: 9 8 7 6 5 4 3 2 1

CONTENTS

CONTRIBUTORS

Scott Matthew Austin, DVM, MS, Dip ACVIM
Wisconsin Equine Clinic, Inc., Oconomowoc, Wisconsin

Leanne Mary Begg, BVSc, Dip VCS, MS, MACVSc, Dip ACVIM
Partner, Randwick Equine Centre, Randwick, New South Wales, Australia

Virginia Ann Buechner-Maxwell, DVM, MS, Dip ACVIM
Assistant Professor, Virginia-Maryland Regional College of Veterinary Medicine, Blacksburg, Virginia

Mark V. Crisman, DVM, MS, Dip ACVIM
Associate Professor, Virginia-Maryland Regional College of Veterinary Medicine, Blacksburg, Virginia

David A. Dargatz, DVM, MS, PhD, Dip ACVIM
Analytic Epidemiologist, United States Department of Agriculture, Veterinary Services, Centers for Epidemiology and Animal Health, Fort Collins, Colorado

Charles Edward Dickinson, DVM, MS, Dip ACVIM
Colorado State University Veterinary Teaching Hospital, Fort Collins, Colorado

Melinda Ann Edwards, DVM
Resident, Department of Equine Internal Medicine, Colorado State University College of Veterinary Medicine and Biomedical Sciences, Fort Collins, Colorado

Melissa T. Hines, DVM, PhD, Dip ACVIM
Associate Professor, Washington State University Veterinary Teaching Hospital, Pullman, Washington

David Ross Hodgson, BVSc, PhD, Dip ACVIM, FACSM
Associate Professor and Hospital Director, University of Sydney Veterinary Centre, Camden, New South Wales, Australia

Susan Holcombe, VMD, MS, PhD, Dip ACVS
Assistant Professor, Department of Large Animal Clinical Sciences, Michigan State University, East Lansing, Michigan

Anthony P. Knight, BVSc, MS, MRCVS, Dip ACVIM
Professor, Department of Clinical Sciences, Colorado State University Veterinary Teaching Hospital, Fort Collins, Colorado

Chris Kawcak, DVM, MS, Dip ACVS
Assistant Professor, Department of Clinical Sciences, Colorado State University Veterinary Teaching Hospital, Fort Collins, Colorado

Guy Lester, BVMS, PhD, Dip ACVIM
Assistant Professor, University of Florida College of Veterinary Medicine, Gainesville, Florida

William B. Ley, DVM, MS, Dip ACT
Professor of Equine Production Management Medicine, Virginia-Maryland Regional College of Veterinary Medicine, Blacksburg, Virginia

Jennifer M. MacLeay, DVM, Dip ACVIM
Clinical Instructor, University of Minnesota College of Veterinary Medicine, St. Paul, Minnesota

Jill Johnson McClure, DVM, MS, Dip ACVIM, ABVP
Professor of Equine Medicine, Louisiana State University Veterinary Teaching Hospital and Clinics, Baton Rouge, Louisiana

J. Trenton McClure, DVM, MS, Dip ACVIM
Assistant Professor of Large Animal Medicine, Department of Health Management, University of Prince Edward Island, Charlottetown, Prince Edward Island, Canada

Rebecca S. McConnico, DVM, PhD, Dip ACVIM
Assistant Profesor of Equine Medicine, Department of Clinical Sciences, Oklahoma State University College of Veterinary Medicine, Stillwater, Oklahoma

Mary Rose Paradis, DVM, MS, Dip ACVIM
Associate Professor, Tufts University School of Veterinary Medicine, North Grafton, Massachusetts

Elias E. Perris, DVM
Clinical Instructor, Ohio State University College of Veterinary Medicine, Columbus, Ohio

Richard J. Piercy, MA, Vet MB
Clinical Instructor, Ohio State University College of Veterinary Medicine, Columbus, Ohio

Stephen M. Reed, DVM, Dip ACVIM
Professor and Head, Department of Equine Medicine and Surgery, Ohio State University College of Veterinary Medicine, Columbus, Ohio

Laura K. Reilly, VMD, Dip ACVIM
Adjunct Assistant Professor of Medicine, University of Pennsylvania School of Veterinary Medicine, Parkesburg, Pennsylvania

Catherine J. Savage, BVSc, MS, PhD, Dip ACVIM
Assistant Professor, Department of Equine Internal Medicine, Colorado State University College of Veterinary Medicine and Biomedical Sciences, Fort Collins, Colorado

Harold C. Schott, II, DVM, PhD, Dip ACVIM
Assistant Professor, Department of Large Animal Clinical Sciences, Michigan State University, East Lansing, Michigan

Debra C. Sellon, DVM, PhD, Dip ACVIM
Department of Veterinary Clinical Sciences, Washington State University, Pullman, Washington

William S. Swecker, Jr, DVM, PhD, Dip ACVN
Associate Professor, Virginia-Maryland Regional College of Veterinary Medicine, Blacksburg, Virginia

Corinne R. Sweeney, DVM, Dip ACVIM
Associate Professor of Medicine, University of Pennsylvania New Bolton Center, Kennett Square, Pennsylvania

Craig D. Thatcher, DVM, MS, PhD, Dip ACVN
Professor, Virginia-Maryland Regional College of Veterinary Medicine, Blacksburg, Virginia

Josie L. Traub-Dargatz, DVM, MS, Dip ACVIM
Professor, Equine Internal Medicine, Colorado State University Veterinary Teaching Hospital, Fort Collins, Colorado

Stephanie J. Valberg, DVM, PhD, Dip ACVIM
Associate Professor, University of Minnesota College of Veterinary Medicine, St. Paul, Minnesota

PREFACE

Equine Internal Medicine is an art as well as a science. It involves questioning clients (owners, trainers, and grooms) to get a full medical history, as our patients cannot talk. It involves introspection as we formulate a differential diagnosis and rationalize which diagnostic tests make sense and in what order they should be performed. More questions need to be asked when therapeutic or management plans are being formulated. We must take into account the degree of medical treatment required, patient comfort, client desires and compliance, economics, and prognosis for survival versus prognosis for desired performance level.

Veterinary students are taught through a question-and-answer format in rounds, on clinics, and during examinations. The education continues through professional veterinary medicine courses, National Boards, and specialization (e.g., internal medicine boards, American College of Veterinary Internal Medicine). The question-and-answer format in this book is a valuable method of focusing on important information that is topic-related. The text provides key material on topics so that those who have difficulty selecting essential knowledge from that which is pertinent but supplementary are able to focus on topic-related questions. It can be of great assistance to students during their clinical years, as well as a great source of easily assimilated, direct information for veterinarians, veterinary technicians and nurses, and trainers and owners of horses.

I am indebted to the collaborators of this text for their great contributions in undertaking this novel approach to the continuing education of veterinary students, veterinarians, and other people interested in the health and well-being of horses.

Kate (C. J.) Savage, BVSC, MS, PhD, Dip. ACVIM

Dedication

To my husband, Charles Kuntz, our son, Nicholas, and my parents, Lan and Ted Savage, without whose love and support this book and everything else of importance would never have been achieved.

1. GENERAL MEDICINE

Catherine J. Savage, B.V.Sc., M.S., Ph.D., Dip. ACVIM

1. What is Cushing's syndrome?

Cushing described a syndrome of edema, hirsutism, osteoporosis, truncal obesity, weakness, amenorrhea, hypertension, glucosuria, and a basophilic tumor of the pituitary in humans. Since the first description and naming of the disease (for the pituitary adenoma), the complex of endogenous Cushing's syndrome has been broadened to include all cases with increased production of cortisol by the adrenal gland, including (1) adrenal hyperplasia secondary to pituitary overproduction of adrenocorticotropic hormone (ACTH); (2) adrenal hyperplasias secondary to nonpituitary, paraneoplastic ACTH production by some nonendocrine tumors; (3) adrenal neoplasia; and (4) adrenal nodular hyperplasia. Exogenous, iatrogenic causes such as prolonged use of corticosteroids or ACTH have been described as iatrogenic Cushing's syndrome.

In horses, Cushing's syndrome is also termed pituitary adenoma, diffuse adenomatous hyperplasia, pituitary hyperplasia, and chromophobe adenoma. It differs from the human and small animal syndromes because the tumor or hyperplasia of the pituitary involves the pars intermedia rather than the accessory lobe of the pituitary.

2. After rectal palpation of a 13-year-old Thoroughbred mare you discover frank blood on the dorsal surface of your rectal sleeve. How should you proceed?

1. Physically restrain the horse (e.g, stocks, twitch, hindlimb-neck rope).

2. Sedate the horse (e.g,. xylazine, 0.3–0.5 mg/kg intravenously, or detomidine, 0.01 mg/kg intravenously), combined with butorphanol, 0.01 mg/kg intravenously).

3. Perform caudal epidural anesthesia, using 100 mg of mepivacaine for a 500-kg (1100-lb) horse, with a 3–5-cm, 20–22-gauge needle.

4. Attempt bare-handed rectal palpation and rectal speculum examination, using a well-lubricated hand and arm (hydrated methylcellulose) to examine and characterize the tear.

5. Remove feces remaining in the rectum to minimize bulk in the rectum and to reduce contamination at the tear site.

6. Locate the tear by gentle and careful circumferential, progressive palpation of the rectum.

7. Prevent further contamination of the injury, especially for grade 3 and 4 tears. Fill a stockinette with 0.25 kg of rolled cotton moistened with disinfectant such as povidone-iodine solution or chlorhexidine, or wrap 0.25 kg of moistened rolled cotton with soft bandage or gauze. The pack should be about 25 cm in length. Lubricate thoroughly with surgical lubricant (e.g, Surgilube, E. Fougera & Co., Melville, NY). Insert this pack about 10 cm craniad to the tear (not within the tear, thus extending it) so that the pack is in front of, covering, and behind the tear. The pack can be fastened with towel clamps, or a pursestring suture can be placed in the anus to keep it in position.

8. Ensure that the epidural anesthesia is sufficient for the time required to transport the horse to a referral center. Another incremental dose of mepivacaine may be required because the pack will cause substantial rectal straining if the epidural anesthesia wears off and thus may extend the tear.

9. Treat the horse with mineral oil via nasogastric intubation to soften feces.

10. Begin a broad-spectrum antimicrobial regimen to cover anaerobes and gram-negative and gram-positive aerobes. Examples include (1) metronidazole (15 mg/kg orally 4 times/day), procaine penicillin G (40,000 IU/kg intramuscularly 2 times/day) or potassium penicillin (40,000 IU/kg intravenously 4 times/day), and gentamicin (6.6 mg/kg intravenously or intramuscularly every 24 hours) **or** (2) metronidazole (15 mg/kg orally 4 times/day), ceftiofur (2.2 mg/kg intravenously or intramuscularly 2 times/day), and gentamicin (6.6 mg/kg intravenously or intramuscularly every 24 hours). Inform the referral center in writing of the medications that you have administered so that dangerous levels of drugs are not given (i.e., readministered because of poor communication).

11. Give a tetanus toxoid vaccine or tetanus antitoxin, depending on vaccine history.

12. Administer a nonsteroidal antiinflammatory drug (NSAID; e.g., flunixin meglumine, 0.5–1.0 mg/kg intravenously). Ensure that you inform the referral center in writing of the medications that you have administered so that dangerous levels of NSAIDs are not given.

13. Do not allow the horse to be fed. If possible, provide or help the owner manufacture a muzzle from a bucket so that the horse cannot eat straw in the trailer.

14. Client communication is essential, even if it is difficult. The client should be told that inexperience of the examiner does not always contribute to production of a rectal tear. The veterinarian must gauge what the client wants to do with the horse; however, all horses with grade 3 and 4 rectal tears should be examined at a referral center, if possible. It should be ascertained whether the horse is insured, what for, and by whom.

15. Communication with the veterinary association to which you belong is also essential.

16. Inform your malpractice insurance company promptly.

17. Communicate with veterinarians at a referral center (even if the owner does not permit transport of the horse to a referral center) so that everything is done for the horse in a timely fashion. This step improves the veterinarian's chances in court if the owners try to take legal action.

18. Abdominal centesis may be performed in the sedated horse if you wish to ascertain whether there is gross contamination of the peritoneal cavity or whether the protein concentration or total nucleated cell count is rising. This information can be useful for clients in deciding what they want to do and how they wish to proceed.

Baird AN: Rectal tears. In Robinson EN (ed): Current Therapy in Equine Medicine, vol. 3. Philadelphia, W.B. Saunders, 1992, pp 232–236.

Baird AN, Taylor TS, Watkins JP: Rectal packing as initial management of grade 3 rectal tears. Equine Vet J Suppl 7:121, 1989.

3. How are rectal tears graded?

GRADE	DEFINITION	PROGNOSIS/DEGREE OF INTERVENTION REQUIRED
1	Mucosal tear only.	Good prognosis; little or no intervention required.
2	Muscularis layer tear only. Mucosa and serosa are intact. Grade 2 tear feels like dip/diverticulum in mucosa. Usually no blood on glove, but veterinarian may have have felt release in tension over hand as muscularis layer tore.	Good prognosis—seldom of immediate clinical significance, although they may cause chronic changes that impede future palpation. Occasionally a large diverticulum is created (despite its coverage by mucosal layer) and may require suturing (per rectum) so that it does not act as a reservoir for fecal material. Suturing is recommended only if diverticulum is > 4 cm in diameter.
3	Mucosa, submucosa, and muscularis layers are torn.	Prognosis is guarded to poor. Intervention ultimately depends on position (i.e., 3A vs. 3B); however, initial management should be followed as in question 2.
3A	Leaves only serosal layer intact.	Guarded-to-poor prognosis; maximal intervention required.
3B	Occurs in dorsalmost region of rectum (e.g., 10 o'clock to 2 o'clock). Grade 3B tears enter mesocolon (i.e., fat-filled region between two layers of serosa).	Guarded-to-poor prognosis. Tear entering mesocolon prevents contamination into abdomen, but abscess formation is likely because tear into mesocolon causes contaminated pocket. Such pockets can abscessate and may even rupture into abdomen, thus forming grade 4 tear. Maximal intervention is required.
4	Disruption of all layers of rectal wall (i.e., mucosa, submucosa, muscularis, and serosa), causing entrance into abdominal cavity.	Grave prognosis; maximal intervention required.

Baird AN: Rectal tears. In Robinson EN (ed): Current Therapy in Equine Medicine, vol. 3. Philadelphia, W.B. Saunders, 1992, pp 232–236.

4. If you wanted to palpate rectally a 2-year-old Arabian stallion, what should you do before and immediately after insertion of your arm?

To perform a thorough rectal examination, the veterinarian must consider the safety of him/herself and the horse. **Restraint** is essential, whether physical (e.g., stocks, twitch, restraint of a hindlimb, via a rope fixing the pastern of the hindlimb contralateral to the arm that the veterinarian is using to palpate, to the neck of the horse), chemical (e.g., sedation with xylazine or detomidine with or without butorphanol), or a combination of both.

Adequate **lubrication** of the rectum is essential to perform the examination safely. The most commonly used lubricant is hydrated methylcellulose. **Local anesthesia** of the rectum appears to decrease straining by the horse as the rectum is entered and during palpation. Some veterinarians add lidocaine directly into the lubricant bottle, whereas others infuse 50–60 ml of 2% lidocaine (or mepivacaine) directly into the rectum with a well-lubricated syringe. Local anesthesia should be used in all stallions, young horses, and breeds thought to have small rectums (e.g., Arabians) or tight anal sphincters.

It is best to invert the rectal sleeve and to cover it with a **soft latex glove**. The lubricated hand should be massaged slowly through the anal sphincter to enter the rectum. At this stage **fecal material should be evacuated,** assessed (e.g., smell, fluidity, volume, degree of mucus coverage), and collected (e.g., for culture of *Salmonella* or *Clostridium* species or for evaluation of sand content) as needed. The arm can then be moved forward unless a peristaltic contraction is passing over the hand, in which case the hand should be retracted until the contraction passes to minimize the possibility of rectal tear. **Slow and methodical evaluation** can then be made of the left kidney, splenic edge, renosplenic ligament and space, bowel, urinary bladder, urethra, accessory sex organs in male horses, and ovaries, uterus, and cervix in female horses.

5. An owner tells you that her horse died after being hit by lightning. She asks for a death certificate so that the insurance company will pay. What should you do?

Both man-made electricity and lightning are capable of producing electric shock and death in a horse. Lightning is high-voltage electricity (estimates of approximately 1 million volts have been made), whereas the electricity supply to most barns in the U.S. is 110 volts. The voltage varies internationally.

Animals that have been struck by lightning are usually found dead with no evidence of struggle. Death is thought to be instantaneous (e.g., feed may still be in the mouth, the ground surrounding them is smooth). Singe marks are most commonly present on the legs. The horse may be under a tree, but a lightning strike also may occur in an open pasture or barn. Horses can survive lightning strike but usually show clinical signs such as hyperexcitability, nystagmus, evidence of vestibular disease, blindness, obtunded mentation, hyperesthesia, ataxia, and paralysis. The nervous tissue of the body, in comparison with the rest of the body tissues, is thought to be an excellent electrical conductor; clinical signs are usually due to nervous system damage.

Before the veterinarian claims that the death of the horse is due to lightning strike, a complete examination of the horse's immediate environment and external appearance should be made. Then a complete necropsy should be performed to exclude other causes of death.

6. How do you differentiate eosinophils from neutrophils and basophils (i.e., the other granulocytes) in equine blood?

The eosinophils of horses are characterized by a large number of extremely large specific granules, which are visible in the cell cytoplasm on light microscopic evaluation. These granules stain pink (i.e., are strongly eosinophilic; hence the name of the cell) when blood is stained with hematoxylin-eosin.

7. What dermatomycotic infections occur in horses? How can they be diagnosed?

In recent years recognition of equine dermatophytic infections has increased significantly. Many species cause lesions in horses, but the most commonly isolated species include (1) *Microsporum canis*, (2) *Microsporum gypseum*, (3) *Trichophyton mentagrophytes*, and (4) *Trichophyton equinum*. *M. canis* fluoresces under a Wood's lamp; the other three do not. Other species that are isolated frequently include *Trichophyton verrucosum, Trichophyton schoenleinii,* and *Keratinomyces ajelloi.*

The agent usually infects the superficial, keratinized areas of the skin and sometimes hair and hoof. Diagnosis can be made by using the Wood's lamp, which provides ultraviolet light causing greenish-blue fluorescence of hair infected with some dermatophytes, especially *M. canis.* A scraping from the affected skin, examined under light microscopy after mixing with a small volume of a 10–15% solution of potassium hydroxide, assists in recognition of spores and/or mycelia in some cases, although usually it does not assist in making a definitive diagnosis. Since actual speciation helps in understanding the epizootiology of the dermatophyte and thus mitigating the problem, it is important to culture the skin scraping. The best results occur when the medium contains antimicrobials to decrease competition by bacteria and when the inoculated medium is incubated for 2–5 weeks at 77–88° F (25–31° C). Once the culture has grown, microbiologists can identify the species based both on macroscopic colony characteristics and microscopic characteristics, such as shape and size of macro/microconidia, walls, and septation. Sometimes a skin biopsy is useful.

8. What is *Dermatophilus congolensis*? What factors predispose to infection in horses? What lesions does it cause?

D. congolensis is an aerobic, filamentous, branching organism that infects the skin and hair of horses. Predisposing factors to infection in horses include the following:
- Moistened/wet skin (e.g., rain, wet pastures)
- Traumatized skin (e.g., poorly fitting riding equipment, biting insects, maceration due to chronic moisture)
- Contact with infected crusts of another horse, goat, sheep, cattle, whether by direct contact or through fomites (e.g., flies). *D. congolensis* can survive in a crust for 2–4 months.

Lesions appear initially as moist skin with a serous exudate. With time the typical lesions appear as thickened crusts, most commonly affecting the pasterns and dorsum. The lesions are usually not pruritic or painful.

Evans AG: Dermatophilus: Diagnostic approach to nonpruritic, crusting dermatitis in horses. Compend Contin Educ Pract Vet 14:1618, 1992.

9. What is the cause of swamp cancer?

Swamp cancer, also known as pythiosis, phycomycocis, Florida leeches, and Gulf Coast fungus, is caused by an aquatic fungus (*Pythium insidiosum*) found in tropical regions of Australia, South America, and the Gulf Coast states of the United States.

10. Discuss urea poisoning in horses.

Horses cope with urea well and rarely show signs of toxicity. They absorb the urea from the small intestine before it can reach the colon and cecum, where most of the urease-producing bacteria are located in horses. Consequently, horses do not show signs unless the gastrointestinal system is greatly overloaded and urea reaches the large colon in an intact form. Head pressing and other neurologic manifestations of ammonia toxicity were seen in a pony when it was fed over 1 pound (i.e., approximately 2.2 mg/kg) of urea. This amount of urea probably overwhelmed the absorption capacity of the small intestine so that urea was able to reach the pony's large colon and cecum intact.

Urea itself is not toxic. However, if it reaches urease-containing bacteria in the large colon of the horse, it is converted to ammonia. Therefore, ammonia toxicity becomes the problem. Horses show fewer signs of urea toxicity than cattle. Since the rumen of cattle is a source of bacterial urease, urea is converted to ammonia in large amounts immediately. The ammonia is absorbed, and clinical signs develop.

11. What is the overall prevalence of gastric ulcers in foals and adult horses?

Reports about prevalence of gastric ulceration in foals range from 25–50%, depending on the age of the foal, gastric location, and presence or absence of clinical signs. Desquamation (with or without concurrent gastric erosion or ulceration) of gastric squamous epithelium occurs in up to 80% of foals.

Reports about the prevalence of gastric ulceration in adult horses vary. The prevalence appears to depend on the work performed, environment, and clinical signs in young/adult horses:
1. Adult horses with no clinical signs (52%)
2. Young adult horses not in training and with no clinical signs (36%)
3. Young adult horses in training and with no clinical signs (78%)
4. Adult horses with inappetance, colic, weight loss (92%)
5. Racing horses (90–100%)
6. Pleasure horses, including showing and riding lessons (~20–40%)
7. Adult horses on pasture (< 20%)

Murray MJ: Gastric ulcers in adult horses. Compend Contin Educ Pract Vet 16:792–794, 1994.
Murray MJ: Gastrointestinal ulceration. In Reed SM, Bayly WM (eds): Equine Internal Medicine. Philadelphia, W.B. Saunders, 1998, pp 615–623.

12. Is *Giardia* species a major cause of diarrhea in horses?

Members of *Giardia* species are not a major cause of diarrhea in horses, although they have been isolated from the feces of clinically normal horses as well as foals and adults with chronic diarrhea. Most veterinarians believe that adult horses with chronic diarrhea may have an abnormal gastrointestinal environment (e.g., increased fluidity) that predisposes to the presence of *Giardia* and *Trichomonas* species. If no other etiologic agents can be identified in horses with chronic diarrhea, some veterinarians treat the horses with metronidazole; results are variable.

13. What happens to the hemostatic (coagulation) profile in pre- and postparturient mares?

MEASUREMENT	MIDGESTATION	PARTURITION	POSTPARTURIENT STAGE
Plasma fibrinogen	Starts to show gradual increase; concentration increases in last month of gestation.	Concentration increases to approximate maximal concentration.	Decreases gradually.
Factor VIII:C	Starts to show gradual increase.	Reaches maximal level.	Decreases gradually.
von Willebrand factor	Starts to show gradual increase.	Reaches maximal level.	Decreases gradually.
Plasma fibronectin	Concentration increases in last month of gestation.	Concentration increases to approximate maximal concentration.	Concentration decreases.
Fibrinogen degradation products (FDPs)	Concentration increases in last month of gestation.	Concentration increases to approximate maximal concentration.	Concentration decreases.
Antithrombin III	Increases *slightly* in 10 days preceding parturition.	Decreases slightly.	Relatively constant.
Factors VII and IX	Relatively constant.	Relatively constant.	Relatively constant.
One-stage prothrombin time (PT)	Stable until 1 month before parturition, then decreases in last 14 days before parturition.	Increases slightly at parturition but less than before 10 months of gestation.	Increases slowly, but relatively constant.
Activated partial thromboplastin time (PTT)	Relatively constant.	Shortest duration just before parturition.	Increases slowly, but relatively constant.

The shortening of PT and PTT at or immediately before parturition may be an adaptation of the parturient mare, thus decreasing the likelihood of major hemorrhage.

Gentry PA, Feldman BF, O'Neill SL, et al: Evaluation of the haemostatic profile in the pre- and postparturient mare, with particular focus on the perinatal period. Equine Vet J 24:33–36, 1992.

14. If you diagnose thrombocytopenia in a horse with no clinical evidence of a bleeding tendency, what should you suspect?

You should suspect an ethylenediamine tetraacetic acid (EDTA)-dependent pseudothrombocytopenia, which may result from platelet clumping in blood that contains EDTA. To confirm this diagnosis, screen blood films for clumping of platelets and compare the platelet count obtained from whole (EDTA) blood with the platelet count obtained from heparinized blood in the same horse.

Hinchcliff KW, Kociba GI, Mitten LA: Diagnosis of EDTA-dependent pseudothrombocytopenia in a horse. J Am Vet Med Assoc 203:1715–1716, 1993.

15. What should you do if you perform a bone marrow aspirate on a horse and find no megakaryocytes?

Before deciding that the horse has a disorder of the megakaryocytic line, perform either another aspirate at a site distant from the first or perform a bone biopsy (better option). Within the bone marrow are certain discrete areas for the megakaryocytes and even for the myeloid and erythroid series of cells. Consequently, it is advisable to check whether the first aspirate simply missed megakaryocytes because a point sample was taken. A bone biopsy (e.g., wing of ilium) is an excellent method for determining all cell types and their spatial distribution within the bone marrow.

Savage CJ, Jeffcott LB, Melsen F, Ostblom LC: Bone biopsy in the horse. I. Method using the wing of ilium. J Vet Med A 38:776–783, 1991.

16. What are the naturally occurring anticoagulants?
1. Protein C (vitamin K-dependent)
2. Protein S (cofactor for protein C; vitamin K-dependent)
3. Antithrombin III (ATIII)

17. What is DIC?

DIC is disseminated intravascular coagulation, an acquired coagulopathy associated with diseases that cause escape of tissue substances into the circulation, endothelial damage (e.g., heat stroke), and vascular stasis. Most of the changes cause thrombin release into the systemic circulation. Disorders in horses that appear to precipitate DIC include severe medical disease (e.g., colitis, duodenitis-proximal jejunitis, burns, smoke inhalation), heat stroke, and, on rare occasions, surgical procedures (especially with ischemia-reperfusion injury). DIC occurs with generalized, diffuse activation of the hemostatic mechanism, which results in conversion of fibrinogen to fibrin by thrombin. This thrombin-induced conversion results in the generation of fibrinopeptides A and B. After production of a fibrin clot, plasmin lyses fibrin polymer (and even fibrin monomer and fibrinogen). Products of plasmin lysis are termed fragments X, Y, D, and E. DIC may result in consumption coagulopathy and hemorrhagic complications, even though the initial event is thrombotic in nature.

18. What clinicopathologic tests are useful in diagnosing DIC?

Since DIC is a dynamic process, sequential testing is essential. Tests that may be of use (although many have not been validated in horses) include the following:
1. Thrombocytopenia
2. Decreased fibrinogen
3. Increased fibrinogen degradation products (FDPs; especially fragments D and E)
4. Increased fibrinopeptides A and B
5. Decreased ATIII
6. Decreased protein C
7. Decreased plasminogen
8. Increased fibrin monomers
9. Increased PT
10. Increased PTT
11. Presence of red cell fragments (schistocytes)

Although FDPs and fibrinogen concentration are purported to be of use in diagnosing cases of DIC, they are unreliable in horses. In most domestic animals, FDPs are increased and fibrinogen is decreased (because it is consumed to make fibrin monomer and then destroyed by plasmin). FDPs, however, are elevated only in some horses, and fibrinogen is often normal or increased because of the effect of the inflammatory precursor (i.e., primary disease) of DIC.

19. What coagulation proteins are vitamin K-dependent?

The vitamin K-dependent coagulation proteins include (1) coagulation protein II (prothrombin), (2) coagulation protein VII (proconvertin, prothrombinogen), (3) coagulation protein IX (Christmas factor, hemophilic factor B), (4) coagulation protein X (Stuart factor), (5) protein C (an anticoagulant), and (6) protein S (cofactor for protein C and thus an anticoagulant). The easy way to remember the coagulation proteins is 2, 7, 9 (i.e., 2 + 7 = 9), and 10.

20. Are protein C and protein S concentrations normal in neonates (equine and human)?

The levels of protein C and protein S are low in equine and human neonates, presumably because of hepatic immaturity. Adult levels are often not reached until the fourth-to-sixth months of life. ATIII concentrations also may be decreased, but the normal neonate rarely has thromboembolic complications.

21. List the 12 coagulation proteins. Are they involved in the extrinsic, intrinsic, or common pathways?

CLOTTING PROTEIN (FACTOR)	NAME(S)	PATHWAY
I	Fibrinogen	Common
II	Prothrombin	Common
III	Tissue thromboplastin	Extrinsic
IV	Calcium	Required in first, second, and third stages of coagulation
V	Labile factor, plasma converting factor, accelerator factor, possibly platelet factor 1	Common
VI	Used to be called accelerin but no longer considered in scheme of hemostasis	—
VII	Proconvertin, prothrombinogen	Extrinsic
VIII	Hemophilic factor A	Intrinsic
IX	Hemophilic factor B, Christmas factor	Intrinsic
X	Stuart factor	Common
XI	Hemophilic factor C	Intrinsic
XII	Hageman factor	Intrinsic

22. What coagulation proteins are produced by the liver? What are the clinical signs of their dysfunction?

Hepatic production is important for many coagulation proteins, including I, II, V, VII, VIII (in part), IX, X, XI, and XII. Clinical signs of coagulopathy are excessive bleeding and hematoma formation from blood sampling sites (i.e., venipuncture or arterial sites), epistaxis, hemarthrosis (i.e., bleeding into the joint[s]), hemoabdomen, and hemothorax. These signs are consistent with dysfunctional secondary hemostasis (i.e., deficiencies in coagulation proteins).

23. What is the cause of Potomac horse fever?

The cause of Potomac horse fever is the monocytotropic rickettsial organism, *Ehrlichia risticii*. This disease is also termed equine monocytic ehrlichiosis.

Palmer JE: Potomac horse fever. Vet Clin North Am Equine Pract 9:399–410, 1993.

24. What is a common reservoir for the agent of Potomac horse fever, even if it is not a vector?

A pleurocid stream snail (*Juga* species), found in northern California, northern Nevada, Oregon, and Washington, has been identified as secreting *E. risticii*-infected cercariae (i.e., polymerase chain reaction [PCR] identification of *E. risticii* gene fragments from cercariae lysates). Cercariae are released from the snails after environmental warming (e.g., late spring, summer, early fall). This release period mimics the period of clinical cases of Potomac horse fever. It is possible that horses ingest infected cercariae in the water, encysted on vegetation, or even in an another intermediate host, such as an insect.

Recently putative *E. risticii* genes were isolated using PCR techniques in the lymnaeid snail (genus *Stagnicola*). This snail has a much wider distribution throughout the U.S. and may be involved in dissemination of Potomac horse fever in regions with endemic problems.

Barlough JE, Reubel GH, Madigan JE, et al: Detection of *Ehrlichia risticii*, the agent of Potomac horse fever, in freshwater stream snails (Peluroceridae; *Juga* spp.) from Northern California. Appl Environ Microbiol 64:2888–2893, 1998.

Reubel GH, Barough JE, Madigan JE: Production and characterization of *Ehrlichia risticii*, the agent of Potomac horse fever, in freshwater stream snails (Peluroceridae; *Juga* spp.) in aquarium culture and genetic comparison to equine strains. J Clin Microbiol 36:1501–1511, 1998.

25. How can aerosolized drugs be administered to a horse?

Devices available for inhalation therapy include jet and ultrasonic nebulizers and pressurized canisters for metered-dose inhalation. A new equine-friendly delivery device that can be used with either metered-dose inhalation pressurized canisters or nebulizers is the Aeromask. The Aeromask is a face mask with a valved mask and spacer. It comes in small, medium, and large sizes. It is supplied by Canadian Monaghan, 220 Adelaide Street, South London, Ontario, Canada (telephone: (800) 465-3296; facsimile: (519) 685-1202). A hand-held, nostril-adapted, metered-dose aerosol delivery system is under investigation by 3M Animal Care Products (St. Paul, MN) and probably will be useful in the equine industry.

26. What drugs can be given by aerosol delivery devices? Provide dose rates and general information about each.

1. **Corticosteroids**
   - Beclomethasone dipropionate, 42 µg/puff metered-dose inhaler (Beclovent), a surface active corticosteroid, does not cause the same level of adrenal suppression as systemic corticosteroids. Improvement starts at about day 3. It may be prudent to administer an antimicrobial (e.g., trimethoprim-sulfa) while the horse is given inhaled steroids. Dose = 1 puff per 45 kg (100 lb) twice daily (i.e., 10 puffs/450-kg [1000-lb] horse twice daily and 1 puff/newborn foal twice daily).
   - Beclomethasone dipropionate, 250 µg/puff metered-dose inhaler (Becloforte), is a more concentrated form. Dose = 1 puff per 400 lb twice daily (not suitable for foals).
   - Fluticasone, 220 mg/puff metered-dose inhaler (Flovent), is approximately 300 times more lipophilic than beclomethasone; therefore, it has a longer duration of action in the lung. Although it has the lowest risk of adrenal suppression, adrenal suppression may still occur. Dose = 1 puff/45 kg (1000 lb) twice daily (e.g., 10–13 puffs/adult horse twice daily).
2. **Bronchodilators**
   - Albuterol, 90 µg/puff metered-dose inhaler (Ventolin), is a β_2-adrenergic agonist. Dose = 1 puff per 45–70 kg (100–150 lb) 4 times/day (i.e., 1–2 µg/kg = 450 µg – 1000 µg); ~ 5–11 puffs/450-kg [1000-lb] horse 4 times/day and ~ 1 puff/newborn to 3-week-old foal 4 times/day). The duration of action is short (approximately 1 hour).
   - Ipratropium bromide (Atrovent), is an anticholinergic agent (i.e., it causes parasympathetic blockade of M3-muscarinic receptors on smooth muscle). Ipratropium bromide inhibits vagal-mediated cough and bronchoconstriction. Dose = 1.5 µg/kg. Although it has slower onset (30–60 minutes) compared with β_2-adrenergic agonists, its effects tend to last longer (4–6 hours).

- The combination of ipratropium bromide and albuterol (Combivent) has 18 μg of ipratropium bromide and 103 μg of albuterol per puff. This combination is synergistic.The usual dose is 10 puffs per horse, which is 1030 μg/horse of albuterol and 180 μg of ipratropium bromide. The albuterol is dosed at the high end of its dose range (i.e., 2 μg/kg) and the ipratropium bromide at the low end (i.e., 0.36 μg/kg instead of 1.5 μg/kg). Anecdotal evidence suggests benefits to horses.
3. **Mast cell-stabilizing drugs**
   - If bronchoalveolar lavage (BAL) has > 2% mast cells, use of a mast cell stabilizer (cromolyn sodium [Intal] or nedocromil sodium [Tilade]) may be indicated.

Derksen FJ: Inhalation therapy for the treatment of lower airway disease. In Robinson NE (ed): Current Therapy in Equine Medicine, vol. 4. Philadelphia, W.B. Saunders, 1997, pp 429–431.
Rush B: Antiinflammatory inhalation therapy in horses. Proc Am Coll Vet Intern Med 16:220–222, 1998.

27. Provide a protocol for inhalation therapy that may be suitable for a horse with severe heaves.

1. Administer Combivent metered-dose inhaler (combination of ipratropium bromide and albuterol).
2. After 5–10 minutes administer either fluticasone (Flovent) or beclomethasone dipropionate (e.g., Beclovent).

This protocol should be performed twice daily. A third dose of Combivent may be given 30 minutes before exercise and even used prophylactically before movement to a new, noncontrolled environment (e.g., stables at show). (Also see question 26.)

Derksen FJ: Inhalation therapy for the treatment of lower airway disease. In Robinson NE (ed): Current Therapy in Equine Medicine, vol. 4. Philadelphia, W.B. Saunders, 1997, pp 429–431.
Rush B: Antiinflammatory inhalation therapy in horses. Proc Am Coll Vet Intern Med 16:220–222, 1998.

28. What motility modifiers are available for equine ileus? Provide name and general information (e.g., action, dose, side effects) for each. Decide whether you would use the drug in a horse with ileus.

Ileus may be due to a variety of conditions, including sympathetic hyperactivity and dopaminergic hyperactivity.

AGENT	GENERAL INFORMATION	DECISION TO USE IN HORSE
Lidocaine	2% lidocaine is used as stock solution. Current recommendation is 1.3 mg/kg slow IV bolus (32.5 ml of 2% lidocaine) for 450–500-kg (100–1100-lb) horse, then 0.05 mg/kg/min (e.g., 75 ml of 2% lidocaine per liter of fluids, with rate of 1 L/hr for about 10 hr. Horses have been known to collapse with this protocol. Blocks sympathetic pain and is sodium-channel blocker (therefore antiarrhythmic drug).	Yes
Cisapride	40–60 mg per rectum (usual dose), although up to 1 mg/kg in propylene glycol per rectum has been tried. Unfortunately, per rectum route does not appear to achieve reasonable levels in most horses (i.e., poor absorption), although it has not yet been reported whether it has local effect on smooth muscle motility. No commercial intravenous form; however, when used experimentally, plasma levels achieved for about 2 hr.	Maybe* (absorption is major concern with per rectum administration)
Erythromycin	Motilin agonist (in other species) Colic signs 25 mg/kg orally every 6 hr	Maybe* (side effects cause concern)

Table continued on following page

AGENT	GENERAL INFORMATION	DECISION TO USE IN HORSE
Yohimbine	α_2-adrenergic blocker (i.e., opposite to xylazine and detomidine, which may predispose horses to ileus). Somewhat effective in horses experimentally.	Maybe
Neostigmine	Reversibly inactivates cholinesterase enzyme; therefore, acetyl choline accumulates (i.e., parasympathomimetic effects). Increases intestinal contraction. Delays gastric emptying and decreases propulsive activity of jejunum, although intestinal contractions are increased. This may be cause of colic signs commonly seen after administration. May work better on large colon. Short-acting (about 15–30 min). Dose: 0.02 mg/kg subcutaneously. Side effects of colic have been recorded.	Maybe* (side effects cause concern)
Bethanecol	Parasympathetic (pure muscarinic; therefore can be antagonized with atropine). Increases intestinal contraction. Dose: 0.025 mg/kg subcutaneously every 6–8 hr, then 0.03–0.3 mg/kg orally 4 times/day (varying doses have been proposed). Colic signs have been recorded.	Maybe* (side effects cause concern)
Domperidone	Dopaminergic antagonist. Dose: 0.2 mg/kg IV. Appears to work experimentally in horses. Does not cross blood-brain barrier; therefore, no CNS signs have been reported. No colic side effects reported.	Has promise
Metoclopramide	Nonspecific dopaminergic antagonist that may sensitize smooth muscle (especially of small intestine) to acetyl choline. Accelerates gastric emptying and decreases transit time in small intestine. Severe CNS (e.g., extreme excitement) and gastrointestinal side effects in horses. Dose: 0.25 mg/kg IV infusion or subcutaneously.	No (side effects cause concern)
Propranolol	β-adrenergic blockade (i.e., decreases sympathetic tone). Did *not* work in horses (vs. humans).	No

* Depends on clinician's positive and negative experiences.

29. An 18-year-old Thoroughbred mare has a heart rate of 90 beats per minute, respiration rate of 28 breaths per minute, sweating, and signs of abdominal pain (i.e., pawing, trying to lie down, attempting to roll). What should be the first treatment that you institute?

Pass a nasogastric tube, prime the nasogastric tube with water, and attempt to reflux the horse. Tranquilization may be necessary. It is imperative to pass a nasogastric tube to relieve gastric and small intestinal pressure. Gastric rupture may be imminent. Then the veterinarian can perform a rectal examination and ascertain whether loops of small intestine can be palpated.

30. What are the signs of acute uveitis vs. chronic uveitis? How does an owner usually describe the clinical signs of a horse with acute uveitis? Which breed of horse is predisposed to equine recurrent uveitis?

Acute uveitis
Miosis
Blepharospasm
Photophobia
Excessive lacrimation

Chronic uveitis
Posterior synechiae
Pigmentation of anterior lens capsule
Corpora nigra atrophy
Blindness

Conjunctivitis	Peripapillary depigmentation ("butterfly lesions")
Aqueous flare	Phthisis bulbi
Hypopyon	Lens luxation
Keratitic precipitates	Reduced intraocular pressure
Corneal edema	Glaucoma (increased intraocular pressure)
Chorioretinitis	Cataract formation

The owner may describe a horse with a weeping, squinting, red eye, indicating excessive lacrimation, blepharospasm, photophobia, and conjunctivitis. The breed that appears to be predisposed to equine recurrent uveitis (moon blindness, periodic ophthalmia) is the Appaloosa.

31. Is performance of a lung biopsy controversial in horses?

Yes. Lung biopsy is an invasive procedure, and severe complications have been observed by equine specialists. In a survey of the diplomates of the American College of Veterinary Internal Medicine (large animal specialty), 77% of respondents had seen at least one complication. The complication may be as mild as a period of tachycardia or mild epistaxis or as severe as collapse and death. However, most specialists indicated that they would perform lung biopsy in cases in which more information was needed. It remains prudent to warn owners about potential complications before performing percutaneous lung biopsy. Documented complications (% indicates respondents in survey who had seen at least 1 horse with the complication) included:

1. Epistaxis (68%)
2. Pulmonary hemorrhage (52%)
3. Tachypnea (39%)
4. Respiratory distress (32%)
5. Dyspnea (25%)
6. Collapse (23%)
7. Pneumothorax (20%)
8. Tachycardia (20%)
9. Death (18%; this percentage refers to the fact that 8 of 44 respondents reported the death of 12 of approximately 400 horses that underwent percutaneous lung biopsy. Thus the estimated death rate is 12 of 400 horses or 3%.)
10. Pale mucous membranes (14%)
11. Great vessel hemorrhage (5%)
12. One respondent reported peritonitis secondary to inadvertent biopsy of the bowel.

Not all respondents indicated how many times they had seen each complication, and no reliable frequency of occurrence could be determined. Of respondents who reported pulmonary or great vessel hemorrhage, a majority suspected the diagnosis and a minority confirmed its presence at necropsy.

Savage CJ, Traub-Dargatz JL, Mumford EL: Survey of the large animal diplomates of the American College of Veterinary Internal Medicine regarding percutaneous lung biopsy in the horse. J Vet Intern Med 12:8–16, 1998.

32. About what risks should you warn the owner of a horse that is to undergo percutaneous lung biopsy?

Owners should be warned about possible risks of the procedure so that they can make an educated decision about whether they want a lung biopsy performed in their horse. Veterinarians should warn owners about the possibility of coughing, hemothorax, peritonitis, hospitalization for at least 24 hours, unspecified general risks, collapse, fever, sepsis or spread of infection to the pleural cavity, tachypnea, respiratory distress, pneumothorax, hemorrhage (e.g., epistaxis, hemoptysis, pulmonary hemorrhage), and death.

Savage CJ, Traub-Dargatz JL, Mumford EL: Survey of the large animal diplomates of the American College of Veterinary Internal Medicine regarding percutaneous lung biopsy in the horse. J Vet Intern Med 12:8–16, 1998.

33. List the major advantages and disadvantages of percutaneous lung biopsy.

The main **advantages** of a lung biopsy are that diseased lung can be obtained and analyzed histologically with light microscopy techniques or electron microscopy (e.g., for silicon particles in patients with suspected pneumoconiosis). Additional samples may be submitted for culture and sensitivity patterns (i.e., bacterial, fungal, and/or viral isolation). Biopsy improves diagnosis and therefore treatment and prognosis. Many owners elect lung biopsy if previous diagnostic tests have shown disease that is suspected to be severe. Lung biopsy in horses with diffuse disease is useful to obtain a specific etiologic diagnosis and to give an accurate prognosis.

The main **disadvantages** relate to the invasive nature of the biopsy and possible complications (see questions 31 and 32) and the fact that such small samples are removed (thus significant lesions may be overlooked).

Savage CJ, Traub-Dargatz JL, Mumford EL: Survey of the large animal diplomates of the American College of Veterinary Internal Medicine regarding percutaneous lung biopsy in the horse. J Vet Intern Med 12:8–16, 1998.

34. How can the different types of *Clostridium perfringens* be identified?

The different types of *Clostridium perfringens* can be identified by polymerase chain reaction (PCR) techniques. Identification is clinically important, because the pathogenicity of different types causing enterocolitis in foals appears to differ markedly (e.g., type A appears to cause less mortality than type C).

East LM, Savage CJ, Traub-Dagartz JL, et al: Enterocolitis associated with *Clostridium perfringens* infection in neonate foals: 54 cases (1988–1997). J Am Vet Med Assoc 212:1751–1756, 1998.

35. A 5-year-old Quarter Horse mare with a history of esophageal obstruction 7 days ago is now inappetant, and her mucous membranes are pale and possibly slightly cyanotic. The capillary refill time is 2.5–3 seconds. The heart rate is 58 beats per minute, and the respiration rate is 40 breaths per minute. An arterial blood gas reveals the following:

- pH = 7.28
- Partial pressure of oxygen in arterial blood (PaO_2) = 62 mmHg
- Partial pressure of carbon dioxide in arterial blood ($PaCO_2$) = 25 mmHg
- Bicarbonate (HCO_3) = 20 mEq/L
- Barometric pressure (P_B) = 740 mmHg (usually 760 mmHg at sea level)
- Water vapor pressure (P_{H_2O}) = 40 mmHg (47 mmHg when air is fully saturated at 37° C)

Calculate the alveolar-arterial O_2 difference.

To calculate the alveolar-arterial O_2 difference, the alveolar oxygen partial pressure (PAO_2) must be calculated. The PaO_2 (62 mmHg) is provided from the blood gas analysis. Room air contains 21% oxygen. Thus the easiest way to determine PAO_2 is to use the following formula:

$$PAO_2 = FiO_2 \times (P_B - P_{H_2O}) - PaCO_2/R$$

where FiO_2 = fractional concentration of inspired oxygen (i.e., 21% or 0.21 when breathing room air) and R = respiratory quotient (the ratio of CO_2 production to O_2 consumption, generally thought to be 0.8). P_B, P_{H_2O}, and $PaCO_2$ are provided on the blood gas analysis sheet. In a simplified manner:

PAO_2 = % O_2 in air × (barometric pressure – water vapor pressure) – $PaCO_2$/constant

$PAO_2 = 0.21 (740 - 40) - 25/0.8$

$PAO_2 = 147 - 31.25$

$PAO_2 = 115.75$

Thus the alveolar-arterial O_2 difference ($PAO_2 - PaO_2$) = 115.75 – 62 = 53.75 (~54). This value should be 0–10 (definitely < 20). A value of 54 reveals a great difference between oxygen tension in the alveoli (PAO_2) and arteries (PaO_2).

36. Why is the alveolar-arterial O_2 difference so useful?

The alveolar-arterial O_2 difference (also known as alveolar-arterial O_2 gradient, A–a gradient, $PAO_2 - PaO_2$) is useful because it tells us about barriers to oxygen diffusion from the alveoli to the arteries and gives information about the disease process. If we calculate the A–a gradient daily over time, we can prognosticate accurately about the disease process. If the value approaches normal, the barrier to diffusion is decreasing and the disease process (e.g., pneumonia) is improving. If the trend is toward an increase in the A–a gradient, we should reevaluate the treatment schedule; if the value is poor, we should reevaluate the prognosis for the horse.

BIBLIOGRAPHY

1. Baird AN: Rectal tears. In Robinson EN (ed): Current Therapy in Equine Medicine, vol. 3. Philadelphia, W.B. Saunders, 1992, pp 232–236.
2. Baird AN, Taylor TS, Watkins JP: Rectal packing as initial assessment of grade 3 rectal tears. Equine Vet J Suppl 7:121, 1989.
3. Barlough JE, Reubel GH, Madigan JE, et al: Detection of *Ehrlichia risticii*, the agent of Potomac horse fever, in freshwater stream snails (Peluroceridae; *Juga* spp.) from Northern California. Appl Environ Microbiol 64:2888–2893, 1998.
4. Derksen FJ: Inhalation therapy for the treatment of lower airway disease. In Robinson NE (ed): Current Therapy in Equine Medicine, vol. 4. Philadelphia, W.B. Saunders, 1997, pp 429–431.
5. East LM, Savage CJ, Traub-Dagartz JL, et al: Enterocolitis associated with *Clostridium perfringens* infection in neonate foals: 54 cases (1988–1997). J Am Vet Med Assoc 212:1751–1756, 1998.
6. Evans AG: Dermatophilus: Diagnostic approach to nonpruritic, crusting dermatitis in horses. Compend Contin Educ Pract Vet 14:1618, 1992.
7. Gentry PA, Feldman BF, O'Neill SL, et al: Evaluation of the haemostatic profile in the pre- and postparturient mare, with particular focus on the perinatal period. Equine Vet J 24:33–36, 1992.
8. Hinchcliff KW, Kociba GI, Mitten LA: Diagnosis of EDTA-dependent pseudothrombocytopenia in a horse. J Am Vet Med Assoc 203:1715–1716, 1993.
9. Murray MJ: Gastric ulcers in adult horses. Compend Contin Educ Pract Vet 16:792–794, 1994.
10. Murray MJ: Gastrointestinal ulceration. In Reed SM, Bayly WM (eds): Equine Internal Medicine. Philadelphia, W.B. Saunders, 1998, pp 615–623.
11. Palmer JE: Potomac horse fever. Vet Clin North Am Equine Pract 9:399–410, 1993.
12. Reubel GH, Barough JE, Madigan JE: Production and characterization of *Ehrlichia risticii*, the agent of Potomac horse fever, in freshwater stream snails (Peluroceridae; *Juga* spp.) in aquarium culture and genetic comparison to equine strains. J Clin Microbiol 36:1501–1511, 1998.
13. Rush B: Antiinflammatory inhalation therapy in horses. Proc Am Coll Vet Intern Med 16:220–222, 1998.
14. Savage CJ, Jeffcott LB, Melsen F, Ostblom LC: Bone biopsy in the horse. I. Method using the wing of ilium. J Vet Med Am 38:776–783, 1991.
15. Savage CJ, Traub-Dargatz JL, Mumford EL: Survey of the large animal diplomates of the American College of Veterinary Internal Medicine regarding percutaneous lung biopsy in the horse. J Vet Intern Med 12:8–16, 1998.

2. ACID-BASE

David Hodgson, B.V.Sc., Ph.D., Dip. ACVIM, FACSM

1. What are the key determinants of acid-base balance?

1. Acid-base balance is tightly regulated in horses and closely related to fluid and electrolyte balance. For example, diseases altering fluid balance (e.g., diarrhea, endotoxemia) are common causes of alterations in extracellular fluid (ECF) balance and therefore acid-base balance.

2. The hydrogen ion concentration (H^+) of the ECF is maintained within tight limits. The normal concentration of H^+ in the ECF is ~ 40 nmol/L, or about 1×10^6 lower than the other commonly measured electrolytes in the ECF. Nonetheless, H^+ has a profound effect on metabolic processes of the body by virtue of altering protein configurations and function. Because enzymes are proteins, they can be markedly affected by alterations in H^+ concentration.

3. Hydrogen ion concentration can be expressed as nmol/L; however, it is most commonly expressed as pH. The pH of a solution is the negative logarithm of the H^+ concentration: pH = $-\log [H^+]$. Therefore, pH varies inversely with H^+ concentration.

2. What is the common nomenclature relating to acid-base balance?

The three most commonly used terms are acidemia, alkalemia, and compensation.

Acidemia is reflected by a blood pH < 7.35 (acidic blood). *Metabolic acidosis* is an abnormal physiologic process characterized by a primary gain of acid (H^+) or primary loss of base (bicarbonate [HCO_3^-]) from the ECF. *Respiratory acidosis* is an abnormal physiologic process characterized by a primary reduction in alveolar ventilation relative to CO_2 production (i.e., increase in the partial pressure of carbon dioxide in arterial blood [$PaCO_2$]). This process is explained in more detail below.

Alkalemia is reflected by a blood pH > 7.45 (alkaline blood). *Metabolic alkalosis* is an abnormal physiologic process characterized by a primary gain in base (HCO_3^-) or loss of acid (H^+) from the ECF. *Respiratory alkalosis* is an abnormal physiologic process characterized by a primary increase in alveolar ventilation to the rate of CO_2 production, thereby resulting in a decrease in $PaCO_2$.

Compensation is the process by which an abnormal pH is returned toward normal by altering the component that is *not primarily* affected by the acid-base disorder. For example, if the $PaCO_2$ is elevated (respiratory acidosis), HCO_3^- is retained as a compensatory measure. Rules that may be helpful in attempting to assess the degree of compensation include:

1. If the $PaCO_2$ or HCO_3^- values are outside normal limits but the pH is within the normal range, the horse is fully compensated.

2. Because the process of compensation takes time (hours to days) to return the pH within normal limits, the presence of a compensatory process implies a degree of chronicity of the primary problem.

3. What variables should be determined to assess possible alterations in acid-base balance?

1. **pH.** The pH is determined to ascertain whether acidemia or alkalemia is present. The pH is the *most* important variable in determining the horse's acid-base status. The subsequently measured variables should be matched to the pH.

2. **$PaCO_2$.** Respiratory alkalosis is indicated when the $PaCO_2$ is < 35 mmHg; respiratory acidosis is present when the $PaCO_2$ is > 50 mmHg.

3. **HCO_3^- concentration.** Metabolic alkalosis is present when the arterial HCO_3^- is > 30 mEq/L; metabolic acidosis is denoted by an arterial HCO_3^- concentration < 22 mEq/L.

4. The **primary problem** should be determined by matching $PaCO_2$, HCO_3^-, or both with the pH of arterial blood (pHa). It then should be possible to determine whether compensation has occurred.

5. Make **adjustments in HCO_3^-** for acute elevations or decreases in $PaCO_2$. The method for making these adjustments is described below.

6. **PaO$_2$.** When the partial pressure of oxygen in arterial blood (PaO$_2$) is < 80 mmHg, hypoxemia should be suspected. However, if the horse lives at altitudes significantly above sea level, it is usual to find PaO$_2$ of 65–85 mmHg in normal horses.

4. What are the normal values for acid-base balance?
   1. pHa = 7.40 units; range = 7.38–7.45 units
   2. pHv (pH of venous blood) = 7.38 units; range = 7.35–7.42 units
   3. PaO$_2$ = 95–100 mmHg; range = 80–110 mmHg (at sea level). **Note:** Values fall with increasing altitude and therefore need to be corrected according to barometric pressure. The lower the barometric pressure, the lower the PaO$_2$.
   4. PvO$_2$ (partial pressure of oxygen in venous blood) = 40 mmHg; range = 35–45 mmHg
   5. PaCO$_2$ = 40 mmHg; range = 35–45 mmHg
   6. PvCO$_2$ (partial pressure of CO$_2$ in venous blood) = 45 mmHg; range = 40–48 mmHg
   7. HCO$_3$$^-$a = 25 mEq/L; range = 22–28 mEq/L
   8. HCO$_3$$^-$v = 27 mEq/L; range = 24–31 mEq/L

5. What are the common acid-base and electrolyte interrelationships?
   Most CO$_2$ entering the blood passes into red blood cells (RBCs). The majority of CO$_2$ enters into a readily reversible reaction to form H$_2$CO$_3$ (carbonic acid) and then HCO$_3$$^-$ and H$^+$. This process, referred to as the **bicarbonate-carbonic acid buffering system**, is reflected in the following equation:

$$CO_2 + H_2O \leftrightarrow H_2CO_3 \leftrightarrow H^+ + HCO_3^-$$

Carbonic anhydrase, an enzyme in red blood cells, facilitates this reaction. The HCO$_3$$^-$ formed by this reaction diffuses out of RBCs; this movement sets up an electrostatic difference across the cell membrane that is neutralized by the movement of chloride ions (Cl$^-$) from plasma into the RBC to maintain electroneutrality. This process is referred to as the **chloride shift**.

6. What is the Henderson-Hasselbalch equation?
   The Henderson-Hasselbalch equation describes the relationship between the bicarbonate-carbonic acid buffer system and pH:

$$pH = 6.1 + \log \frac{[HCO_3^-]}{[H_2CO_3]}$$

where 6.1 is the pK for the HCO$_3$$^-$/H$_2CO_3$ pair. From a physiologic standpoint the bicarbonate-carbonic acid buffer system is the most important element in acid-base balance. HCO$_3$$^-$ is present in relatively high concentrations, it is easy to measure, and it is the buffer system over which the body has most control.

   Plasma pH is a function of the ratio of the concentrations of HCO$_3$$^-$ and H$_2$CO$_3$ in the plasma. The partial pressure of CO$_2$ in the alveolar air, the partial pressure of gaseous CO$_2$ dissolved in the blood, and the H$_2$CO$_3$ concentration of the blood influence the dynamics of this reaction. H$_2$CO$_3$ concentration is determined by measuring the partial pressure of CO$_2$ (PCO$_2$) and concentration of HCO$_3$$^-$ in blood. The PCO$_2$ is multiplied by the solubility constant for CO$_2$ in plasma (0.03). Thus the Henderson-Hasselbalch equation becomes

$$pH = 6.1 + \log \frac{[HCO_3^-]}{0.03 \times PCO_2}$$

Therefore, the pH can be estimated accurately from measurements of HCO$_3$$^-$ and PCO$_2$.

7. What are the principles of the physiochemical or nontraditional approach to acid-base balance?
   1. In the 1980s Stewart described a quantitative physiochemical approach to acid-base balance. Stewart proposed that the acid-base balance of body fluids was a function of the Henderson-Hasselbalch equation plus the effects of strong ions, weak acids, and carbon dioxide. Acid-base balance is determined as a function of the three independent variables: strong ion difference (SID), PaCO$_2$, and the total concentration of nonvolatile weak acids ([A$_{tot}$]).

2. The location and absolute numbers of positively and negatively charged ions (strong ions) and their difference determine the SID. The principal strong ions are Na^+, K^+, Cl^-, and lactate. Thus $SID = ([Na^+] + [K^+]) - ([Cl^-] + [lactate^-])$.

3. The principal component $[A_{tot}]$ is the total plasma protein concentration.

4. SID in combination with $PaCO_2$ and $[A_{tot}]$ determines the changes in pH ($[H^+]$) and $[HCO_3^-]$, which are dependent variables.

5. The concentration of an independent variable cannot be changed within the system and is unaffected by changes that take place in other systems. The concentration of a dependent variable changes whenever the independent variable changes; its concentration is a function of the interaction among the other systems.

6. Changes in strong ions in various body fluids result in changes in SID, which provide the major mechanism for acid-base interactions. Generally, a decrease in SID is accompanied by a fall in pH. In contrast, when SID increases (e.g., with hypochloremia), the pH tends to increase.

7. To maintain electrical neutrality, electrolyte shifts generally occur simultaneously with acid (H^+) or base (HCO_3^-) shifts. The most important electrolyte shift with acid-base changes is the K^+ shift. For example, when HCO_3^- is added to the ECF, H^+ leaves cells, causing K^+ to move intracellularly to maintain electrical equilibrium. Therefore, as a rule of thumb, when metabolic alkalosis is present, suspect hypokalemia; when metabolic acidosis is present, suspect hyperkalemia or at least correct the K^+ concentration in the ECF/plasma.

8. How is the anion gap calculated? What are the normal values in horses? When should it be determined?

The anion gap (AG) can be calculated by determining the difference between the major cations (Na^+ and K^+) and the measured anions (Cl^- and HCO_3^-), as reflected in the formula:

$$AG = (Na^+ + K^+) - (Cl^- + HCO_3^-)$$

The AG provides an estimate of the unmeasured anions. Unmeasured anions typically consist of negatively charged plasma proteins. The normal anion gap in horses usually falls in the range of 7–15 mEq/L. Foals have a larger anion gap than adults. Common causes of decreases in AG include hypoabluminemia and hyperchloremic metabolic acidosis. Increased AG is common in disorders in which metabolizable acids such as lactic acid are produced. Examples include intense exercise and hypovolemic (and often endotoxemic) shock. Measurement of AG may be useful in attempting to identify mixed acid-base disturbances. For example, a mixed acid-base imbalance should be suspected when the change in anion gap does not approximate the change in HCO_3^-.

9. What do the terms base excess and base deficit mean?

Base excess indicates the alteration of the buffer base from normal; it is referred to as **base deficit** when it has a negative value. This value is usually provided in routine assessments of acid-base balance. The result is generally considered as an alteration in the HCO_3^- value from normal. If the horse is acidotic, calculation of the base deficit gives some indication of the amount of HCO_3^- required to replenish losses. Because extracellular water is approximately 30% of body weight, base deficit × body weight (kg) × 0.3 = an estimation of of the amount of HCO_3^- required for replacement in the first instance. However, the bicarbonate space is likely to approximate the total body water (i.e., ~ 60% of the bodyweight). Therefore, although it is recommended to use the 30% value in estimating requirements after equilibration, more HCO_3^- may be required because this ion equilibrates across all fluid spaces in the body.

10. How should samples for acid-base analysis be collected and stored?

1. Samples should be drawn anaerobically and sealed to prevent alterations due to atmospheric exposure. Samples should be collected into heparin as the anticoagulant.

2. If a delay between sampling and analysis is likely, samples should be stored on ice—an ice slurry is ideal. In this medium, samples maintain accurate values for blood gases and acid-base variables for at least 4 hours after collection.

3. Samples should be corrected for body temperature. In general, alterations in temperature have the greatest effect on PaO_2 and $PaCO_2$ and are much more profound than the effects on HCO_3^- or base deficit/excess. Arterial blood samples are ideal, particularly if primary respiratory disorders are evaluated or if the horse is under general anesthesia. In contrast, venous blood samples provide information about acid-base balance and therefore may be used routinely if one wishes to determine the presence of acidosis or alkalosis.

4. Collection of blood from different sampling sites affects the values achieved. There are consistent variations between values for arterial and venous blood; the values for pH and PCO_2 are lower in arterial blood than in venous blood (see question 4). In contrast HCO_3^- concentration and the base deficit/base excess are similar in arterial and venous blood samples.

11. What is metabolic acidosis?

Metabolic acidosis is characterized by a decrease in pH and HCO_3^-. It may be caused by a loss of HCO_3^- or a gain in H^+ ions. Initially the change in pH is buffered by ECF buffers and the exchange of extracellular H^+ for intracellular K^+. This process helps to ameliorate against an excessive increase in H^+ in the ECF and is referred to as the **cation shift**.

12. What are the most common causes of metabolic acidosis?

1. Metabolic acidosis most commonly results from gastrointestinal loss of HCO_3^- due to diarrhea or an accumulation of lactate (plus H^+) associated with endotoxemia.

2. Renal failure may result in a reduced ability to retain HCO_3^-.

3. Intense exercise also results in transient metabolic acidosis in horses due to an increase in lactate production. This process usually reverses with 60 minutes after cessation of exercise.

13. What is respiratory acidosis? What causes it in horses?

Respiratory acidosis is characterized by a decrease in pH due to an increase in $PaCO_2$. It results from decreased effective alveolar ventilation. General anesthesia is the most common cause of respiratory acidosis. However, pneumonia, chronic obstructive pulmonary disease, and drugs that suppress the respiratory center may result in respiratory acidosis. Respiratory acidosis is commonly associated with hypoxemia because CO_2 is ~ 40 times more diffusable than O_2. Therefore, any process that impedes ventilation, even to a small degree, is likely to result in hypoxemia. The increase in $PaCO_2$ is a potent stimulus for the respiratory center, providing a strong drive for ventilation. The sensitivity of the respiratory center to hypoxemia is much lower than its sensitivity to hypocapnia. Therefore, when primary hypoxemia exists, the respiratory center does not respond until the PaO_2 falls to 70–80 mmHg. Horses respond to intense exercise by experiencing mild-to-moderate hypercapnia, which leads to respiratory acidosis that is rapidly reversible after cessation of exercise.

14. What are the partial pressures of inspired gases at the different parts of the respiratory tract?

The table below relates to a conscious standing horse inspiring ambient air. The partial pressures (mmHg) of the different gases (oxygen, carbon dioxide, water, nitrogen [N]) and of the total of all gases in the inspired air (i.e., ambient air), conducting airways, terminal alveoli, and arterial and mixed venous blood are as follows:

	AMBIENT AIR	CONDUCTING AIRWAYS	TERMINAL ALVEOLI	ARTERIAL BLOOD	MIXED VENOUS BLOOD
PO_2	156	149	100	95	40
PCO_2	0	0	40	40	46
PH_2O	15*	47	47	47	47
PN_2	589	564	573	573	573
P total	760	760	760	755	706

* PH_2O varies according to humidity and has a proportionate effect on PO_2 and PN_2.

15. What happens to the partial pressure of oxygen in arterial blood as the percentage of oxygen in the inspired air is increased?

Effect of Increasing the Percentage of Oxygen in Inspired Gas (FiO_2) on the Predicted (Ideal) PaO_2

FiO_2 (%)	PREDICTED PaO_2 (MMHG)
20	95–100
30	150
40	200
50	250
80	400
100	500

16. What is metabolic alkalosis? What causes it in horses?

Metabolic alkalosis is characterized by an increase in pH and HCO_3^-. In horses, a disease process commonly associated with metabolic alkalosis is loss of H^+ from the gastrointestinal tract in response to anterior/posterior enteritis (i.e., duodenitis-proximal jejunitis). Metabolic alkalosis also may be caused by administration of the loop diuretic, furosemide, which results in increased losses of HCO_3^-, thereby resulting in metabolic alkalosis. Similarly, losses of chloride-rich sweat in response to prolonged exercise may result in metabolic alkalosis in horses. Exogenous administration of HCO_3^- via intravenous or oral routes also may result in metabolic alkalosis. This practice has been undertaken in some parts of the world where $NaHCO_3$ is administered as an ergogenic agent to racehorses before competition. The agent is usually given via nasogastric tube at doses of up to 0.5–1 gm/kg. This practice is illegal in many states.

17. With what is respiratory alkalosis associated? Does it occur in horses?

Respiratory alkalosis is associated with an increase in pH and a decrease in $PaCO_2$. Hyperventilation is the most common cause of respiratory alkalosis. Other causes include hypoxemia associated with pulmonary disease, heart failure, or severe anemia. Neurologic disorders may stimulate the respiratory center and thereby cause respiratory alkalosis. An example is gram-negative sepsis. Although not considered a panting mammal, horses exposed to severe heat stress or exercise-induced hyperthermia are likely to hyperventilate in an attempt to reduce core temperature and thereby experience respiratory alkalosis.

18. How are primary acid-base and blood gas classifications made?

Disorders of alterations in acid-base balance can be assessed in terms of the primary disorder, which in most instances can be determined by measuring and correlating values for $PaCO_2$, pH, HCO_3^-, and base excess (BE).

Effects of the Most Common Primary Acid-Base Disorders

DISORDER	$PaCO_2$ (mmHg)	pH (UNITS)	HCO_3^- (mEq/L)	BE (mEq/L)
Acute ventilatory failure	↑	↓	N	N
Chronic ventilatory failure	↑	N	↑	↑
Acute alveolar hyperventilation	↓	↑	N	N
Chronic alveolar hyperventilation	↓	N	↓	↓
Uncompensated metabolic acidosis	N	↓	↓	↓
Compensated metabolic acidosis	↓	N	↓	↓
Uncompensated metabolic alkalosis	N	↑	↑	↑
Compensated metabolic alkalosis	↑	N	↑	↑

↑ = increase, ↓ = decrease, N = normal or no change.

Note: Mixed respiratory and metabolic conditions may coexist. In such cases, individual values for pH, $PaCO_2$, and HCO_3^- should be assessed to determine the severity of the admixture of the respiratory and metabolic components.

19. What are mixed acid-base disturbances? How are they distinguished from compensatory mechanisms?

Mixed acid-base disturbances occur when several primary acid-base disturbances coexist. For example, metabolic acidosis and metabolic alkalosis may coexist in combination with respiratory acidosis or alkalosis. The following points should be considered in evaluating mixed acid-base disturbances:

1. Compensating mechanisms do not result in overcompensation.
2. Rarely is pH corrected to normal.
3. A change in pH in the opposite direction expected for the primary disorder reflects a mixed acid-base disturbance.
4. In a primary disturbance with compensation, HCO_3^- and $PaCO_2$ always deviate in the same direction. Therefore, if these variables deviate in opposite directions, a mixed acid-base disturbance must be present.

20. What are the common compensatory mechanisms for primary alterations in acid-base balance?

1. The HCO_3^- concentration rises about 1–2 mEq/L for each acute 10-mmHg increase in $PaCO_2$ above 40 mmHg. The maximal change in HCO_3^- concentration is about 4 mEq/L.
2. The HCO_3^- concentration falls ~ 1–2 mEq/L for each acute 10-mmHg decrease in $PaCO_2$ below 40 mmHg. The maximal expected change is about 6 mEq/L.
3. Acute respiratory and nonrespiratory disorders can be distinguished by studying the values for $PaCO_2$ and HCO_3^-. A HCO_3^- concentration above 30 or below 15 mEq/L implies a nonrespiratory (metabolic) component. In response to chronic elevations of $PaCO_2$ (hypercapnia), each 10-mmHg increase in $PaCO_2$ causes an increase of ~ 4 mEq/L in HCO_3^- concentration.
4. An acute 10-mmHg increase in $PaCO_2$ results in a decrease of ~ 0.05 units in pH. An acute 10-mmHg decrease in $PaCO_2$ results in an increase of ~ 0.10 units in pH.
5. To calculate the predicted respiratory pH, determine the difference between the measured $PaCO_2$ and 40 mmHg, then move the decimal point two places to the left. If the $PaCO_2$ is > 40, subtract *half the difference* from 7.40; if the $PaCO_2$ is < 40, add the *whole difference* to 7.40. Consider the following examples:
   - Measured pH = 7.01 and $PaCO_2$ = 75 mmHg (i.e., $PaCO_2$ > 40 mmHg). The predicted effect of the respiratory component (acidosis) on overall pH is 75 – 40 = 35. Then move the decimal point two places to the left and divide by half: $0.35 \times 0.5 = 0.175$ (i.e., ~ 0.18). Subtract this value from the normal pH (i.e., 7.40). The predicted pH is 7.40 – 0.18 = 7.22. Metabolic acidosis contributes to the measured pH of 7.01.
   - Measured pH = 7.43 and $PaCO_2$ = 23 (i.e., $PaCO_2$ < 40 mmHg). The predicted effect of the respiratory alkalosis on overall pH is calculated by subtracting the measured $PaCO_2$ from 40 (i.e., 40 – 23 = 17). Then move the decimal point two places to the left (i.e., 0.17) and add to the normal pH value. Therefore, the predicted pH is 7.40 + 0.17 = 7.57. In this case the predicted pH has been compensated, returning the measured pH to the near-normal range.
6. To calculate the metabolic component of an acid-base disturbance: A 10-mEq/L change in HCO_3^- concentration changes pH by 0.15 units. Therefore, if the decimal point for the pH value is moved two places to the right, a 10:15 ratio or two-thirds relationship exists between HCO_3^- and pH. The absolute difference between measured pH and predicted respiratory pH is the metabolic component of the pH change. Moving the decimal two points to the right and multiplying by two-thirds (i.e., 0.66) will yield an estimate of mEq/L variation of the buffer baseline, which usually is assumed to be represented by the change in HCO_3^-.

7. One of best methods for making quantitative clinical determinations of acid-base changes involves two steps: (1) determination of predicted respiratory pH and (2) estimation of base excess or deficit. Consider the following examples:
- If the measured pH = 7.02 and $PaCO_2$ = 75 mmHg, the predicted contribution of the respiratory component to the pH is as follows:

$$75 - 40 = 35$$
$$0.35 \times 0.5 = 0.175$$
$$7.40 - 0.18 = 7.22$$

The metabolic contribution to the overall pH is as follows:

$$7.22 - 7.02 = 20 \times 0.66 = \text{base deficit of 13.3 mEq/L}$$

- If the measured pH = 7.64 and $PaCO_2$ = 25, the predicted pH on the basis of $PaCO_2$ is as follows:

$$40 - 25 = 15$$
$$7.40 + 0.15 = 7.55$$

The metabolic contribution to the overall pH is as follows:

$$7.64 - 7.55 = 9 \times 0.66 = \text{base excess of 6.0 mEq/L}$$

21. What are the effects of exercise on acid-base balance?

High-intensity exercise leads to an increase in $PaCO_2$, a decrease in pH, and a decrease in HCO_3^-. Examples of expected changes in arterial and venous blood variables in response to intense exercise are reflected in the table below.

	Arterial			Venous		
	pH	$[HCO_3^-]$	PCO_2	pH	$[HCO_3^-]$	PCO_2
Before exercise	7.40	26	43	7.36	27	49
After exercise	7.10	18	60	6.95	30	145

Prolonged low-intensity exercise tends to produce a decrease in plasma chloride concentration because chloride is lost in sweat. As a consequence, HCO_3^- is retained with a resultant metabolic alkalosis.

22. What are the commonly accepted approaches to treatment of acid-base disturbances?

Therapy usually involves correction of the primary problem with supportive therapy tailored to address the disturbance in acid-base balance. Most therapies are discussed in the relevant chapters on fluids and electrolytes/hematology. However, important rules of thumb include the following:
1. Base deficits of less than 10 mEq/L are not treated routinely.
2. If the pH is above 7.20, routine treatment is not required unless there is evidence of shock.
3. In cases of endotoxemia, plasma volume expansion with polyionic solutions should be the main aim of treatment. Correction of such deficits is likely to result in correction of the acid-base disturbance.

23. What happens to $PaCO_2$, PaO_2, and pH if the blood sample for blood gas analysis is exposed to room air (e.g., an air bubble)?

Because the CO_2 level is higher in the blood sample than in the ambient air, CO_2 diffuses into the air from the blood sample, thus decreasing $PaCO_2$. Consequently, the pH increases. PaO_2 also increases because of the concentration gradient.

24. What happens to $PaCO_2$, PaO_2, and pH if the blood sample for blood gas analysis sits for a prolonged period at room temperature?

Because of metabolism of cells, $PaCO_2$ increases (i.e., production), PaO_2 decreases (i.e., consumption), and pH decreases.

BIBLIOGRAPHY

1. Carlson GP: Fluid, electrolyte, and acid-base balance. In Kaneko JJ (ed): Clinical Biochemistry of Domestic Animals, 4th ed. San Diego, Academic Press, 1989, pp 543–575.
2. Kingston JK, Bayly WM: Effect of exercise in acid-base status of horses. Vet Clin North Am Large Animal 14:61–73, 1998.
3. Rose BD: Clinical Physiology of Acid-Base and Electrolyte Disorders, 2nd ed. New York, McGraw-Hill, 1984.

3. HEMATOLOGY AND ELECTROLYTES

R. McConnico, D.V.M., Ph.D., Dip. ACVIM, and
D. Sellon, D.V.M., Ph.D., Dip. ACVIM

REGENERATIVE ANEMIA

1. How do you assess red cell regenerative responses in anemic horses?

Unlike other domestic animal species, horses do not release reticulocytes into circulation in response to an acute hemorrhagic or hemolytic episode. Sometimes horses demonstrate an increased mean cell volume (MCV, mean corpuscular volume) or red cell distribution width (RDW) after hemorrhage or hemolysis, but neither finding is a reliable indicator of regeneration. The best method of assessing the equine erythroid regenerative response is determination of the bone marrow myeloid-to-erythroid (M:E) ratio and/or bone marrow reticulocyte count. A bone marrow M:E ratio of 0.5 (1:2) is consistent with erythrocyte regeneration (normal M:E ratio = 1:1). Normal equine marrow contains approximately 3% reticulocytes, but after acute severe hemorrhage, reticulocytes may increase to 66%. If bone marrow analysis is not an option, peripheral blood packed cell volume (PCV) may be monitored to assess regeneration. Accelerated bone marrow red cell production should be evident by 3–7 days after acute hemorrhage, with an average increase in PCV of 0.5–1.0% per day.

2. How do you treat acute severe hemorrhage (i.e., loss of 15–30% of total blood volume)?

The most important aspects of therapy are controlling the hemorrhage and replacing blood volume. External hemorrhage may be stopped by applying direct pressure to the site or ligating the offending vessel(s). Control of internal hemorrhage can be more problematic. Some form of volume replacement therapy is indicated if the horse is tachycardic with poor peripheral perfusion. Volume replacement may be accomplished with hypertonic saline, isotonic fluids, and/or whole blood transfusion. Hypertonic saline at 4–6 ml/kg administered intravenously over 15 minutes rapidly increases cardiac output and peripheral perfusion. This therapy should be followed within a few hours by isotonic fluid administration in sufficient quantity to replace estimated total body fluid deficits. Hypertonic saline therapy is controversial when hemorrhage cannot be adequately controlled. If isotonic fluids are administered as a sole therapy, total volume should exceed the estimated volume of blood loss by a factor of 2–3. Blood transfusions are indicated with persistent severe tachycardia (> 72 beats/minute), profound hypotension (mean arterial pressure < 65 mmHg), or extreme weakness. Assuming a donor PCV of approximately 40%, 1 ml of whole blood/lb of body weight (1 kg = 2.2 lb) should increase the recipient horse's PCV by 1%. Therefore, one liter of whole blood should increase the PCV of a 450-kg (1000-lb) horse by approximately 1%.

3. How do you differentiate between intravascular and extravascular hemolysis?

During intravascular hemolysis, hemoglobin from the lysed erythrocytes is released directly into the plasma. Initially this excessive hemoglobin is bound to haptoglobin. As the binding capacity of haptoglobin is exceeded, gross hemoglobinemia develops. Some excessive hemoglobin is taken up by mononuclear phagocytes and metabolized to bilirubin. Other hemoglobin is filtered through the renal glomerulus, resulting in hemoglobinuria and potential renal tubular damage. As a general rule, plasma hemoglobin concentrations are normally approximately one-third of the PCV. In cases of intravascular hemolysis, the plasma hemoglobin concentration exceeds one-third of the PCV and plasma bilirubin concentrations are increased. Intravascular hemolysis also results in an increased mean cell hemoglobin (MCH) and mean cell hemoglobin concentration (MCHC). During extravascular hemolysis, damaged red blood cells are removed from circulation by mononuclear phagocytes, and gross hemoglobinemia and hemoglobinuria do not occur. Hemoglobin is directly degraded into bilirubin inside the phagocytic cell, and serum bilirubin concentrations increase.

4. What is the pathogenesis of anemia in red maple (*Acer rubrum*) leaf toxicity?

Wilted leaves and bark of *A. rubrum* contain an uncharacterized toxin that oxidizes ferrous (Fe^{2+}) iron in the normal hemoglobin molecule to the ferric (Fe^{3+}) form. The ferric form of hemoglobin, known as methemoglobin, is incapable of carrying oxygen to the tissues. Normal blood methemoglobin concentration is $< 2\%$. Horses that have ingested wilted red maple leaves may have methemoglobin concentrations of $> 25\%$. Excessive methemoglobin results in a brownish discoloration to blood and tissues. Oxidant stress to erythrocytes also results in formation of disulfide linkages in the protein component of the hemoglobin molecule with resultant denaturation and precipitation of the molecule. Denatured hemoglobin is visualized as spherical, refractile Heinz bodies attached to the erythrocyte membrane. Heinz bodies increase osmotic fragility, resulting in intravascular hemolysis, and also may enhance cell clearance from circulation by mononuclear phagocytes (i.e., extravascular hemolysis).

5. Describe the pathogenesis of neonatal isoerythrolysis (NI) in horses.

The blood type or antigenic components on the surface of a horse's red blood cells (alloantigens) are derived from the combined genetic input of the sire and dam. These genes are codominant: the alloantigens inherited from each parent are simultaneously expressed in the offspring. If a mare is exposed to blood factors that are not normally present on her own blood cells, she will develop antibodies against the foreign antigen. Exposure to foreign group antigens may occur at birth, during pregnancy, during parturition, after a transfusion, or as the result of administration of biologic agents of equine origin. Exposure at birth or after a transfusion and administration of an equine biologic agent (e.g., plasma) are the main reasons that a primiparous mare may have a foal with NI, although NI is more common in foals of multiparous mares. As parturition approaches, the mare concentrates immunoglobulin (including alloantibodies) in her colostrum. After the foal is born, the immunoglobulin-rich colostrum is ingested, and alloantibodies reach the foal's blood. If the foal has inherited an incompatible alloantigen from the sire, absorbed antibodies attach to circulating red blood cells. The result is severe intravascular and/or extravascular hemolytic anemia in the foal. There are seven major blood group systems in horses, but the vast majority of NI is due to the incompatibility of blood types Aa and Qa (i.e., mares that are Aa- or Qa-negative are at risk of exposure to Aa- or Qa-positive factors and therefore produce anti-Aa or anti-Qa antibodies).

6. How do you confirm a diagnosis of immune-mediated hemolytic anemia (IMHA)?

IMHA is the result of immunoglobulin and/or complement attachment to the surface of circulating red blood cells. Immunoglobulin attachment results in destruction of affected erythrocytes by tissue mononuclear phagocytes (i.e., extravascular hemolysis). Most IMHA is extravascular, but if the antibody fixes and activates complement, intravascular complement-mediated hemolysis may occur. Antibody attachment to red blood cells may result in autoagglutination of cells, which is grossly or microscopically visible with ethylenediamine tetraacetic acid (EDTA)-anticoagulated blood samples. Although autoagglutination is considered diagnostic of IMHA, it must be differentiated from Rouleaux formation, a normal characteristic of equine blood. Unlike Rouleaux formation, autoagglutinated erythrocytes do not disperse when the blood is mixed with normal saline. When autoagglutination is not apparent, a direct antiglobulin (Coombs') test may be used to confirm IMHA. This test detects the presence of antibody on the surface of the patient's red blood cells. The Coombs reagent should contain antisera to equine IgG, IgM, and C3 (third component of complement).

7. How do you treat IMHA?

Most cases of IMHA in horses occur secondary to an underlying disease or drug therapy. Viral, bacterial, neoplastic, and inflammatory diseases have been linked to IMHA. When IMHA is suspected, any previously administered drug therapy should be discontinued. Underlying primary disease processes should be specifically treated. Whole blood transfusion from a compatible donor may be necessary if tissue oxygenation is inadequate because of the severity of the hemolysis.

Parenteral corticosteroids are beneficial in suppressing the horse's immune response. Dexamethasone, 0.05–0.2 mg/kg intravenously or intramuscularly once or twice daily, is recommended in acute, severe IMHA. After the PCV has stabilized, corticosteroid doses should be gradually decreased to the lowest dose necessary for maintenance and eventually discontinued. If long-term therapy is needed, oral prednisolone may be administered with a diminishing dose every other dose. Caution is recommended in administering prolonged or high-dose corticosteroids because of the risk of laminitis or exacerbation of any primary underlying infectious disease process.

8. What causes transfusion reactions? What are the clinical signs?

Transfusion reactions most frequently occur because of immune reactions to antigens in the transfused blood product or because of contamination of blood products with bacteria or endotoxin. Donor horses should be previously tested to ensure that they are Aa- and Qa-negative and lack detectable circulating alloantibodies against erythrocyte antigens that may be present in the recipient. Aa- and Qa-negative geldings are less likely to have been exposed to Aa- and Qa-positive factors; thus, Aa- and Qa-negative geldings without anti-Aa and anti-Qa antibodies make ideal and convenient donors in numerous situations. Cross-matching may be used to detect existing antibody. A major cross-match detects incompatibilities between donor erythrocytes and alloantibodies that may be present in the recipient. A minor cross-match detects incompatibilities between recipient erythrocytes and alloantibodies that may be present in the donor. Cross-matching decreases but does not eliminate the likelihood of an in vivo transfusion reaction. Immune reactions may occur if the recipient is allergic to other blood protein components (e.g., white blood cell or platelet antigens, blood proteins). Blood product transfusions should always be administered through a blood administration set with an in-line filter.

Signs of an immediate transfusion reaction include trembling, tachypnea, tachycardia, piloerection, urticaria, restlessness, cardiac arrhythmia, hypotension, collapse, and abdominal pain. If alloantibodies against recipient red blood cells are present in the transfused blood, a hemolytic crisis may be observed after the transfusion.

NONREGENERATIVE ANEMIA

9. What is the pathogenesis of anemia of chronic disease?

Chronic infectious, inflammatory, or neoplastic diseases are frequently associated with mild-to-moderate normocytic normochromic nonregenerative anemia. Three mechanisms have been implicated in the pathogenesis of anemia of chronic disease:

1. Inhibition of iron release from reticuloendothelial storage inhibits heme synthesis.
2. Defective response of the bone marrow to circulating erythropoietin
3. Decreased red blood cell life span

10. How do red cell indices differ between young (< 2 years) and mature (>5 years) horses?

Young horses normally have a lower MCV of erythrocytes than mature horses. Mean cell hemoglobin (MCH) is decreased in younger horses because of the smaller size of their red cells; however, mean cell hemoglobin concentration (MCHC) is the same.

11. How do you differentiate between anemia of chronic disease and iron deficiency anemia?

PARAMETER	ANEMIA OF CHRONIC DISEASE	IRON DEFICIENCY ANEMIA*
Total iron-binding capacity (TIBC)	Normal to decreased	Normal to increased
Serum ferritin	Normal to increased	Normal to decreased
Bone marrow iron stores†	Normal to increased	Normal to decreased
Percent saturation of transferrin	Normal to decreased	Normal to decreased
Serum iron	Normal to decreased	Normal to decreased

* For example, chronic blood loss anemia.
† Evaluated by Prussian blue staining.

12. What is the most common cause of iron deficiency anemia in horses?

The majority of the body's iron is present as a complex with hemoglobin in red blood cells (~ 66% of total iron reserves in the body). The remaining iron stores are distributed in the liver, spleen, and bone marrow. Consequently, chronic external blood loss is the most common cause of iron deficiency anemia in horses. The equine diet normally contains ample iron for maintenance of body functions, and gastrointestinal absorption of iron is rarely impaired. Therefore, dietary iron deficiency is extremely rare. Congenital iron deficiency described in calves has not been described in foals.

13. How does erythropoietin administration result in pure red cell aplasia (nonregenerative anemia) in horses?

Erythropoietin stimulates red blood cell production in the bone marrow. Because maximal athletic performance is often limited by the ability to deliver adequate oxygen to tissues, recombinant human erythropoietin (rHuEpo) is occasionally administered to horses to increase their total red blood cell mass and oxygen-carrying capacity. After multiple rHuEpo injections, some horses develop life-threatening nonregenerative anemia, which is thought to result from production of antierythropoietin antibodies. Bone marrow biopsies reveal a pure red cell aplasia with normal production and maturation of white blood cells and platelets.

14. When is a bone marrow aspirate/biopsy indicated? How should it be obtained?

Bone marrow evaluation is indicated for any hematopoietic disorder that cannot be diagnosed from information gathered by history, physical examination, and routine laboratory analysis. It may be helpful in characterization of anemia, evaluation of iron stores, definition of abnormal blood cell populations, or diagnosis of cytopenic conditions. Bone marrow aspirates are most reliably obtained from the sternebrae. An aspirate is obtained by inserting a bone marrow needle into the marrow cavity and aspirating spicular contents into a syringe containing an anticoagulant. These contents are placed on a clean glass microscope slide and examined after appropriate staining procedures (e.g., Wright's-Giemsa, Prussian blue stains). A bone marrow core biopsy is obtained either by inserting a manual bone marrow biopsy needle through the cortex of the bone (e.g., sternebrae, wing of ilium, rib) and advancing the needle into the marrow cavity or by using a bone biopsy drill. A rotary motion is used to facilitate detachment of the base of the biopsy specimen. The needle is removed from the bone, and the core biopsy specimen is placed in appropriate histologic fixative.

15. What are the causes of erythrocytosis? How are they differentiated?

Erythrocytosis may result from one of several pathogenetic mechanisms and diseases. Relative erythrocytosis is an apparent increase in red cell mass caused by an absolute decrease in plasma volume (dehydration) or splenic contraction with release of stored red cells in to the circulation. Absolute erythrocytosis is a true increase in the total circulating red blood cell mass and may be either primary or secondary. Primary erythrocytosis is a myeloproliferative disorder in which erythropoiesis occurs despite normal or decreased concentrations of erythropoietin in the blood. Secondary erythrocytosis occurs because of appropriate (chronic hypoxia) or inappropriate excessive production of erythropoietin.

Causes of Erythrocytosis

Relative erythrocytosis
    Excitement (splenic contraction)
    Dehydration
    Laboratory error

Absolute erythrocytosis
    Primary
        Polycythemia vera
        Hereditary primary erythrocytosis

Table continued on facing page

Causes of Erythrocytosis (Continued)

Secondary
- Appropriate
  High altitude
  Chronic lung disease
  Cardiopulmonary disease with right-to-left shunting
  Low-output congestive heart failure
  High-oxygen affinity hemogloginopathy
- Inappropriate
  Neoplasia (hepatic, renal, ovarian, uterine, central nervous system carcinoma)
  Renal disease (hydronephrosis, polycystic kidneys)
  Hereditary secondary erythrocytosis

INFECTIOUS DISEASES

16. What is the etiologic agent of equine infectious anemia (EIA)? What are the most common clinical signs

EIA is caused by a virus classified in the lentivirus genus of the Retroviridae family. Once infected with this virus, a horse remains infected for life, which is the hallmark of a retrovirus. Acute infection is associated with fever and lethargy. Some horses exhibit anemia and thrombocytopenia. Most horses recover from the initial febrile episode but may undergo recurring febrile episodes associated with periodic emergence of novel antigenic variants of the virus. In some horses these episodes become more severe, and the horse develops classic clinical signs of EIA: weight loss, ventral edema, fever, lethargy, anemia, thrombocytopenia, and hyperglobulinemia. In most horses, however, the febrile episodes become less frequent and less severe, and the horse becomes an inapparent carrier of the virus. Inapparent carriers are normal on physical examination but often have subtle clinicopathologic alterations suggestive of ongoing viral activity (increased serum globulin concentrations, decreased albumin:globulin ratio, intermittent thrombocytopenia, or mild anemia).

17. How is EIA transmitted?

EIA virus is most commonly transmitted by the intermittent feeding of hematophagous insects, especially biting flies of the genus *Tabanus* (horseflies) or *Chrysops* (deerflies). Flies are strictly mechanical vectors, and the virus does not live long outside the horse. Mosquitoes are *unlikely* to transmit EIA virus for the following reasons: (1) because mosquitoes do not produce a painful bite to a horse, the feeding pattern is not interrupted; (2) mosquito saliva adversely affects EIA virus viability; and (3) the mosquito mouthparts are not large enough to contain an infective dose of EIA virus. For transmission to occur, a fly must begin a blood meal on an infected horse, be interrupted, and immediately resume feeding on an uninfected horse. EIA virus also may be transmitted transplacentally, especially if a pregnant mare experiences febrile episodes during gestation. Transmission via ingestion of colostrum or milk from an infected mare is possible but not likely. Venereal transmission is rare. Iatrogenic transmission may occur through the use of shared needles for injections or use of improperly sterilized surgical instruments or other devices that contact equine blood.

18. What recommendations would you make for prevention of EIA on a horse farm?

All horses on a farm should be tested at least yearly for the presence of antibodies to EIA virus. Presence of antibodies indicates that the horse is infected and will remain infected for life. Infected horses should be permanently quarantined or euthanized. All new horses should have recently tested negative before arrival on the farm. Farm management practices should attempt to minimize fly populations through appropriate rubbish and manure disposal and judicious use of chemical or nonchemical insect control programs. Horsefly bites are usually most numerous during daylight hours in wooded areas. Pasture turnout schedules should take these facts into consideration. Horse owners and veterinarians should strictly adhere to the "one needle, one horse" rule. All instruments that come into contact with equine blood should be thoroughly disinfected before use on another horse. Horse owners and veterinarians should encourage organizers of equestrian events to require proof of a negative EIA test (e.g., agar gel immunodiffusion test or enzyme-linked immunosorbent assay) for all horses before participation.

19. Discuss the etiologic agent, clinical signs, and treatment of equine piroplasmosis.

Equine piroplasmosis (babesiosis) is caused by one of two species of hemoprotozoal parasites: (1) *Babesia caballi* or (2) *Babesia equi*. These intraerythrocytic parasites are transmitted primarily by tick vectors. Within 1–4 weeks of exposure, previously unexposed horses develop signs of fever, depression, dyspnea, pale or icteric mucous membranes, ecchymoses of the nictitating membrane, constipation, colic, and dependent edema. Massive infection results in classic signs of intravascular hemolysis: icterus, hemoglobinemia, anemia, hemoglobinuria, and hyperbilirubinemia. Clinical signs in horses infected with *B. caballi* last a few days to a few weeks; the mortality rate is low. Most horses spontaneously clear the organism after 12–42 months of infection. Infection with *B. equi* is more severe, and horses may die within 24–48 hours of the onset of clinical signs. Infection is usually life-long unless the horse is treated. In endemic areas, it is desirable to suppress clinical signs of disease without eliminating the organism from the horse. As with some other protozoal infections, effective immunity depends on continual exposure to the organism (premunity). Imidocarb dipropionate or buparvaquone is effective for treatment of clinical signs of babesiosis in horses. *B. caballi* infections are easier to eliminate than *B. equi* infections.

20. Discuss the causative agent and clinical signs of equine granulocytic ehrlichiosis.

Equine granulocytic ehrlichiosis is caused by *Ehrlichia equi*, a rickettsial organism that resides in equine neutrophils and eosinophils. Infection results in fever, anorexia, depression, petechia and ecchymoses, icterus, ventral edema, and ataxia that lasts 3–16 days. Infected horses are usually thrombocytopenic, leukopenic, and anemic. Clinical signs are most severe in adult horses; foals may experience only a mild fever.

21. How is equine granulocytic ehrlichiosis diagnosed and treated?

During acute stages of infection, granular inclusion bodies may be seen in the cytoplasm of neutrophils and eosinophils on blood smears routinely stained with a Wright's-Giemsa stain. The inclusions are pleomorphic, blue-gray to dark blue spoke-wheel shapes representing a cluster of coccobacillary organisms with cytoplasmic membrane-bound vesicles. A fluorescent antibody test is available for detection of antibody to *E. equi*. A four-fold change in acute and convalescent titers is considered diagnostic of infection. Mortality is rare, and most untreated horses recover over a period of 2 weeks. Recovery may be hastened by treatment with oxytetracycline at 7 mg/kg intravenously once or twice daily for up to 7 days. To avoid development of hypocalcemia, the oxytetracycline should be diluted in 500–1000 ml of 0.9% saline and infused intravenously.

DISORDERS OF HEMOSTASIS

22. What is disseminated intravascular coagulation (DIC)? What are its causes?

DIC is a condition of pathologic activation of coagulative and fibrinolytic systems throughout the body with resultant deposition of microthrombi in small vessels, ischemia, and secondary organ dysfunction. Paradoxically, the severest form of DIC is characterized by hemorrhage due to overwhelming consumption of coagulation factors. DIC may occur as a complication of many types of disorders. In horses, DIC is frequently associated with gastrointestinal disease or sepsis. The common initiating factor in most cases is endotoxin, the external cell wall lipopolysaccharide component of gram-negative bacteria. Endotoxin may directly activate factor XII and the intrinsic coagulation system. It also may cause widespread vascular endothelial cell damage, exposing subendothelial collagen and releasing tissue thromboplastin to trigger both intrinsic and extrinsic coagulation systems. Other conditions that may be associated with DIC include intravascular hemolysis, bacteremia, viremia, neoplasia, immune-mediated diseases, fetal autolysis in utero, hepatic disease, and renal disease.

23. What coagulation abnormalities are commonly present in horses with DIC?

A wide variety of coagulation parameters may be abnormal in horses with DIC. The most commonly evaluated parameters are platelet count, prothrombin time (PT), partial thromboplastin time (PTT), and fibrin degradation products (FDPs). Early in the disease process a horse may be hypercoagulable with decreased PT and PTT. However, by the time most horses are examined they have reached a stage of increased bleeding due to consumption of coagulative elements. Such horses generally have decreased platelet counts and prolonged PT and PTT. FDPs are often increased as a result of extensive fibrinolysis. In contrast to some other species, horses with DIC almost always have normal to increased plasma fibrinogen concentration, probably because fibrinogen acts as an acute-phase reactant in horses and the underlying disease process in most horses is inflammatory and stimulates accelerated hepatic production.

24. Define primary and secondary hemostasis. How do their clinical presentations differ?

The immediate or primary response to disruption of a blood vessel wall is vasoconstriction, followed by adherence of platelets to the disrupted endothelium to form a temporary "plug" of the defect and prevent additional hemorrhage. Secondary hemostasis is the interaction of soluble coagulation factors to produce a stable fibrin clot to reinforce the platelet plug. Thrombocytopenia, platelet function defects, and vasculitis are primary hemostatic abnormalities. Affected horses present with petechia and ecchymoses, epistaxis and hyphema, prolonged bleeding from venipuncture sites, and sometimes melena. Secondary hemostatic defects include disorders in quantity or function of soluble coagulation factors. Affected horses present with spontaneous or excessive hemorrhage in response to surgery or trauma, hemorrhage into body cavities, epistaxis, hemarthroses, or excessive hemorrhage.

25. How does aspirin impair platelet function?

All nonsteroid antiinflammatory drugs (NSAIDs), including aspirin, inhibit cyclooxygenase, the enzyme responsible for prostaglandin, thromboxane, and prostacyclin synthesis from arachidonic acid. Thromboxane A2 is a potent vasoconstrictive agent and stimulates platelet aggregation and release reactions. Aspirin covalently acetylates cyclooxygenase, thus permanently inhibiting the enzyme. Platelets are anucleate cells and as such lack the capacity to produce more cyclooxygenase enzyme; thus circulating platelets are rendered permanently dysfunctional. Platelet function is restored only when aspirin is cleared from the circulation and new platelets with functional cyclooxygenase are released from the bone marrow. Most other NSAIDs (e.g, flunixin, phenylbutazone) reversibly inhibit cyclooxygenase function; as blood concentrations of the drug decline, cyclooxygenase activity returns.

26. What are the differential diagnoses for thrombocytopenia in horses?

Pseudothrombocytopenia is common in horses as a result of in vitro clumping of platelets in EDTA-anticoagulated blood. In such cases, platelet clumps are usually observed on the feathered edge of a blood smear. Thrombocytopenia should be confirmed by repeating the platelet count using whole blood anticoagulated with sodium citrate. The most common causes of true thrombocytopenia in horses are DIC and immune-mediated platelet destruction. Less common causes of thrombocytopenia in horses include bone marrow failure (myelophthisis, myeloproliferative disease, myelosuppressive drugs, idiopathic pancytopenia), recent thrombosis or hemorrhage, platelet sequestration in an enlarged spleen, and drug reactions. Many horses with equine infectious anemia or equine granulocytic ehrlichiosis are thrombocytopenic. Any acute viral infection also may be associated with mild-to-moderate thrombocytopenia.

27. What are the most common causes of thrombocytosis?

Thrombocytosis is most commonly a response to a chronic infectious, inflammatory, or neoplastic disease. Thrombocytosis also may occur as a rebound response to severe thrombocytopenia,

hemorrhage, or hemolytic anemia or as a primary myeloproliferative disorder. Exercise or excitement may be associated with mild thrombocytosis. Young male horses tend to have higher
platelet counts than other types of horses.

28. Describe the clinical signs associated with vasculitis. What are the differential diagnoses for this clinical presentation?

Vasculitis (inflammation of blood vessels) is characterized by increased microvascular permeability with hemorrhage and edema as fluid and cellular components of blood escape from
vessels. Petechial hemorrhages may be visible on mucous membranes, sclera, pinnae of the ear,
and external surfaces of the viscera. Edema of the distal limbs, ventral abdomen, and head may
occur. Untreated vasculitis may result in ischemia and necrosis with extensive skin sloughing, especially on the distal limbs. Vasculitis usually occurs as a secondary complication of infectious,
immunologic, toxic, or neoplastic disorders. Infectious diseases associated with vasculitis include equine viral arteritis, equine infectious anemia, equine granulocytic ehrlichiosis, and
African horse sickness. Purpura hemorrhagica is a form of immune-mediated vasculitis classically associated with previous or concurrent *Streptococcus equi* infection but may be preceded
by other types of viral or bacterial respiratory tract infections. Immune complexes are deposited
in the walls of small subcutaneous vessels, resulting in complement activation, leukocyte chemotaxis, and inflammation (type III hypersensitivity reaction). Fever is common, and affected
horses are often reluctant to move because of pain.

29. What hereditary disorders of coagulation have been described in horses?

Hereditary Disorders of Coagulation in Horses

DISORDER	ABNORMALITY	BREED(S) AFFECTED	CLINICAL PATHOLOGY
von Willebrand disease	Prolonged bleeding after minor trauma because of abnormal vWF	Quarter Horse	Normal clotting times Abnormal quantity or function of vWF
Prekallikrein (Pk) deficiency	Abnormal intrinsic coagulation because Pk is not available for control phase	Belgian Miniature Horse	Prolonged PTT Definitive diagnosis requires specific factor assay
Hemophilia A	Factor VIII deficiency transmitted as X-linked recessive trait	Thoroughbred Arabian Standardbred Quarter Horse	Prolonged PTT Normal PT Definitive diagnosis requires specific factor assay
Protein C deficiency	Deficiency of important inhibitor of coagulation, resulting in hyper-coagulable state with thrombus formation	Thoroughbred	Abnormal quantity or activity of protein C

vWF = von Willebrand factor, PTT = partial thromboplastin time, PT = prothrombin time.

30. Why does bleeding diathesis occur with severe liver disease?

The liver is the major site of production for all soluble blood coagulation factors except
vWF, several regulatory proteins (antithrombin III, protein C, protein S), and important components of the fibrinolytic system (plasminogen, α-2 antiplasmin). If cholestasis is severe, absorption of fat-soluble vitamins is impaired, and production of of the vitamin K-dependent clotting
actors (II, VII, IX, X) is decreased. Hepatic Kupffer cells remove any activated coagulation factors and fibrinolytic products from circulation, and impaired clearance of these factors may contribute to development of DIC. Significant changes in aPTT and PT with severe bleeding are a
poor prognostic indicator in horses with hepatic disease.

31. How do anticoagulant rodenticides cause hemorrhage? How is this toxicity treated?

Most anticoagulant rodenticides contain dicoumarol derivatives similar to warfarin as their active ingredient. These agents act as antagonists of vitamin K, a fat-soluble vitamin essential for a final α-carboxylation step in the hepatic synthesis of several coagulation factors. The serine proteases (factors II, VII, IX, and X) require α-carboxylation before they are fully functional. Because factor VII has the shortest half-life of the susceptible coagulation factors, PT is prolonged earlier in the disease process than aPTT. Concurrent administration of phenylbutazone exacerbates the toxic effects of warfarin. Phenylbutazone displaces the protein-bound warfarin, increasing the concentration of toxic unbound warfarin in plasma. Toxic doses of dicoumarol derivatives may result in spontaneous life-threatening hemorrhage.

Vitamin K1 may be administered at up to 1.0 mg/kg subcutaneously to reverse toxicity. The dose may be repeated every 4–6 hours until the PT is within normal limits (usually within 24 hours). In cases of accidental ingestion of a second-generation anticoagulant (such as brodifacoum, the most popular ingredient in rodenticides in the 1990s), the half-life is much longer than warfarin's, and vitamin K1 treatment may need to be continued for as long as 3–4 weeks. In such cases, oral vitamin K1 (2.5 mg/kg every 12 hr) may be more practical, although it is expensive. High-quality alfalfa hay is an excellent source of vitamin K1 and should be provided to any horse with anticoagulant rodenticide toxicity. In horses with severe hemorrhage whole blood transfusions may be necessary. Vitamin K3 (menadione sodium bisulfite) should *never* be administered to horses because it has been associated with acute, fatal renal failure.

IMMUNE DISORDERS

32. Describe the most common clinical signs in horses with lymphoma.

The clinical signs of lymphoma (i.e., lymphosarcoma) in horses are diverse and usually reflect the primary tumor sites in an individual animal. Four forms of lymphoma have been described in horses: multicentric, alimentary, mediastinal, and extranodal. **Multicentric lymphoma** is the most common form and typically involves multiple lymph nodes and organs, including liver, kidney, and spleen. Bone marrow involvement may result in secondary "leukemia" with circulating neoplastic lymphocytes. The horse with **alimentary lymphoma** usually presents with weight loss, decreased appetite, dependent edema, and hypoproteinemia. Diarrhea and intermittent abdominal pain also may occur. Alimentary lymphoma may occur in horses of any age, but many affected horses are < 5 years old. Horses with **mediastinal lymphoma** often present with pleural effusion, tachypnea, dyspnea, and dependent edema. If a large cranial mediastinal mass is present, the horse may have jugular venous distention and forelimb lameness. **Extranodal lymphoma** may affect the skin, ocular structures, upper respiratory tract (nasal passages, larynx, pharynx), or central nervous system. Lesions may be nonpainful, firm, well-circumscribed masses or ulcerated painful lesions.

33. What is combined immunodeficiency (CID)? How is it diagnosed?

CID is a lethal primary immunodeficiency disorder of horses characterized by a failure to produce functional B or T lymphocytes. It occurs as an autosomal recessive disorder of Arabian horses. Affected horses have a five nucleotide mutation in DNA-dependent protein kinase (DNA-PKCS), a gene required for effective recombination of variable, diverse, and joining gene segments of lymphocytes. Affected foals usually die by 5 months of age as result of secondary infections that are unresponsive to appropriate antimicrobial therapy. Three criteria have traditionally been required for a diagnosis of CID: persistent lymphopenia (< 1,000/L), absence of IgM, and thymic hypoplasia. A genetic test is now available for specific diagnosis and identification of homozygous affected foals and heterozygous carrier horses.

34. What other primary immune deficiencies have been described in horses?

Transient hypogammaglobulinemia, agammaglobulinemia, and selective IgM deficiency have been described in horses. **Transient hypogammaglobulinemia** is characterized by a delay in the onset of immunoglobulin production until approximately 3 months of age. Supportive care with appropriate antimicrobial therapy or plasma transfusions is usually successful at maintaining affected foals until their endogenous immunoglobulin production improves. Prognosis for full recovery is good. **Agammaglobulinemia** is characterized by an absence of B lymphocytes and failure to produce immunoglobulins of any isotype. Cell-mediated immune function is normal in affected foals. This disorder has been described only in males and may be inherited as an X-linked trait. Supportive care may result in transient improvement, but long-term prognosis is poor. **Selective IgM deficiency** may occur in young horses, presumably as an inherited disorder, or in older horses secondary to lymphoma. Prognosis is poor.

35. What clinical signs and laboratory abnormalities are associated with multiple myeloma?

Multiple myeloma is a rare myeloproliferative disorder of terminally differentiated B cells. Clinical signs include limb edema, lameness, epistaxis, weight loss, lymphadenopathy, and decreased appetite. Clinicopathologic abnormalities include anemia, thrombocytopenia, hypoalbuminemia, and monoclonal gammopathy. Occasionally hypercalcemia occurs.

ELECTROLYTES

36. What are the normal electrolyte concentrations (mEq/L) in equine plasma and commercially available balanced crystalloid solutions?

SOLUTION	SODIUM	CHLORIDE	POTASSIUM	BICARBONATE	CALCIUM
Equine plasma	140	100	4.0	25	5.5
0.9% Saline	154	154			
Plasmalyte	140	98	5	50 (A, G)	
Normosol	140	98	5	50 (A, G)	
Lactated Ringer's solution	130	109	4	28 (L)	3

A = acetate, G= gluconate, L = lactate.

37. Which electrolyte is the major determinant of extracellular fluid volume?

Sodium has the most potent influence on blood volume (much of the extracellular fluid volume). The concentration of sodium, multiplied by 2, is equal to the osmolality of extracellular fluid because sodium (Na^+), chloride (Cl^-), and bicarbonate (HCO_3^- anion) exert enough osmotic pressure to maintain most of the extracellular volume.

38. What clinical signs are associated with sodium excess? With sodium depletion?

Sodium excess results in increased extracellular fluid volume; thus ascites and edema are common clinical signs. **Sodium depletion** is most commonly associated with hypovolemia.

39. How does potassium (K^+) depletion affect total body water?

The sum of exchangeable Na^+ and exchangeable K^+ divided by total body water (TBW) is approximately equal to the plasma sodium concentration {plasma $[Na^+] \cong (Na^+ + K^+)$}. Potassium loss from the cell causes movement of sodium into the cell to maintain electroneutrality, inducing hyponatremia. Potassium depletion causes a decrease in intracellular osmolarity, and without a comcomitant decrease (movement) of sodium out of the cell water will leave the cell, causing dilution of sodium in the extracellular space. The third way that potassium depletion affects sodium concentration is via hormonal mechanisms, specifically through the action of antidiuretic hormone (ADH, also known as vasopressin). ADH release results in water retention during sodium excess, increasing water reabsorption in the renal collecting tubules and ducts. ADH release occurs when cells in the supraoptic nuclei shrink because of loss of free body water, increased extracellular fluid osmolarity, or loss of intracellular K^+. All of these mechanisms result in movement of free water out of the cell. Sudden increases in serum K^+ concentration (8–9 mEq/L) are the result of transcellular movement of potassium and are associated with profound electrocardiographic abnormalities, fluid shifts, and acid-base abnormalities.

40. Where is K^+ concentrated in the body?
The potassium ion is located predominantly in the intracellular space. The sodium-potassium-adenosine triphosphate (ATP) pump is located in the cell wall and is responsible for maintaining high intracellular levels of potassium. Therefore, plasmas potassium levels are not a good reflection of body K^+ levels.

41. What happens to plasma potassium levels during acidemia?
Plasma levels of potassium may be increased (hyperkalemia) during states of acidemia, even in the presence of normal or reduced total body potassium. Hypokalemia, on the other hand, occurs in association with elevated levels of plasma insulin or during total body potassium depletion. These changes occur in acidemia, because as hydrogen (H^+) moves intracellularly, K^+ moves into the extracellular fluid to maintain electroneutrality.

42. What role does potassium play in maintaining homeostasis?
Potassium plays a critical role in muscle and nerve responsiveness. Hypokalemia may cause cardiac arrhythmias, myocardial dysfunction, muscular weakness, and intestinal ileus.

43. What is hyperkalemic periodic paralysis (HYPP)?
HYPP is a familial disease described in humans and horses (Quarter Horse and Quarter Horse crosses) that causes episodic weakness. The disease is autosomal dominant and is due to a point mutation resulting in a phenylalanine/leucine substitution in a key part of the skeletal muscle sodium channel alpha subunit. The imbalance in sodium and potassium fluxes causes a persistent depolarization of muscle cells and temporary weakness. Depending on the the affected muscle groups, clinical signs may vary (e.g., laryngeal paralysis, muscle fasciculations, prolapse of the third eyelid, generalized weakness, and recumbency). Episodes may last from minutes to hours. More severe episodes and often death are associated with the homozygous animals. Diagnosis is made by DNA testing (mane/tail hair roots or nucleated blood cells).

44. Is there any way to measure total body potassium levels?
Some laboratories have measured erythrocyte potassium levels, but further studies have shown that they are a poor indicator of total body potassium. Therefore, estimation (e) is based on a formula using total plasma Na^+ levels and estimating total body water (TBW) volume:

$$K^+_e = (plasma\ [Na^+] \times TBW) - Na^+_e$$

45. What are the sources of potassium for horses?
Roughage diets, in particular alfalfa and good-quality grass hays.

46. In what types of disease conditions are horses most prone to potassium loss?
Heavy sweating (endurance horses in competition) causes loss of Na, K, Cl, calcium, and magnesium and is usually associated with metabolic alkalosis. Salivary loss (esophageal obstruction, pharyngeal/laryngeal dysfunction) causes metabolic acidosis with loss of Na and HCO_3 predominantly. Diarrhea in horses causes loss of Na, K, Cl, and HCO_3.

47. Hyperkalemia is reported commonly in humans and animals with massive muscle necrosis. What about horses?
Horses do *not* routinely become hyperkalemic with massive muscle inflammation or necrosis. Vigorous short-term exercise causes short-lived transient hyperkalemia associated with lactic acidosis from anaerobic exercise.

48. What are the causes of hyperkalemia in horses?

True hyperkalemia	False hyperkalemia
Hypovolemia with renal failure	In vitro hemolysis (red blood cell breakdown)
Metabolic acidosis	Prolonged storage
Vigorous exercise	Markedly elevated white blood cell or platelet
HYPP	count
Renal disease	
Diabetes mellitus	
Addison's disease	

49. How do changes in chloride affect total body water?

Chloride usually parallels sodium imbalances, and loss of both sodium and chloride are related to loss or gain of free water.

50. What happens when chloride changes without a parallel change in sodium?

Decreases in plasma chloride concentration without an accompanied change in Na ion lead to nonrespiratory alkalosis caused by an increase in the strong ion difference. Associated conditions involve losses of gastric reflux, sweat, or saliva. The reverse also may occur—acidosis may result from hyperchloremia due to the strong ion difference. Cases of renal tubular acidosis may occur in horses associated with hyperchloremia and acidosis with or without hypernatremia.

51. What controls calcium and phosphorus regulation?

Parathyroid hormone (PTH) and calcitonin are the major regulatory hormones of calcium and phosphorus. The net effect of PTH is to increase ionized serum calcium levels and decrease serum phosphorus levels by (1) increasing the absorption of calcium from the intestinal tract, (2) enhancing resorption of calcium from renal tubules, (3) increasing resorption of calcium from bones, and (4) increasing the loss of phosphorus through the renal tubules by decreasing reabsorption of phosphorus. The major stimulus for PTH is decreased levels of ionized serum calcium. Since PTH plays a major role in homeostasis of calcium, ionized serum calcium is seldom decreased for long periods.

52. What are the clinical manifestations of acute hypocalcemia in horses?

Horses respond to hypocalcemia similarly to dogs and humans by manifesting tetany rather than paresis. Hypocalcemia allows spontaneous diffusion of sodium into nerve cells, causing depolarization. Overheating, exhaustion, heavy sweating, and pain are common causes of respiratory alkalosis that may trigger hypocalcemic tetany or synchronous diaphragmatic flutter in horses with marginally low serum calcium levels. Acute life-threatening hypocalcemic tetany is reason for immediate treatment.

53. How do you treat hypocalcemia in horses?

Horses may be treated similarly to cows with milk fever (postparturient paresis). Calcium borogluconate (23% solution in 0.9% saline, 5% dextrose, or Normasol, Plasmalyte, or Multisol and diluted 1:4 to 1:20) is recommended. If an arrhythmia or change in heart rate develops, the calcium infusion should be discontinued. Horses that are prone to episodes of hypocalcemia should have calcium restricted in their diet before an endurance ride. Infrequently, lactating mares also may become hypocalcemic after stress.

54. What is synchronous diaphragmatic flutter? How do you treat it?

Synchronous diaphragmatic flutter, also known as "thumps," occurs when the diaphragm contracts in synchrony with the heart. There is often a contraction or twitching in the flank region. Severe cases are associated with a characteristic "thumping" sound. In addition to hypocalcemia, synchronous diaphragmatic flutter has been associated with hypochloremic metabolic alkalosis with hypomagnesemia (most common abnormality). It is postulated that fluid, electrolyte, and acid-base derangements may disrupt the normal membrane potential of the phrenic nerve, resulting in nerve discharges in response to atrial depolarization.

Signs usually abate when the underlying cause no longer exists. Most horses undergo rapid improvement after treatment directed at the electrolyte or acid-base disturbance. Intravenous fluid therapy (23% calcium borogluconate at 250–500 ml/500 kg adult horse, diluted 1:4 to 1:20 with 0.9% saline solution) is recommended.

BIBLIOGRAPHY

1. Johnson PJ: Physiology of body fluids in the horse. Vet Clin North Am Equine Practice 14(1):1–22, 1998.
2. Whitehair KJ, Haskins SC, Whitehair JG, Pascoe JG: Clinical applications of quantitative acid-base chemistry. J Vet Int Med 1(9):1–11, 1995.

4. CLINICOPATHOLOGY

Catherine J. Savage, B.V.Sc., M.S., Ph.D., Dip. ACVIM

1. What clinicopathologic changes may be seen in a horse with exocrine pancreatic disease?
Gamma glutamyl transferase (GGT). GGT is found in high concentration in the pancreas. Thus, pancreatic damage may result in elevated serum/plasma concentrations of GGT.

Aspartate aminotransferase (AST). AST is found in high concentration within pancreatic tissue and may be elevated in horses with pancreatic damage.

Creatine kinase (CK). The BB dimer isoenzyme of CK is found in greatest concentration within the equine pancreas; however, it is of little clinical benefit because CK isoenzymes are rarely measured on an individual basis. Since the BB dimer of CK contributes relatively little to the overall CK concentration, elevation is not always noted in pancreatic disease.

Lactate dehydrogenase (LDH). The most prevalent isoenzyme of LDH in the pancreas is LDH-1, which contributes to approximately 20% of the total serum concentration and may be elevated in horses with pancreatic disease.

Amylase. Normal equine amylase concentration has been reported as 14–35 IU/L and increases dramatically in some cases of pancreatic disease (e.g., > 700 IU/L). Comparison of amylase values in serum and peritoneal fluid may be useful in horses suspected of pancreatic involvement; in normal horses the amylase concentration should be higher in serum than in peritoneal fluid (normal range of amylase within peritoneal fluid: 0–14 IU/L). In horses with acute pancreatitis, peritoneal concentrations may exceed serum levels. However, analysis of peritoneal fluid amylase concentration is unhelpful in horses with chronic, insidious, nonnecrotizing pancreatic disease. The specificity of serum amylase is poor, and false-positive elevations occur in horses with duodenitis-proximal jejunitis/small intestinal ileus, when glomerular filtration rate is reduced, and after administration of narcotic drugs. Fractional excretion of amylase has been used to determine its origin. Amylase concentrations, however, can be misleading because they may be low or normal in the face of severe pancreatic disease.

Lipase. The normal range for equine serum lipase has been reported as 23–87 IU/L, whereas the range for equine peritoneal fluid lipase is 0–36 IU/L. Peritoneal fluid for analysis of lipase concentrations should be collected in a plain tube without anticoagulant. Lipase concentrations are usually elevated in horses with acute pancreatic necrosis; however, they may be low or normal (and thus unhelpful).

Lipemia. In some cases lipemia may be visualized grossly in the plasma. It may be a sign of pancreatic exocrine or endocrine failure or hepatic disease.

Calcium. It is important to evaluate the calcium concentration and to correct it for hypoalbuminemia. Horses with pancreatic problems (especially acute, necrotizing pancreatitis) may have moderate-to-severe hypocalcemia, presumably secondary to calcium deposition after fat necrosis. Although hypocalcemia is more characteristic of pancreatic disease, it is also possible for horses to have hypercalcemia.

Fibrinogen. Hyperfibrinogenemia may occur in cases of pancreatitis, since fibrinogen is an acute-phase inflammatory protein. However, values may be difficult to interpret if severe disease precipitates disseminated intravascular coagulation (DIC). DIC differs in horses and small animals; fibrinogen levels are rarely decreased because of the preexisting, predisposing inflammatory condition that precipitated the coagulopathy.

Globulin. Concentrations of globulin also may be elevated as a result of inflammation.

Furr MO, Robertson J: Two cases of equine pancreatic disease and a review of the literature. Equine Vet Educ 4:55–58, 1992.

McClure JJ: Acute pancreatitis. In Robinson NE (ed): Current Therapy in Equine Medicine , vol. 2. Philadelphia, W.B. Saunders, 1987, pp 46–47.

Parry BW, Crisman MV: Serum and peritoneal fluid amylase and lipase reference values in horses. Equine Vet J 23:390–391, 1991.

2. Why is exocrine pancreatic disease difficult to distinguish from hepatic disease ?

Hepatic disease and exocrine pancreatic disease may be difficult to distinguish clinicopatho-logically because elevations of enzymes, including GGT, AST, and LDH, may be similar. Although the isoenzyme configuration of LDH varies between hepatic and pancreatic diseases, an isoenzyme analysis is seldom performed. If the isoenzymes are analyzed, the pancreas has more LDH-1, which may be elevated in disease states. The liver's predominant isoenzyme is LDH-5, which is usually found in the serum only during hepatic disease. Lipemia, visualized grossly in the plasma, may be a sign of hepatic disease or pancreatic exocrine or endocrine failure in horses.

3. What clinicopathologic changes may be seen in a horse with hepatic failure?

- Low albumin (hypoalbuminemia)
- Low fibrinogen (hypofibrinogenemia)
- Low glucose (hypoglycemia)
- Low blood urea nitrogen (BUN)
- Increased ammonia (hyperammonemia)
- Prolonged prothrombin time (PT)
- Prolonged partial thromboplastin time (PTT, aPTT)
- Low packed cell volume (PCV) (i.e., < 18 %)
- Profound polycythemia (i.e. PCV > 55 %)

Jeffcott LB: Primary liver cell carcinoma in a young thoroughbred horse. J Pathol 97:394–397, 1969.

Messer NT, Johnson PJ: Idiopathic acute hepatic disease in horses: 12 cases (1982–1992). J Am Vet Med Assoc 204:1934–1937, 1994.

Roby KAW, et al: Hepatocellular carcinoma associated with erythrocytosis and hypoglycemia in a yearling filly. J Am Vet Med Assoc 180:1422–1424, 1982.

4. What enzymology tests can be used to assess hepatic disease? What information do they reveal?

PARAMETER	SIGNIFICANCE
AST	Liver (hepatocellular); also an enzyme of muscle and pancreas
L-iditol dehydrogenase (sorbitol dehydrogenase, L-iDH, SDH)	Sensitive hepatocellular enzyme
LDH-5	Liver isoenzyme; useful and stable indicator of hepatocellular damage
Total LDH	Not hepatic-specific and of limited use
Arginase	Liver enzyme; specific indicator of hepatic disease because minimal concentrations exist in other organs; may increase mildly with fasting
GGT	Membrane-bound enzyme on canalicular surface of hepatocytes and biliary epithelial surface; significant increases recognized in cases of biliary disease/cholestasis
Alkaline phosphatase (AP, ALP)	Membrane-bound enzyme on canalicular surface of hepatocytes and biliary epithelial surface; significant increases predominantly recognized in cases of biliary disease

5. What causes hyperbilirubinemia and thus icterus in horses?

The most classic sign alerting the veterinarian to the possibility of hepatobiliary disease is icterus. However, icterus may be due to a variety of causes:

1. **Inappetance.** Decreased nutritional intake by the horse (e.g., in cases of pneumonia, peritonitis) is often mistaken for a primary hepatic problem, because peripheral indirect-reacting (i.e., unconjugated) bilirubin increases. Hyperbilirubinemia due to inappetance is probably

caused by diminished uptake of indirect-reacting bilirubin by hepatocytes because of a decrease in a cell surface protein termed ligandin. Its decreased concentration is induced by protein deprivation. Ligandin is one of the proteins responsible for transport and uptake of bilirubin. In general, hyperbilirubinemia due to fasting does not exceed 5 mg/dl, although higher concentrations (e.g., 8–9 mg/dl) occur occasionally.

2. **Hemolysis of red blood cells.** Hyperbilirubinemia due to hemolysis is diagnosed easily as long as a packed cell volume (PCV) is measured concurrently. The PCV is often less than 18–20%. A confounding situation may exist when horses in terminal hepatic failure progress into an hemolytic event. Because such horses show evidence of both hepatic disease and hemolysis, the bilirubin concentration may be very high.

3. **Hepatic compromise.** Hepatic disease may cause increases in indirect- and direct-reacting bilirubin, depending on the primary and secondary hepatic dysfunctions. Other situations in which hyperbilirubinemia may be confusing are cases of endotoxemia secondary to colitis/colotyphlitis, enteritis/enterocolitis, and ischemia-reperfusion. Horses with endotoxemia usually have moderately elevated bilirubin levels and may have mild-to-moderate elevations in hepatic enzyme concentrations. These changes are presumably caused by the exposure of the liver to high concentrations of endotoxin (i.e., lipopolysaccharide) from gram-negative bacteria travelling from compromised intestine to the liver via the portal circulation. Although the liver has mechanisms for detoxification, it may be damaged by the toxins. Because endotoxemic horses are often inappetant, the hyperbilirubinemia is often compounded by fasting. Hyperbilirubinemia and elevation of liver enzymes may be seen in cases of colonic torsion secondary to extreme distention of the large intestine and cause hepatocellular damage and biliary stasis. Horses with colonic torsion may suffer from endotoxemia before and after surgery, which also may cause hyperbilirubinemia.

4. **Extrahepatic problems.** If the biliary ducts are obstructed or disrupted, large increases in direct-reacting bilirubin (direct hyperbilirubinemia) are present. In general, there is much more indirect-reacting bilirubin than direct-reacting bilirubin in horses; thus, hyperbilirubinemia consisting of > 20% direct-reacting bilirubin indicates a posthepatic disorder.

6. What reasons have been given for hepatoencephalopathy?

Although theories abound, the pathophysiologic mechanisms for hepatoencephalopathy in horses are not known. Extrapolations from work in other species suggest that numerous disorders are involved. The following theories are currently thought to be most accurate:

1. Hypoglycemia.

2. Hyperammonemia, with ammonia acting as a neurotoxin on the cerebrum.

3. Increased concentrations of an endogenous benzodiazepine-like substance; for this reason, diazepam is no longer considered the best drug for sedating horses with hepatoencephalopathy, although it appears to be effective.

4. Altered plasma amino acid metabolism results in deranged monoamine neurotransmission (i.e., serotonin and tryptophan).

5. An imbalance of excitatory neurotransmission (mediated by glutamate and aspartate) and inhibitory neurotransmission (mediated by gamma-aminobutyric acid [GABA] and glycine).

6. Abnormal and/or excessive production of substances derived from bacterial or protein metabolism in the intestine. If the concentration of these substances is reduced by therapeutic agents, which diminish intestinal flora, or by a low protein diet, cerebral function may improve without a primary effect of therapeutic agents on the liver.

Maddison JE: Hepatic encephalopathy. Current concepts of the pathogenesis. J Vet Intern Med 6:341–353, 1992.

7. What is the difference between unconjugated and conjugated bilirubin?

Unconjugated bilirubin is indirect-reacting, and has not passed through the hepatocyte for conjugation. Conjugated bilirubin is direct-reacting, has undergone uptake by the hepatocyte and conjugation, and is released into the canaliculi of the biliary system. Conjugated bilirubin is more water-soluble and more likely to be passed into the urine in states of hyperbilirubinemia.

8. Why do sclera appear so icteric in patients with hyperbilirubinemia?

The sclera are an excellent site for assessment of icterus because they are unpigmented, and bilirubin has a high affinity for elastin, which exists in high concentration within the sclera.

9. What happens to urobilinogen and conjugated bilirubin in patients with complete blockage of the common hepatic duct?

If blockage occurs, both unconjugated and conjugated bilirubin increase. A concentration of conjugated bilirubin exceeding 20% of the total bilirubin is a significant elevation. In normal horses, urobilinogen is excreted into the urine and should be detected on a urinary reagent strip; however, bile flow is obstructed in patients with complete blockage of the common hepatic duct. Thus, conjugated bilirubin does not reach the intestine, and there is no substrate from which anaerobic bacteria can produce urobilinogen. Consequently, the urobilinogen may be abnormally absent in the urine after a short time. Some of the excessive amount of conjugated bilirubin may be excreted into the urine, because it is water-soluble. Its concentration can be measured on a urinary reagent strip or in the laboratory. A crude estimate can be gained by shaking the urine; if bilirubin is present in the urine, a yellow-to-green froth forms.

10. How are bilirubin, urobilinogen, and stercobilin manufactured in horses?

Aged red blood cells
↓
Hemoglobin
(phagocytozed via monocyte-phagocyte system)
↓
Heme and globin
↓
Pyrrole chain and free iron
↓
Biliverdin
↓
Indirect-reacting bilirubin (i.e., unconjugated)
(released from macrophages into plasma in an insoluble form; i.e., not water-soluble)
↓
Indirect-reacting bilirubin—albumin complex for plasma transfer
(cannot be removed by the kidneys because of its large size and because it is not water-soluble)
↓
Arrives at liver
↓
Hepatocyte uptake
↓
Conjugation with glucose and diglucuronide in the hepatocyte
↓
Direct-reacting bilirubin (i.e., conjugated) secreted into canaliculi
↓
Transported into bile duct
(horses have no gallbladder for storage of bile)
↓
Small intestine (anaerobic bacterial activity)
↓
Urobilinogen and stercobilin
↓   ↓
Absorbed from intestine   Incorporated into feces
and excreted in urine
↓
Reexcreted by the liver

11. What are the functions of bile acids?

Bile acids (i.e., bile salts) are an important component of bile in horses. They function as detergents in the intestinal tract to emulsify fat particles, thus reducing the surface tension. They also assist in the formation of micelles and therefore the absorption of fatty acids.

12. How are bile acids conjugated in horses?

In contrast to small animals and humans, most equine bile acids are conjugated with taurine rather than glycine. One should be sure that the laboratory can test for tauroconjugated as well as glycoconjugated bile acids.

13. What level of bile acids indicates hepatobiliary disease? Why is one sample sufficient for bile acid measurement in horses? In what diseases have very high bile acid concentrations been demonstrated?

Total bile acid measurements > 14–20 μM/l indicate hepatobiliary disease. Because the horse does not have a gallbladder, there is no postprandial increase in circulating bile acids (as in small animals). Consequently, a single sample may be taken for bile acid analysis, regardless of the timing of the horse's last meal. Exceedingly high values have been recorded in cases of cholelithiasis and portosystemic shunts.

Traub-Dargatz JL: Biliary disorders. In Robinson NE (ed): Current Therapy in Equine Medicine, vol. 3. Philadelphia, W.B. Saunders, 1992, p 260.

14. List the reasons why an adult horse may be hypoglycemic or hyperglycemic.

Hypoglycemia in adult horses indicates (1) failure of gluconeogenesis pathways of the liver in hepatic disease/failure, (2) bacteremia and consumption of glucose, (3) endotoxemia, or (4) in vitro glycolysis (by erythrocytes).

Hyperglycemia in adult horses reflects (1) stress and excitement, (2) pain (e.g., colic), (3) diabetes mellitus (primary types I and II and secondary), (4) pituitary adenoma (which causes secondary diabetes mellitus), (5) exogenous glucocorticoid administration, or (6) iatrogenic rapid administration of dextrose. Hyperglycemia secondary to stress and pain may be seen in horses with hepatic disease, or stress and pain may artificially elevate a low glucose measurement (from decreased gluconeogenesis). For this reason even low normal glucose concentrations should be viewed with suspicion in horses with severe hepatic disease.

15. Explain the use of the hepatic enzyme, alanine aspartate transferase (ALT).

ALT is *not* useful in assessing the liver of horses and should be ignored if a value is provided on the biochemical profile. Laboratories specializing in human or small animal analyses may provide the ALT value.

16. What is L-iditol dehydrogenase (L-iDH)?

L-iDH was known until recently as sorbitol dehydrogenase (SDH). It is an hepatocellular enzyme and is the most sensitive indicator of hepatocyte health and therefore damage in horses. L-iDH is a labile enzyme and has a short half-life in the plasma. Blood should be transported to the laboratory quickly if the measurement is to be accurate. Unfortunately, some laboratories do not analyze for L-iDH because of its instability. However, if measurement can be performed, serial samples are especially useful.

17. Is lactate dehydrogenase (LDH) a useful indicator of hepatic damage?

It is not useful to measure total LDH because it is not specific for the liver. However, the isoenzyme LDH-5 is a specific indicator of hepatocellular damage and can be measured by laboratories with relative ease; a specific assay is now available. Because LDH-5 is stable at room temperature for over 24 hours, it is a useful test for the practitioner in the field.

18. List the reasons why a horse may have a decreased BUN concentration.

1. Hepatic failure (most common reason for decreased BUN value in adult horses)
2. Intravenous fluid administration (overhydration)

3. Neonatal foals (lower value than adult horses)
4. Low protein diet (uncommon)
5. Administration of anabolic steroid drugs

19. Why is it important to understand the urea cycle in a horse with liver failure?

If the liver is failing, the urea cycle does not function; thus, urea and BUN are not formed from ammonia. As a result, ammonia increases (which may be important in the pathogenesis of hepatoencephalopathy) and BUN decreases.

20. How should ammonia be measured?

A heparin tube should be used to obtain a blood sample and then placed on ice or an ice water slurry. The heparin tube should be centrifuged as soon as possible. Because of its instability the plasma still must be maintained on ice or an ice water slurry until final transport to the laboratory performing the ammonia analysis. It is prudent to warn the laboratory about the sample's arrival. It is imperative to obtain blood (treated in the same manner) from a control horse (i.e. age- and sex-matched) for concurrent ammonia analysis.

21. What causes hyperammonemia?

Hyperammonemia results from malfunction of the hepatic-based urea cycle; ammonia is not converted through the cycle to urea. Hyperammonemia is associated with a poor prognosis in horses with hepatic disease or failure and also has also been associated with the onset and signs of hepatoencephalopathy. It has been described in a woodchuck and in one horse with renal encephalopathy.

22. How do starvation, burn wounds, and diseases with significant fever result in increased BUN?

These processes are associated with rapid tissue catabolism. The subsequent increase in BUN is usually small.

23. What mechanisms can cause hypoalbuminemia? List differential diagnoses for each mechanism.

MECHANISMS	DIFFERENTIAL DIAGNOSES
Insufficient production	Liver failure
Protein losing enteropathy (i.e., gastrointestinal loss)	Intestinal infiltration (e.g., lymphoma, inflammatory intestinal disease) and other causes of malabsorption
	Intestinal mucosal integrity compromise (e.g., colitis, enterocolitis, ulceration, endoparasitism)
Protein-losing nephropathy (i.e., renal loss)	Nephrosis
	Glomerular nephritis
Protein loss into body spaces	Peritonitis
	Pleuropneumonia/pleuritis
	Wounds
Malnutrition	Poor dentition
	Inadequate feed
Hemodilution	Subsequent to hemorrhage

24. Which protein provides the greatest oncotic pressure support to the vascular space?

Albumin. Under normal circumstances albumin is produced by the liver and is responsible, in conjunction with assistance from sodium and chloride ions (i.e., the Donnan effect) and other plasma proteins, for maintaining oncotic pressure within the circulatory system. Albumin concentrations < 2.2 g/dl are associated with an increased risk of edema, which occurs commonly in the areas of the prepuce, ventrum, and distal limbs. Ascites occurs secondary to imbalances in Starling's law (governing the movement between the circulatory system and peritoneal cavity).

25. What is the significance of the globulin concentration of a horse?

The globulin fraction of the plasma protein concentration provides information about the degree of inflammatory response. The globulin fraction of plasma protein is composed of α-globulin (lipoproteins, acute-phase proteins), β-globulin (iron-containing proteins, complement), and γ-globulin (immunoglobulins) fractions. Serum electrophoresis should be performed to examine the individual fractions. This information can be useful (1) to ascertain the presence of a monoclonal gammopathy (e.g., in cases of plasma cell myeloma, multiple myeloma, and possibly lymphoma [γ-globulin increase]); (2) to assess degree of inflammation (e.g., α-globulin and γ-globulin involvement); (3) to assess tissue damage (e.g., α-globulin increase); and (4) to support a tentative diagnosis of immune-mediated disease (e.g., possible γ-globulin increase). It is rare for the β-globulin fraction to be increased alone.

26. What enzymes are sometimes used to assess myocardial damage? How reliable are they in horses?

The myocardial fraction of CK, CK-MB, and isoenzymes LDH-1 and LDH-2 may be used to assess acute myocardial damage in horses. Unfortunately, further studies are needed to assess the predictive value of elevations of these enzymes in horses with myocardial injury and necrosis. They are most likely elevated in cases of myocardial necrosis. Currently, normal levels do not rule out the presence of significant (even acute) myocardial damage.

Bonagura JD, Reef VB: Cardiovascular diseases. In Reed SM, Bayly WM (eds): Equine Internal Medicine. Philadelphia, W.B. Saunders, 1998, pp 342–345.

Eaded SC, Bounous DI: Laboratory Profiles of Equine Disease. St. Louis, Mosby, 1997, pp 7, 88.

27. What ratio is performed on equine urine to provide information about renal disease or dysfunction?

The urinary GGT-to-creatinine ratio (urinary GGT:Cr) is performed on equine urine, *not* the protein-to-creatinine ratio, as in small animals. GGT is an enzyme found in the brush border of the proximal renal tubular epithelium as well as in the liver and pancreas of horses. GGT from the liver and pancreas, however, is not filtered by the glomerulus unless significant proteinuria is present. The urinary GGT-to-creatinine ratio is calculated using the following formula:

$$\text{Urinary GGT:Cr ratio} = \text{GGT}_U/\text{creatinine}_U \times 0.01$$

If the value is < 25, the brush border of the renal tubules (especially proximal tubules) is not affected (i.e., normal renal tubular function generally may be assumed). If the value is 25–60, however, it is possible that the horse is normal or has been azotemic, probably because of prerenal mechanisms (e.g., dehydration). There may have been a minor increase in the GGT released from the brush border into the urine filtrate. Of interest, when researchers held horses off water for 48 hours, no differences were seen in GGT activity. Some veterinarians believe that ratio values < 60 are normal.

If the value is > 60–100, it is likely that the kidney has undergone some degree of damage and that GGT has been released from the renal tubule brush border into the urine filtrate. The limitation of this ratio is that it does not appear to be a good prognostic indicator. A lower abnormal value (e.g., 120 vs. 200) does not guarantee that renal damage is less severe. However, if a trend is established (i.e., if the ratio value is increasing or decreasing),it may be of some prognostic use.

Bayly WM: Urinary enzymes. In Reed SM, Bayly WM (eds): Equine Internal Medicine. Philadelphia, W.B. Saunders, 1998. pp 845–847.

Hinchcliff KW, McGuirk SM, MacWilliams PS: Gentamicin nephrotoxicity. Proc Am Assoc Equine Pract 33:67, 1987.

28. What system should you assess in an inappetant, possibly "foundered" horse that was ridden on a long trail ride 3 days ago? You learn in a telephone conversation with the owner that the patient is an unconditioned, 6-year-old Quarter Horse mare.

Assessment of the urinary system, specifically of renal damage, is warranted. It is advisable to take a blood sample for a biochemical profile (especially creatinine, BUN, sodium, chloride, potassium, calcium, and total carbon dioxide), a urine sample to evaluate specific gravity, and a reagent stick analysis for blood (includes pigment), glucose, and protein. If the specific gravity is isosthenuric (i.e., 1.008–1.014) and/or blood is present, a complete urinalysis at a laboratory should be performed. The patient potentially has had three nephrotoxic insults:

1. Dehydration may be present. Inappetance often means that the horse stops drinking.

2. The owner may have given phenylbutazone, believing that the horse has "foundered" (i.e. has laminitis). Nonsteroidal antiinflammatory drugs (NSAIDs) may cause renal papillary necrosis, especially if the horse is dehydrated.

3. Myoglobinemia may have led to myoglobinuria. Trail riding of an unconditioned horse may result in a rhabdomyolytic episode.

29. What is azotemia? Discuss prerenal, renal, and postrenal azotemia.

Azotemia refers to an increase in BUN and creatinine in plasma or serum.

Prerenal azotemia is the reversible increase in BUN and creatinine due to decreased renal perfusion. The horse retains its urine-concentrating ability (i.e., specific gravity > 1.020). Even if renal damage has occurred (as in certain diseases or after surgery), the terms prerenal azotemia and prerenal failure are still used when azotemia is reversible and urine is not isosthenuric. Therefore, prerenal azotemia may lead to a permanent decrease in functional renal mass. This loss remains clinically silent unless further compromise occurs. Usually the increases in BUN and creatinine are small in comparison to horses with renal or postrenal azotemia. In many species the BUN-to-creatinine ratio is very high in prerenal azotemia because of an increased absorption of urea when tubular flow rates are low. However, this phenomenon does not appear to occur in all horses.

Renal azotemia is an increase in BUN and creatinine due to primary renal disease. The horse loses its ability to concentrate urine, even in the presence of dehydration. Specific gravity is < 1.020 and often becomes isosthenuric (specific gravity of 1.008–1.014). Azotemia occurs in both acute renal failure and chronic renal failure, although in horses the creatinine and BUN vary. Usually the BUN-to-creatinine ratio is < 10:1 in acute renal failure and > 10:1 in chronic renal failure. History, physical examination, other clinicopathologic measurements, and even ultrasonographic evaluations can also differentiate the two syndromes.

Postrenal azotemia occurs in diseases in which the urinary tract is obstructed, disrupted, or ruptured past the point of the renal tubules. Postrenal azotemia due to bladder rupture usually causes a high BUN-to-creatinine ratio due to preferential diffusion of urea (compared with creatinine) across the peritoneal surface.

Schott HC II: Examination of the urinary system. In Reed SM, Bayly WM (eds): Equine Internal Medicine Philadelphia, W.B. Saunders, 1998, pp 830–845.

30. What clinicopathologic parameters should you assess in a horse with suspected acute renal failure?

It is advisable to obtain a blood sample for a biochemical profile (especially creatinine, BUN, sodium, chloride, potassium, calcium, and bicarbonate/total carbon dioxide [tCO_2]). A urine sample should be obtained for urinalysis or at least to evaluate the specific gravity and perform a reagent strip analysis for blood (includes pigment), glucose, and protein.

31. What clinicopathologic changes are associated with acute renal failure in horses?

Alterations associated with acute renal failure include the following:

1. Increased creatinine (Cr) (substantial increases often measured)
2. Increased BUN
3. BUN:Cr ratio < 10:1 (usually)
4. Hyponatremia
5. Hypochloremia
6. Hyperkalemia (variable; also depends on bicarbonate/total carbon dioxide concentration; may require correction)

7. Hypocalcemia (calcium values may be normal)
8. Bicarbonate/total carbon dioxide decreased to normal
9. Specific gravity isosthenuric (i.e., 1.008–1.014)
Other changes that may be present include the following:
1. Urinary gross blood and microscopic red blood cells
2. Urinary gross pigmentation (with no/few microscopic red blood cells)
3. Urinary protein
4. White blood cells on urinalysis
5. Urinary casts
6. Urinary crystals (usually a normal finding)
7. Packed cell volume may be decreased in horses with hematuria. If you believe that the horse is in chronic renal failure, it is advisable to check the packed cell volume. Horses with chronic renal failure are frequently anemic because of a decrease in erythropoietin production.

32. If a horse experiences an episode of equine rhabdomyolytic syndrome (ERS) or "tying-up" at 0 hours, when will increases and decreases in the concentrations of CK and AST occur? Why do they differ in the time to peak concentrations?

CK is a sensitive and specific indicator of muscle damage. The half-life is short (2 hours), and peak CK levels are reached by approximately 6 hours. If the muscle disease is a single event, CK levels may decrease to normal by 24 hours. However, if the insult is massive or myolysis/myonecrosis continues, CK may remain elevated for many days. Challenging aspects of the assessment of CK are its short half-life, its ability to increase continually in the face of an ongoing myolytic episode, and the fact that hemolysis may cause an elevated CK level.

AST (also known as serum glutamic oxaloacetic transaminase [SGOT]) is a less specific indicator of muscle damage because large concentrations are also found in the liver, along with smaller concentrations within the erythrocytes, kidney, and pancreas. The half-life of AST is 18 hours (much longer than the half-life of CK), and peak concentrations after a single myolytic event are usually attained after approximately 24 hours (vs. 6 hours for CK). The AST may persist at elevated concentrations in the plasma for approximately 10–14 days after the most recent muscle damage. AST is slower to rise in concentration, because it is associated with hepatocyte and myocyte mitochondria; therefore, its concentration in the plasma takes some time to increase.

33. What are the three isoenzymes of CK?
1. CK-MM (found in skeletal muscle)
2. CK-MB (found in cardiac muscle)
3. CK-BB (found in brain and other central neurologic tissue)

34. Give the advantages and disadvantages of measuring CK concentration in the cerebrospinal fluid (CSF) of a horse.
   Advantages
   • CK may be increased in neurologic disease associated with myelin degeneration and neuronal cell damage (e.g., equine protozoal myeloencephalitis [EPM], equine degenerative myelopathy [EDM], equine motor neuron disease [EMND], and polyneuritis equi [cauda equina syndrome]).
   • Horses with the neurologic form of EHV-1 may have alterations in the permeability of the blood-brain barrier and thus increases in CSF CK.
   • CK has been used as an adjunct to differentiate EPM from compressive spinal cord disease because CK concentration is higher in EPM.
   • Persistently elevated CSF CK in horses with EPM is associated with poor prognosis.
   Disadvantages
   • If the blood-brain barrier is damaged, CK may leak into the CSF from the peripheral blood and give an erroneously elevated value.
   • The test is neither specific nor sensitive.

35. In what disease has elevated LDH been recognized in CSF? What concentration of LDH is normal in the CSF of horses ?

Elevated levels of LDH in the CSF have been recognized in horses with spinal lymphoma. In normal horses, CSF from either the atlantooccipital space or the lumbosacral space may have an LDH concentration of 0–8 IU/L.

BIBLIOGRAPHY

Bayly WM: Urinary enzymes. In Reed SM, Bayly WM (eds): Equine Internal Medicine. Philadelphia, W.B. Saunders, 1998. pp 845–847.

Bonagura JD, Reef VB: Cardiovascular diseases. In Reed SM, Bayly WM (eds): Equine Internal Medicine. Philadelphia, W.B. Saunders, 1998, pp 342–345.

Eaded SC, Bounous DI: Laboratory Profiles of Equine Disease. St. Louis, Mosby, 1997, pp 7, 88.

Furr MO, Robertson J: Two cases of equine pancreatic disease and a review of the literature. Equine Vet Educ 4:55–58, 1992.

Hinchcliff KW, McGuirk SM, MacWilliams PS: Gentamicin nephrotoxicity. Proc Am Assoc Equine Pract 33:67, 1987.

Jeffcott LB: Primary liver cell carcinoma in a young thoroughbred horse. J Pathol 97:394–397, 1969.

Maddison JE: Hepatic encephalopathy. Current concepts of the pathogenesis. J Vet Intern Med 6:341–353, 1992.

McClure JJ: Acute pancreatitis. In Robinson NE (ed): Current Therapy in Equine Medicine , vol. 2. Philadelphia, W.B. Saunders, 1987, pp 46–47.

Messer NT, Johnson PJ: Idiopathic acute hepatic disease in horses: 12 cases (1982–1992). J Am Vet Med Assoc 204:1934–1937, 1994.

Parry BW, Crisman MV: Serum and peritoneal fluid amylase and lipase reference values in horses. Equine Vet J 23:390–391, 1991.

Roby KAW, et al: Hepatocellular carcinoma associated with erythrocytosis and hypoglycemia in a yearling filly. J Am Vet Med Assoc 180:1422–1424, 1982.

Schott HC II: Examination of the urinary system. In Reed SM, Bayly WM (eds): Equine Internal Medicine Philadelphia, W.B. Saunders, 1998, pp 830–845.

Traub-Dargatz JL: Biliary disorders. In Robinson NE (ed): Current Therapy in Equine Medicine, vol. 3. Philadelphia, W.B. Saunders, 1992, p 260.

5. ENDOCRINOLOGY

Mary Rose Paradis, D.V.M., M.S., Dip. ACVIM, and
Melissa T. Hines, D.V.M., Ph.D., Dip. ACVIM

1. What is the most common endocrinologic problem in horses?

Equine Cushing-like syndrome is the most common endocrinologic problem in horses. It is caused by adenomatous/hyperplastic changes in the pars intermedia of the pituitary gland. It is known as equine pituitary adenoma, equine pituitary hyperplasia, equine Cushing's disease/syndrome, and pituitary pars intermedia dysfunction.

2. What is the normal anatomy of the equine pituitary?

The pituitary gland is formed embryonically from extensions of both nervous tissue from the brain and epithelia from the oral cavity, which form the neurohypophysis and the adenohypophysis. The adenohypophysis is composed of the pars distalis, pars tuberalis, and pars intermedia. In horses the pars intermedia surrounds the neurohypophysis.

3. What is the signalment of animals most likely to have equine Cushing's disease?

Equine Cushing's disease affects the elderly horse. The average age in one study of 21 cases of pituitary adenoma in horses was 21 years. The youngest reported case was a 7-year-old horse. There is no breed or gender predilection.

van der Kolk JH, Kalsbeek HC, van Garderen E, et al: Equine pituitary neoplasia: A clinical report of 21 cases (1990–1992). Vet Rec 133:594–597, 1993.

4. What are the clinical signs of equine Cushing's disease?

The most common clinical sign of equine Cushing's disease is hirsutism, an excessively long, curly haircoat (see figure on following page). It may be present over the entire body, found in patches, or represented by long guard hairs in the jugular furrow. Affected horses may have delayed shedding or may not shed their haircoat in the summer. Owners remark that animals feel damp because of increased sweating. Other clinical signs include polyuria/polydipsia, muscle wasting, laminitis, blindness (rare), seizures (rare), and increased susceptibility to infections (e.g., parasitism, pneumonia, subsolar abscesses).

5. What are the more common clinicopathologic abnormalities, as determined by biochemical profile and complete blood count, in horses with Cushing's disease?

Hyperglycemia has been reported in 26–85% of affected horses. Elevations of alkaline phosphatase also have been noted. Less commonly neutrophilia with lymphopenia has been seen and diagnosed as a stress leukogram.

Dybdal N: Pituitary pars intermedia dysfunction (equine Cushing's-like disease). In Robinson E (ed): Current Therapy in Equine Medicine, 4th ed. Philadelphia, W.B. Saunders, 1997, pp 499–501.

van der Kolk JH, Kalsbeek HC, van Garderen E, et al: Equine pituitary neoplasia: A clinical report of 21 cases (1990–1992). Vet Rec 133:594–597, 1993.

6. Why are Cushingnoid horses hyperglycemic?

The hyperglycemia in Cushingnoid horses is probably related to the development of an insulin resistance. Affected horses often have elevated insulin levels and do not respond appropriately to an intravenous glucose tolerance test.

Garcia MC, Beech J: Equine intravenous glucose tolerance tests: Glucose and insulin responses of healthy horses fed grain or hay and of horses with pituitary adenoma. Am J Vet Res 47:570–572, 1986.

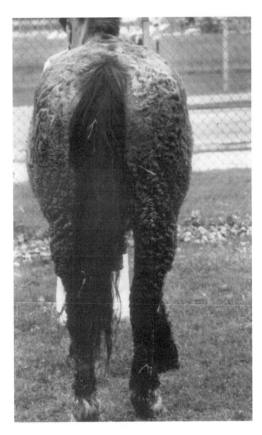

Hirsutism in an aged horse with Cushing's syndrome (pituitary adenoma). Note the long curly hair.

7. What is the mechanism of polydipsia/polyuria in some horses with Cushing's syndrome?

Several mechanisms may contribute to the polydipsia/polyuria seen in some Cushingnoid horses. Osmotic diuresis may result from the hyperglycemia. In addition, enlargement of the pars intermedia may compress the neurohypophysis, which normally produces antidiuretic hormone. Elevated cortisol also may increase glomerular filtration rate.

8. Name six tests used to diagnose equine Cushing's disease.
1. Adrenocorticotrophic hormone (ACTH) stimulation test
2. Dexamethasone suppression test
3. Measurement of endogenous ACTH levels
4. Measurement of insulin levels
5. Intravenous glucose tolerance test
6. Thyrotropin-releasing hormone test

9. Which of the above tests is least helpful in determining the presence of pituitary dysfunction?

The ACTH stimulation test has *not* been consistently helpful in the diagnosis of equine Cushing's disease. The expected result in normal horses is a 2–3-fold increase of plasma cortisol after stimulation with ACTH. The horse with a pituitary adenoma would be expected to have an exaggerated response 4 times greater than baseline cortisol. Unfortunately, the results from each group may overlap considerably.

10. Which of the above tests are the most helpful?

Probably the most helpful tests are the dexamethasone suppression test, endogenous ACTH level test, and measurement of insulin levels. Often the combination of these tests yields the most reliable diagnosis.

11. Describe how the overnight dexamethasone suppression test is performed.

Dexamethasone, 40 µg/kg (i.e., 20-mg dose in a 500-kg [1100-lb] horse), is administered intramuscularly at 5 PM after a baseline blood sample for cortisol measurement has been drawn. A second blood sample for cortisol measurement is drawn between 8 AM and noon on the next day. The expected response in normal horses is suppression of cortisol levels below 1 µg/ml. The horse with a pituitary adenoma will *not* suppress, and the cortisol level will be above 1 µg/ml. This test is safe for most animals; however, it should not be performed in a horse that has recurrent laminitis (which may be a complication of pituitary adenoma).

Dybdal NO, Hargreaves KM, Madigan JE, et al: Diagnostic testing for pituitary pars intermedia dysfunction in horses. J Am Vet Med Assoc 204:627–632, 1994.

12. Compare the endogenous ACTH levels in normal horses and ponies with levels in horses or ponies with pituitary adenomas.

ACTH levels in normal horses and ponies are significantly different. The ACTH level in normal horses is 18.68 ± 6.79 pg/ml, whereas in normal ponies it is 8.35 ± 2.92 pg/ml. In horses and ponies with pituitary dysfunction the ACTH levels are elevated to a mean of 199.18 ± 182.8 and 206.21 ± 319.56, respectively. The range in both groups is wide; therefore, endogenous ACTH levels > 27 pg/ml in ponies and > 50 pg/ml in horses should be considered diagnostic of a pituitary adenoma.

Couetil L, Paradis MR, Knoll J: Plasma adrenocorticotropin concentration in healthy horses and in horses with clinical signs of hyperadrenocorticism. J Vet Intern Med 10:1–6, 1996.

13. ACTH can be quite labile after collection. Describe the handling protocol necessary to obtain a valid sample.

Blood is collected in an ethylenediamine tetraacetic acid (EDTA)-coated tube. Recently it was found that plasma ACTH remains stable at room temperature (19° C) for up to 3 hours. During this time the blood must be spun down and separated into a plastic (polypropylene) tube and frozen. It should be shipped on dry ice to the laboratory. In the unlikely circumstance that it is not possible to obtain dry ice, one may freeze the plastic tube in a cup of water for transportation. However, if the sample thaws, it is useless.

Couteil L, Paradis MR, Knoll J: Plasma adrenocorticotropin concentration in healthy horses and in horses with clinical signs of hyperadrenocorticism. J Vet Intern Med 10:1–6, 1996.

14. Compare insulin levels in normal horses and horses with pituitary adenoma.

Plasma insulin levels are consistently higher in horses with pituitary adenomas. The normal levels in hay- and grain-fed horses are 11.9 ± 2.0 µU/ml and 16.4 ± 3.2 µU/ml, respectively. In one study, horses with pituitary adenomas had average insulin levels of 105.1 ± 20.2 µU/ml. Usually they are insulin-resistant.

Garcia MC, Beech J: Equine intravenous glucose tolerance tests: Glucose and insulin responses of healthy horses fed grain or hay and of horses with pituitary adenoma. Am J Vet Res 47:570–572, 1986.

15. Describe the thyrotropin-releasing hormone (TRH) stimulation test.

The TRH stimulation test may be used instead of the dexamethasone suppression test in animals with laminitis. One milligram of TRH is administered intravenously after baseline cortisol levels have been taken. In horses with pituitary adenomas, the cortisol levels should increase by 15 minutes and remain elevated for 90 minutes. No significant change occurs in normal animals. The disadvantage is that TRH is difficult to obtain.

Beech J, Garcia M: Hormonal response to thyrotropin-releasing hormone in healthy horses and in horses with pituitary adenoma. Am J Vet Res 46:1941–1943, 1985.

16. How does equine Cushing's disease differ from pituitary-related Cushing's disease in humans?

In horses with equine Cushing's disease, the lesion is located in the pars intermedia of the pituitary gland. In humans with pituitary-related Cushing's disease, the lesions are most often ACTH-secreting microadenomas of the pars distalis.

17. Contrast the cortisol levels and rhythm of secretion in normal horses vs. horses with Cushing's disease.

The normal horse has a circadian rhythm of cortisol release; the highest level occurs between 8 AM and noon and the lowest level in the late evening. Cushingnoid horses show no circadian rhythm in cortisol levels, which generally remain constant within the normal of slightly higher-than-normal range.

Dybdal NO, Hargreaves KM, Madigan JE, et al: Diagnostic testing for pituitary pars intermedia dysfunction in horses. J Am Vet Med Assoc 204:627–632, 1994.

18. Proopiolipomelanocortin (POMC) peptides are produced by the pars intermedia of the equine pituitary. What changes affect POMC peptides in equine Cushing's disease?

The processing of POMC peptides in the pars intermedia of the pituitary gland of normal horses yields α-melanocyte-stimulating hormone (αMSH), βMSH, β-endorphin (βEND), and corticotropin-like intermediate lobe peptide (CLIP). ACTH is the prohormone for βEND and CLIP and is not normally an end-product of the pars intermedia. In horses with Cushing's disease the production of these peptides is altered. ACTH levels in the tumor increase by 6-fold. The levels of the other resultant hormones, MSH, CLIP, and βEND, are increased by a far greater proportion—40 times that of ACTH.

Wilson MG, Nicholson WE, Holscher MA, et al: Proopiolipomelanocortin peptides in normal pituitary, pituitary tumor, and plasma of normal and Cushing's horses. Endocrinology 110:941–954, 1982.

19. Why do these peptide changes occur?

It has been suggested that the processing of POMC peptides in the pars intermedia is inhibited by dopaminergic innervation. In pars intermedia tumors, the levels of dopamine are markedly decreased. This decrease is consistent with the release of dopaminergic inhibition, which results in increased production of end-hormones.

Orth DN, Holscher MA, Wilson MG, et al: Equine Cushing's disease: Plasma immunoreactive proopiolipomelanocortin peptide and cortisol levels basally and in response to diagnostic tests. Endocrinology 110:1430–1441, 1982.

20. Why is the ACTH level in Cushingnoid horses not controlled by the negative feedback of increased cortisol levels?

Glucocorticoids do not appear to have an effect on the pars intermedia secretion of POMC peptides. It is believed that these melanotropes (i.e., cells in the equine pars intermedia) lack glucocorticoid receptors.

21. What is seen on gross pathologic examination of horses with Cushing's disease?

The pituitary gland has been remodeled in horses with Cushing's disease. The pars intermedia is grossly enlarged and often compresses the pars nervosa and the rest of the adenohypophysis. The mass grows by expansion. No metastasis has been noted. Bilateral hyperplasia of the adrenal glands is often seen (see figure at top of facing page).

22. What is seen on histopathologic examination of the pituitary gland of a horse with Cushing's disease?

On histopathologic evaluation the "neoplastic" cells are polyhedral, spindle-shaped, or cylindrical. They are usually arranged in columns or rosettes around capillary beds and connective tissue septa. The mitotic index is low. Some investigators believe that this architecture is reminiscent of the normal pars intermedia of the horse; hence the confusion over whether the disease is truly a neoplastic syndrome or merely hyperplasia of normal tissue.

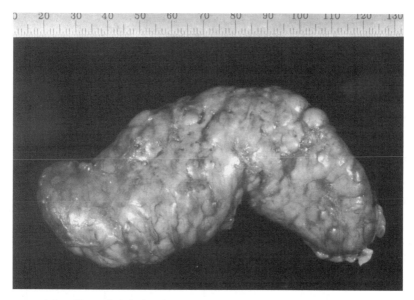

Adrenal hyperplasia in the adrenal glands of a horse with a pituitary adenoma.

23. What management precautions should an owner of a horse with Cushing's syndrome take?

Management of horses with Cushing's syndrome is an important part of their treatment. Whole body clipping may be necessary in animals with severe hirsutism. The immune system of the affected horse is thought to be somewhat suppressed because of the constant levels of cortisol (i.e., abolition of circadian rhythm). Consequently the horses are more prone to infection and heal more slowly. Any injuries or infections should be treated aggressively. Other nonspecific management practices, such as good dental and nutritional care and an adequate vaccination and deworming schedule, are important in all older horses, not just horses with pituitary adenomas.

24. Describe the possible medical protocols for treatment of Cushing's disease.

Currently two drugs are used to treat equine Cushing's disease: cyproheptadine and pergolide. One protocol for cyproheptadine is one dose of 0.25 mg/kg/day orally once for 6–8 weeks. If there is no response, the dose may be increased to 0.5 mg/kg divided into twice-daily doses. The cost per day at the initial dose level is approximately $1.20.

Pergolide may be given at the rate of 0.5 mg/horse orally once daily for 4–6 weeks. If there is no response, the dose should be increased in increments of 0.25–0.5 mg/day. Doses as high as 3 mg/day have been given, but the dose should be increased slowly because side effects of sweating and dyspnea have been noted. The cost per day of the 0.5-mg dose is approximately $3.70.

Dybdal NO, Levy M: Pituitary pars intermedia dysfunction in the horse. Part II: Diagnosis and Treatment. Proceedings ACVIM, Lake Buena Vista, FL, 1997, pp 470–471.

van der Kolk JH: Equine Cushing's disease. Equine Vet Educ 9:209–214, 1997.

25. Describe the rationale for use of pergolide in the treatment of equine Cushing's disease.

Pergolide is a dopaminergic agonist used as replacement therapy for the decreased dopaminergic inhibition of the pars intermedia. Although the pharmacodynamic profile is unknown in horses, pergolide appears to decrease POMC peptides.

26. Describe the rationale for using cyproheptadine in Cushingnoid horses.

Cyproheptadine is an antiserotonergic drug that was reported to induce remission of pituitary-associated Cushing's disease in 3 women. Its use in horses has produced varying reports of efficacy. Because the drug appears to have some anecdotal results and is safe and inexpensive, many use it as the initial treatment of equine Cushing's disease.

27. Bromocriptine has been used to treat equine Cushing's disease. Why may it be helpful?

Bromocriptine is similar to pergolide in action as a dopaminergic agonist. Some reports say that it is unpalatable and poorly absorbed orally. It may be administered subcutaneously. Some swelling at the site may occur. Some veterinarians believe that it may exacerbate preexisting laminitis.

DIABETES INSIPIDUS

28. What is diabetes insipidus?

Diabetes insipidus is a syndrome of polyuria/polydipsia resulting from one of two general mechanisms: (1) neurogenic diabetes insipidus, caused by a deficiency of antidiuretic hormone (ADH, vasopressin) or (2) nephrogenic diabetes insipidus, caused by decreased sensitivity of the renal collecting duct epithelial cells to ADH. ADH, which is the primary determinant of renal water excretion, is synthesized in the hypothalamus and then transported to the posterior pituitary (neurohypophysis), where it is stored for release.

29. Does diabetes insipidus occur in horses?

Both neurogenic and nephrogenic diabetes insipidus have been reported in horses, although infrequently. Neurogenic diabetes insipidus probably results most often from destruction of the posterior pituitary secondary to enlargement of the pars intermedia. In addition, cases of neurogenic diabetes insipidus that are idiopathic or acquired secondary to encephalitis have been described. Primary nephrogenic diabetes insipidus has been reported in sibling Thoroughbred colts, suggesting a possible inherited form of the disease as in humans. Nephrogenic diabetes insipidus also may be acquired secondary to various renal disorders.

Breukink HJ, Van Wegen P, Schotman AJH: Idiopathic diabetes insipidus in a Welsh pony. Equine Vet J 15:284–287, 1983.

Schott HC: Diabetes insipidus. In Reed SM, Bayly WM (ed): Equine Internal Medicine. Philadelphia, W.B. Saunders, 1998, pp 898–899.

Schott HC, Bayly WM, Reed SM, Brobst DF: Nephrogenic diabetes insipidus in sibling colts. J Vet Intern Med 7:68–72, 1993.

30. How does diabetes insipidus present?

Horses with diabetes insipidus have polyuria/polydipsia with dilute urine (urine specific gravity = 1.008–1.010). The water deprivation test reveals inability to concentrate urine. In neurogenic diabetes insipidus, the plasma concentration of ADH may be low and does not increase in response to water deprivation. Animals with nephrogenic diabetes insipidus demonstrate an appropriate increase in ADH after water deprivation but remain unable to concentrate urine. Such animals also do not respond to exogenous ADH.

31. What is the protocol for the water deprivation test?

1. Before starting the test, measure the blood urea nitrogen (BUN) and creatinine levels. A water deprivation test should not be performed on a horse that is azotemic or dehydrated. Then collect a baseline urinalysis (collected by catheterization to empty the bladder at the start of the test), and determine the body weight, if possible.

2. Remove the horse's water supply. Although it is not necessary to remove the feed, limiting feed intake may help to prevent some of the gastrointestinal complications that occasionally accompany water deprivation.

3. Measure the urine specific gravity and weight loss after 12 and 24 hours. Normal horses typically produce urine with a specific gravity above 1.045 after 24–72 hours of water deprivation. If the urine specific gravity reaches 1.025 or greater, the test may be stopped. In addition, the test should be discontinued if the horse loses more than 5% of its body weight or shows signs of dehydration.

32. Can diabetes insipidus be treated?

Cases of neurogenic diabetes insipidus may respond to ADH replacement therapy. In one case, intramuscular injections of 40 units of pitressin tannate in oil every 2–3 days was successful in limiting polydipsia/polyuria. Potential complications of therapy include resistance or allergic reactions. The potent ADH analog, desmopressin, may be of future use in the diagnosis and treatment of diabetes insipidus. Hormone replacement is ineffective for nephrogenic diabetes insipidus. The only practical form of treatment has been restriction of sodium and water intake. Although the mechanism is poorly understood, thiazide diuretics may be of benefit.

Breukink HJ, Van Wegen P, Schotman AJH: Idiopathic diabetes insipidus in a Welsh pony. Equine Vet J 15: 284–287, 1983.

ADRENAL GLANDS

33. Describe the normal anatomy and function of the equine adrenal glands.

The equine adrenals are paired glands that sit craniomedial to the kidneys. They normally weigh approximately 15–17 gm each and are about 9–10 cm × 3–4 cm × 1–2 cm in size. They are composed of two functionally distinct regions:

1. **Adrenal cortex**
   - *Zona glomerulosa,* which produces mineralocorticoids primarily in response to angiotensin II and serum concentrations of potassium and sodium.
   - *Zona fasciculata,* which produces glucocorticoids and adrenal androgens in response to stimulation by ACTH.
   - *Zona reticularis,* which functions with the zona fasciculata in the production of adrenal androgens and glucocorticoids in response to ACTH.

2. **Adrenal medulla**, which produces catecholamines (predominantly epinephrine, with some norepinephrine and dopamine).

34. Are disorders of the adrenal glands common in horses?

The adrenal glands are important shock organs in horses as in other species. Therefore, hemorrhage and necrosis are recognized as common sequelae to endotoxemia and septic shock. Primary disorders of the adrenal gland, including pheochromocytomas, hypoadrenocorticism, and hyperadrenocorticism, have been recognized in horses but are uncommon.

35. What are pheochromocytomas?

Pheochromocytomas are tumors of the chromaffin cells of the adrenal medulla; if functional, they secrete sufficient catecholamines to cause clinical signs. As in other species, most pheochromocytomas in horses are probably nonfunctional and therefore do not cause clinical signs. Functional pheochromocytomas have been reported in horses and are thought to produce either epinephrine or norepinephrine. Pheochromocytomas do not appear to metastasize and are usually unilateral but may be bilateral.

Johnson PJ, Goetz TE, Foreman JH, Zachary JF: Pheochromocytoma in two horses. J Am Vet Med Assoc 206:837–841, 1995.

Rivas L: Diseases of the adrenal glands. In Reed SM, Bayly WM (eds): Equine Internal Medicine. Philadelphia, W.B. Saunders, 1998, pp 934–936.

Yovich JV, Ducharme NG: Ruptured pheochromocytoma in a mare with colic. J Am Vet Med Assoc 183:462–464, 1983.

36. Is there a particular signalment for horses with functional pheochromocytomas?

Pheochromocytomas are generally a disease of older horses; only one case has been described in a horse less than 12 years of age. There is no breed or gender predilection.

37. Describe the common clinical signs of a functional pheochromocytoma.

The clinical signs are usually acute in onset and appear to progress rapidly. They are attributable to adrenergic stimulation from increased catecholamines and vary considerably. Frequently observed signs include anxiety, tachycardia, tachypnea, profuse sweating, muscle fasciculations, and mydriasis with an intact pupillary light response. Abdominal pain is also common. Pheochromocytomas are predisposed to hemorrhage and rupture, and retroperitoneal swelling on palpation per rectum or hemoperitoneum may be detected. Other reported signs include hyperthermia; dry, pale mucous membranes with an increased capillary refill time; bladder paralysis; and ataxia. Noninfectious abortion at 271 days' gestation was reported in one case.

Johnson PJ, Goetz TE, Foreman JH, Zachary JF: Pheochromocytoma in two horses. J Am Vet Med Assoc 206:837–841, 1995.

38. What clinicopathologic abnormalities are seen in horses with functional pheochromocytomas?

The hematologic abnormalities vary. An increase in hematocrit may be seen, most likely as a result of epinephrine-mediated splenic contraction. Both a stress leukogram (mature neutrophilia with lymphopenia) and leukopenia due to neutropenia with a left shift have been seen. Changes in the serum biochemical profile are also variable and nonspecific. Azotemia and metabolic acidosis with hyperkalemia are among the most consistent clinicopathologic findings. Hyponatremia, hypocalcemia, and hyperphosphatemia also have been reported. Hyperglycemia and glycosuria are common and probably result from the glycogenolytic action of epinephrine.

39. How is functional pheochromocytoma diagnosed?

Antemortem diagnosis of pheochromocytomas is difficult because the disease is rare and the clinical and laboratory finding are nonspecific. Therefore, most cases are diagnosed at necropsy. In a horse with consistent signs, it is important to rule out other diseases. Documentation of high serum concentrations of catecholamines or their metabolites in urine is useful in the diagnosis but unfortunately is difficult in horses. The presence of hypertension may support the diagnosis.

Treatment by surgical removal of the affected adrenal gland after preoperative management with alpha-adrenergic receptor blockers has an excellent prognosis in humans. Theoretically, adrenalectomy may be attempted in horses if an antemortem diagnosis is made, although the procedure would be technically difficult.

40. What is Addison's disease? Is it seen in horses?

Addison's disease is primary adrenal insufficiency or hypoadrenocorticism. True Addison's disease as seen in other species probably does not occur in horses; if it does, it is very rare. Theoretically, however, the adrenal glands may be damaged after endotoxemia or shock. In addition, poorly defined syndromes of adrenal insufficiency or exhaustion have been recognized in horses either in association with discontinuance of iatrogenic steroids or ACTH or after intense training programs. These syndromes are sometimes referred to as steroid letdown syndrome or turn-out syndrome. The amount and duration of exogenous steroid treatment required to induce adrenocortical atrophy are uncertain.

Dybdal NO: Endocrine disorders. In Smith BP (ed): Large Animal Internal Medicine, 2nd ed. St. Louis, Mosby, 1996, pp 1444–1454.

Rivas L: Diseases of the adrenal glands. In Reed SM, Bayly WM (eds): Equine Internal Medicine. Philadelphia, W.B. Saunders, 1998, pp 934–936.

41. What clinical signs and laboratory abnormalities are associated with adrenal insufficiency?

Horses with apparent adrenal insufficiency demonstrate nonspecific signs such as depression, anorexia, weight loss, mild abdominal discomfort, poor hair coat, and lameness. If hypoaldosteronism is present, polyuria/polydipsia may be seen. Laboratory analyses are variable. Results may be normal or reveal hyponatremia, hypochloremia, hyperkalemia, and hypoglycemia.

42. How is adrenal insufficiency diagnosed?

The clinical presentation of adrenal insufficiency in horses is fairly nonspecific; therefore, it is important to rule out other more common disorders. However, the condition should be considered in horses with consistent clinical and laboratory findings, especially with a history of prolonged steroid administration, intensive training, or recent severe illness. If one has suspected chronic renal disease (because of weight loss, intermittent abdominal pain, polyuria/polydipsia, hyponatremia, hypochloremia, and hyperkalemia) but renal size, ultrasonographic evaluation, and even biopsy results are normal, one should ascertain whether any steroids have been administered.

Serum cortisol concentrations are not a reliable indicator of adrenal cortical function because of the short half-life and daily fluctuation (i.e., circadian rhythm) of cortisol. However, horses with adrenal insufficiency generally fail to respond to the ACTH stimulation test.

43. What is the protocol for the ACTH stimulation test?

At least two protocols have been used for the ACTH stimulation test:

1. ACTH gel test
   - Collect pre-ACTH heparinized sample for cortisol determination between 8–10 AM.
   - Administer 1 IU/kg of ACTH gel intramuscularly.
   - Collect heparinized samples for cortisol determination 2 and 4 hours later.
2. Aqueous ACTH test
   - Collect pre-ACTH heparinized sample between 8 AM and noon.
   - Administer 100 IU (or 1 mg) synthetic aqueous ACTH intravenously.
   - Collect heparinized sample 2 hours later.

The baseline concentration of cortisol is generally at least 1 μg/ml. Both protocols should result in a twofold or greater increase in the concentration of cortisol over baseline.

Dybdal NO: Endocrine disorders. In Smith BP (ed): Large Animal Internal Medicine, 2nd ed. St. Louis, Mosby, 1996, pp 1444–1454.

44. Is any treatment available for adrenal insufficiency?

Treatment for adrenal insufficiency has not been well defined. Rest and avoidance of stress are recommended. Steroid supplementation may be indicated in some cases.

45. Does hyperadrenocorticism occur in horses other than in association with pituitary dysfunction?

Both iatrogenic and adrenal hyperadrenocorticism have been reported in horses, although they are rare. As with pituitary dysfunction, the clinical signs often include polyuria/polydipsia, weight loss, and depression. Iatrogenic hyperadrenocorticism was induced in a 10-year-old Quarter Horse gelding after repeated administration of triamcinolone. The horse also demonstrated a reversible steroid hepatopathy.

Cohen ND, Carter GK: Steroid hepatopathy in a horse with glucocorticoid-induced hyperadrenocorticism. J Am Vet Med Assoc 200:1682–1684, 1992.

THYROID GLAND

46. Describe the anatomy of the thyroid gland.

The equine thyroid gland is composed of two lobes (located at the caudal aspect of the larynx) and the thyroid gland body or isthmus. In adult horses, each lobe has an average size of 5 cm × 2.5 cm × 2 cm; the isthmus is generally present only as a fibrous remnant connecting the caudal poles. The isthmus may be more prominent in foals, donkeys, and mules. The thyroid gland is highly vascular, with a blood flow approximating 5 times the weight of the gland each minute.

The thyroid gland is composed of large numbers of closed follicles filled with a secretory substance called colloid. The major constituent of colloid is the large glycoprotein thyroglobulin, which contains the thyroid hormones. Interspersed among the thyroid follicles are the C cells, which produce calcitonin, a hormone involved in calcium homeostasis.

47. How are the thyroid hormones formed?

The basal membrane of the thyroid cell has the ability to pump iodide to the interior of the cell in a process called iodide trapping. Once within the thyroid, the iodine is oxidized and then bound to tyrosyl residues within the thyroglobulin molecule, forming monoiodotyrosine and diiodotyrosine. These then undergo coupling to form the thyroid hormones, thyroxine (T_4) and triiodothyronine (T_3), which remain part of thyroglobulin for storage within the follicles.

48. What factors regulate the production of thyroid hormones?

The synthesis and release of thyroid hormones are under the control of thyroid-stimulating hormone (TSH), which is released from the anterior pituitary gland under the influence of thyrotropin-releasing hormone (TRH) from the hypothalamus. The circulating concentrations of thyroid hormones give feedback to both the anterior pituitary and hypothalamus to alter hormone release. Iodine availability also influences the production of thyroid hormones.

49. How are the thyroid hormones released?

Thyroglobulin is not released into the circulation in significant amounts. Instead, T_4 and T_3, when needed, are cleaved from thyroglobulin and transported into the circulation. Once in the circulation, most thyroid hormones are bound to transport proteins, primarily thyroid-binding globulin, but also T_4-binding prealbumin and albumin. The protein binding is reversible, and the thyroid hormones are released slowly. Unbound or free thyroid hormones cross the capillary endothelium to exert biologic effects in the tissues.

50. What thyroid hormones are found in the circulation?

1. **T_4 (thyroxine).** Approximately 90% of thyroid hormone released from the thyroid gland is T_4. Compared with T_3, T_4 has a greater protein binding affinity and longer half-life, which is approximately 50 hours in horses. However, T_4 has less biologic activity and is often considered a prohormone; most T_4 is converted to T_3 by peripheral deiodination in the process of T_3 neogenesis.

2. **T_3 (triiodothyronine).** Only about 10% of thyroid hormone secreted by the thyroid gland is T_3; thus, the majority of T_3 is formed by peripheral deiodination of T_4. T_3 is estimated to be 3–5 times as potent as T_4.

3. **Reverse T_3 (rT_3).** Although T_3 is the major product of peripheral deiodination of T_4, some rT_3 is formed by deiodination at the carboxyl end. The functional significance of rT_3 is not fully understood, but concentrations of rT_3 are high in the fetus and in humans with systemic illness.

4. **Free T_4 and free T_3 (fT_4 and fT_3).** Only 1% of the total concentration of thyroid hormones circulates in the free state, unbound to carrier proteins. Free T_3 and free T_4 are biologically active and interact in the feedback loop to regulate thyroid hormone synthesis and release.

51. What is the function of the thyroid hormones?

The general effect of the thyroid hormones is to increase nuclear transcription of multiple genes. This increase, in turn, results in the increased synthesis of numerous proteins and ultimately in a generalized increase in the metabolic activities of most tissues. There is no question that thyroid function is essential throughout the body. Important thyroid functions include maintenance of the basal metabolic rate, thermogenesis, neural transmission, and stimulation of heart rate, cardiac output, and blood flow. In the fetus and neonate, the thyroid hormones promote differentiation and proliferative growth and play an important role in overall growth and development, particularly of skeletal, cerebral, and neuronal tissues.

52. Hypothyroidism is frequently reported in other species and is the most commonly diagnosed endocrinopathy in dogs. Does it occur in horses?

Hypothyroidism occurs in foals. However, the frequency of true hypothyroidism in adult horses remains controversial because of numerous factors, including difficulties in accurately assessing thyroid function and the number of nonthyroidal factors that affect thyroid hormone concentrations. When histologic examination or stimulation tests are performed, few equine thyroid glands are abnormal, and hypothyroidism is probably an uncommon endocrine disease in adult horses.

Duckett WM: Thyroid gland. In Reed SM, Bayly WM (eds): Equine Internal Medicine. Philadelphia, W.B. Saunders, 1998, pp 916–925.

Messer NT: Thyroid dysfunction in horses. Proc Am Assoc Equine Pract 153–154, 1994.

53. Define the basic mechanisms that can lead to hypothyroidism.

1. Primary hypothyroidism, due to pathologic processes intrinsic to the thyroid gland, results in defective production of thyroid hormones.

2. Secondary (hypophyseal) and tertiary (hypothalamic) hypothyroidism are due to a deficiency of TSH or TRH, respectively; they are sometimes referred to as central hypothyroidism.

3. Peripheral resistance to the action of thyroid hormones is rare.

In both dogs and humans, most cases of hypothyroidism are primary and characterized by low concentrations of thyroid hormones with elevated concentrations of TSH. In horses, the frequency of these conditions in unknown.

54. What clinical signs may be seen in adult horses with hypothyroidism?

Experimental models in horses have established that various signs may be associated with hypothyroidism, including lethargy, diminished appetite, failure to grow, decreased exercise tolerance, muscular problems, hypothermia, poor hair coat, and edema. Clinically, hypothyroidism has been suspected but generally not confirmed in horses with alopecia, anhidrosis, exercise intolerance, exertional rhabdomyolysis, obesity, and laminitis.

55. How is hypothyroidism diagnosed?

Unfortunately, practical and reliable means of assessing thyroid function in horses remain elusive, making the diagnosis of hypothyroidism difficult. The difficulties stem from a number of factors, such as the availability of tests, the wide variation in normal values, and the influence of extrathyroidal factors. It is therefore important to interpret test results carefully while considering all differentials. As the understanding of equine thyroid disease increases and additional tests become available, documentation of thyroid dysfunction should improve.

1. **Hormone levels.** The concentrations of total T_4, total T_3, fT_4, fT_3, and rT_3 can be measured in horses. Normal values vary widely with the laboratory and specific technique. Because the concentrations of thyroid hormones may be influenced by a number of factors, it is generally not possible to make a clinical diagnosis of thyroid dysfunction solely on the basis of baseline serum thyroid hormone concentrations in horses.

2. **Trophic response tests.** Both TSH and TRH stimulation tests have been performed in horses. Although responsiveness is somewhat variable, these tests remain among the most accurate methods of determining thyroid function. However, the unavailability of economically priced, approved TSH and TRH currently limits their usefulness.

3. **TSH concentration.** In humans, determination of TSH concentration, often in conjunction with T_4 concentration, has been the most sensitive test for diagnosing primary hypothyroidism. TSH concentrations are generally higher than control values in primary hypothyroidism and lower in centrally mediated hypothyroidism. A commercial assay for equine TSH may be available in the near future; its accuracy in diagnosing equine thyroid dysfunction must be evaluated.

4. **Aspirate or biopsy.** These procedures help to establish the pathologic process within the thyroid gland but do not determine thyroid function. The thyroid gland is highly vascular, and complications may result from this fact.

5. **Others.** The basal metabolic rate is the most direct measure of metabolic activity, but routine clinical determination is not practical. Ultrasonographic imaging may help to define structural abnormalities but does not aid in the assessment of function. Scintigraphic imaging has been used primarily to evaluate thyroid carcinomas.

Duckett WM: Thyroid gland. In Reed SM, Bayly WM (eds): Equine Internal Medicine. Philadelphia, W.B. Saunders, 1998, pp 916–925.
Messer NT: Thyroid dysfunction in horses. Proc Am Assoc Equine Pract 153–154, 1994.

56. What extrathyroidal factors affect thyroid function and therefore influence testing?

Consideration of nonthyroidal factors may help to explain low concentrations of thyroid hormones in otherwise healthy horses:

1. **Age.** Neonatal foals typically have high concentrations of circulating thyroid hormones (10–20 times those of adults). These concentrations decrease rapidly within the first few weeks of life and then slowly thereafter.

2. **Climate.** Thyroid activity tends to increase as horses become acclimatized to colder temperatures.

3. **Diet.** Many dietary factors influence thyroid hormone concentrations. Both deficient and excessive levels of dietary iodine can depress the concentrations of thyroid hormones. Selenium plays a role in the conversion of T_4 to T_3. In addition, diets high in carbohydrates, especially when fed as two large meals, tend to decrease thyroid hormone concentrations. Fasting or anorexia also decreases circulating concentrations of T_3, T_4, fT_3, and fT_4 while increasing concentrations of rT_3.

4. **Activity.** Studies investigating the effects of exercise on thyroid hormone concentrations have yielded variable results. One study suggested that T_4 concentrations increased with training, whereas another study of Thoroughbreds in training found that concentrations of thyroid hormones were low compared with normal ranges. After a single exercise bout, thyroid hormone concentrations have been shown either to increase or to decrease.

5. **Exogenous compounds.** Various substances decrease thyroid hormone concentrations, including iodine-containing drugs, corticosteroids, and nonsteroidal antiinflammatory drugs.

Duckett WM: Thyroid gland. In Reed SM, Bayly WM (eds): Equine Internal Medicine. Philadelphia, W.B. Saunders, 1998, pp 916–925.

Glade MJ, Gupta S, Reimers JJ: Hormonal response to high and low planes of nutrition in weanling Thoroughbreds. J Animal Sci 59:658–665, 1984.

Messer NT: Thyroid dysfunction in horses. Proc Am Assoc Equine Pract 153–154, 1994.

57. What is euthyroid sick syndrome?

Euthyroid sick syndrome develops when the circulating concentrations of thyroid hormones are low in response to a catabolic state. The animal may lower its resting metabolic rate to conserve calories and energy. Thus, any debilitated horse or horse with chronic disease may have low thyroid hormone concentrations. However, affected animals should respond to exogenous TSH because the thyroid gland is normal. Euthyroid sick syndrome may explain why some horses with pituitary adenomas have low thyroid hormone concentrations.

58. How is hypothyroidism treated?

Various protocols have been used for oral thyroid hormone replacement therapy, including iodinated casein (5–10 gm/day), dessicated thyroid extract (2 mg/kg/day), T_4 supplementation (20 mg/kg/day), and T_3 (1 mg/kg/day). Monitoring of both clinical response and thyroid hormone concentrations has been recommended. Anecdotally, many horses appear to improve with thyroid supplementation. However, such reports are a poor basis for making a diagnosis of hypothyroidism; even euthyroid animals may appear to improve because metabolic rate and general activity level are enhanced by additional thyroid hormone.

Duckett WM: Thyroid gland. In Reed SM, Bayly WM (eds): Equine Internal Medicine. Philadelphia, W.B. Saunders, 1998, pp 916–925.

59. In view of the difficulty in determining thyroid status, are any risks associated with empirical supplementation of thyroid hormones?

Little information is available about the long-term effects of thyroid supplementation in horses. In other species, however, supplementation may suppress endogenous TSH and result in varying degrees of thyroid gland atrophy.

60. What are the clinical characteristics of hypothyroidism in foals?

Hypothyroidism in foals has been associated with a hypometabolic state characterized by incoordination, poor suckling and righting reflexes, hypothermia, and goiter. In addition, a distinct syndrome, known as either congenital hypothyroidism and dysmaturity syndrome (CHD) or thyroid hyperplasia and musculoskeletal deformities, has been described. Originally reported in foals from the western provinces of Canada, the condition now appears to be more widespread. Clinical features include mandibular prognathism, incomplete skeletal ossification, prolonged gestation, and marked flexural deformities, such as contracted tendons and rupture of the common digital extensor. Of importance, most foals show no palpable enlargement of the thyroid glands, despite histologic evidence of thyroid hyperplasia. The underlying cause of the hypothyroidism has not been determined, although exposure to nitrates and other possible goitrogens may play a role.

Allen AL, Townsend HGG, Doige CE, Fretz PB: A case-control study of the congenital hypothyroidism and dysmaturity syndrome of foals. Can Vet J 37:349–358, 1996.

Hines MT, Gay C, Talcott T: Congenital hypothyroidism and dysmaturity syndrome of foals: Diagnosis and possible risk factors. Proceedings ACVIM, Lake Buena Vista, FL, 1997, pp 363–364.

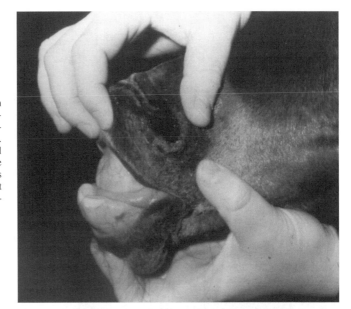

Mandibular prognathism in a foal with congenital hypothyroidism and dysmaturity syndrome (CHD). Although not present in all affected foals, this is one of the classic clinical signs of CHD and should alert the clinician to the possibility of hypothyroidism.

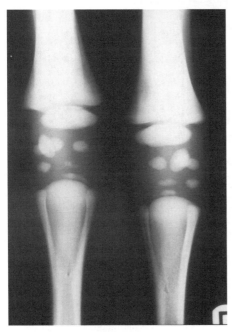 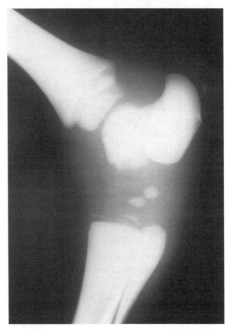

Radiographs demonstrating incomplete ossification of the cuboidal bones in the carpi *(left)* and tarsus *(right)* of a foal severely affected with CHD. Although flexural deformities are usually most evident in the forelimbs, poor ossification is generally present in all limbs. This foal survived but is unsound as a result of tarsal collapse.

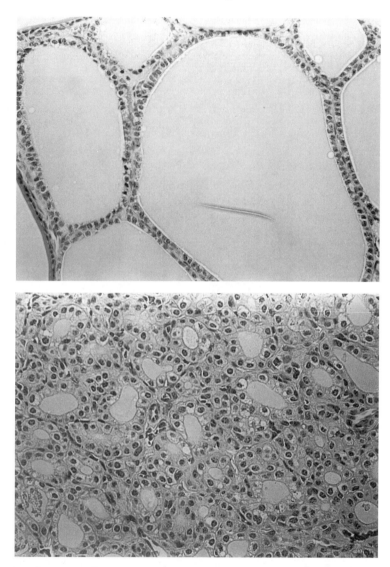

Top, The thyroid gland from a normal neonatal foal with colloid containing follicles. *Bottom,* The thyroid gland from a foal with CHD. Note the diffuse, severe hyperplasia of thyroid follicular epithelial cells and lack of normal colloid.

61. Is there a treatment for CHD? What is the prognosis?

Treatment of CHD has been largely supportive: prevention of failure of passive transfer, splints, physical therapy, and nutritional support. It is unclear whether administration of a thyroid supplement is beneficial. Limited data suggest that the surviving foals become euthyroid over time even without exogenous supplementation.

The prognosis tends to vary with the severity of the condition, particularly skeletal abnormalities. Because of musculoskeletal problems present at birth, affected foals often have difficulty in standing to suckle and therefore are at increased risk for failure of passive transfer. The prognosis is worse in foals that develop concurrent septicemia. Various orthopedic problems have been identified in surviving foals, although some mildly affected foals have become successful performance animals.

62. Have cases of hyperthyroidism been described in horses?

Well-documented cases of hyperthyroidism have yet to be reported in horses. However, a syndrome that may be associated with increased thyroid function has been described in race-horses. Signs include tremors, excitability, tachycardia, sweating, and weight loss despite good appetite. Affected horses responded to antithyroid treatment with 1 gm potassium iodide/day.

Duckett WM: Thyroid gland. In Reed SM, Bayly WM (eds): Equine Internal Medicine. Philadelphia, W.B. Saunders, 1998, pp 916–925.

63. Define goiter.

Goiter is defined as any enlargement of the thyroid gland.

64. What types of thyroid tumors have been demonstrated in horses?

Three types of thyroid tumors have been recognized: adenomas, adenocarcinomas, and medullary carcinomas. Tumors generally can be diagnosed by fine-needle aspirate or biopsy, but one must remember that the thyroid gland is highly vascular.

The most common thyroid tumor is the **adenoma**, which is seen predominantly in horses over 16 years of age. These tumors are benign and generally unilateral and are not associated with thyroid dysfunction. Occasionally their size may warrant surgical excision.

Thyroid **adenocarcinomas** have been reported with less frequency. Serum concentrations of T_3 and T_4 may be normal or decreased. Systemic metastasis has been reported in one horse that had a concurrent pituitary adenoma.

Medullary carcinomas (C-cell or parafollicular cell tumors) also have been reported, although infrequently. Other than persistent gulping due to the size of the enlarged glands, these tumors have not been associated with clinical problems in horses.

PARATHYROID GLANDS

65. Describe the anatomy of the parathyroid glands in horses.

Horses are generally considered to have four parathyroid glands, which are located in the region of the thyroid. The precise location of these glands varies, and the glands are extremely difficult to distinguish grossly.

66. What is parathyroid hormone (PTH)?

PTH (also called parathormone) is produced by the chief cells of the parathyroid gland primarily in response to decreased plasma concentrations of ionized calcium. PTH acts to increase plasma calcium concentrations by three basic mechanisms: (1) stimulating bone resorption in the presence of vitamin D, (2) increasing formation of the active form of vitamin D (calcitriol), and (3) increasing active renal reabsorption of ionized calcium.

67. Has parathyroid dysfunction been recognized in horses?

Parathyroid dysfunction should be considered as a differential diagnosis in animals exhibiting calcium abnormalities. Primary, secondary, and pseudohyperparathyroidism have been reported in horses, although primary hyperparathyroidism appears to be quite rare. Affected animals typically exhibit hypercalcemia or a calcium-to-phosphorus imbalance. Recently, hypoparathyroidism was described in a horse with hypocalcemia. It is now possible to measure PTH concentrations to aid in the diagnosis of parathyroid dysfunction.

Couetil L, Sojka JE, Nachreiner RF: Primary hypoparathyroidism in a horse. J Vet Intern Med 12:45–49, 1998.

Dybdal NO: Endocrine disorders. In Smith BP (ed): Large Animal Internal Medicine, 2nd ed. St. Louis, Mosby, 1996, pp 1444–1454.

68. How may secondary hyperparathyroidism develop?

1. **Nutritional hyperparathyroidism.** Also known as big head or bran disease, nutritional hyperparathyroidism was once common, but the incidence has decreased significantly as knowledge of proper nutrition has improved. It is caused by either an absolute calcium deficiency or, more often, a relative calcium deficiency secondary to excessive dietary phosphorus (calcium-to-phosphorus ratio < 1). It also may be seen in association with the chronic ingestion of oxalate-containing plants, because oxalates interfere with calcium absorption. The absolute or relative calcium deficiency results in excessive PTH and subsequently excessive osteoclast activity with increased bone absorption. As the weakened bone remodels, the classic sign of enlargement of the maxilla often develops. A stiff gait or shifting leg lameness also may be recognized. Although the serum concentrations of calcium and phosphorus may be normal, the urinary concentration of phosphorus is elevated. Once the diet is corrected, the prognosis for improvement depends on the severity of the skeletal lesions.

2. **Renal failure.** Hypercalcemia is seen in some cases of renal failure, but the exact mechanism is not understood. Investigations of some hypercalcemic horses with renal failure have found low concentrations of PTH, suggesting that a mechanism other than hyperparathyroidism is responsible for the hypercalcemia. Acute nephrosis, however, is associated with an increase in PTH concentration and hypercalcemia that appear to be transient.

69. What is pseudohyperparathyroidism?

Pseudohyperparathyroidism results from elaboration of a PTH-like substance by a neoplasm. This process is responsible for the hypercalcemia of malignancy that has been recognized in some horses with neoplastic conditions, including lymphosarcoma, squamous cell carcinoma, and mesothelioma.

PANCREAS

70. Define diabetes mellitus.

Diabetes mellitus is defined by the presence of chronic hyperglycemia with glucosuria. Clinical signs often include weight loss and polyuria/polydipsia. A metabolic disorder characterized by the inability to oxidize carbohydrates, diabetes mellitus generally results from either a lack of insulin or a failure of the tissues to respond to insulin (insulin resistance). The terminology surrounding diabetes mellitus can be confusing. One classification scheme is as follows:

1. **Primary diabetes mellitus** refers to cases with no distinct underlying disease to account for the carbohydrate intolerance. In some reports, the term diabetes mellitus is meant to imply a primary condition. Primary diabetes mellitus is further subdivided into two types:
   - Type I—primary disease of insulin-producing beta cells; associated with a decreased concentration of circulating insulin.
   - Type II—resistance to the activity of insulin for uncertain reasons.

2. **Secondary diabetes mellitus** refers to cases in which an established underlying disease accounts for the carbohydrate intolerance.

Diabetes mellitus also may be classified as insulin-dependent or non–insulin-dependent. Despite some overlap, most cases of primary type one diabetes mellitus are insulin-dependent, whereas most cases of type two and secondary diabetes mellitus are non–insulin-dependent.

71. Does diabetes mellitus occur in horses?

By far the most common form of diabetes mellitus recognized in horses is secondary diabetes mellitus due to the insulin resistance associated with pituitary adenomas. Secondary diabetes mellitus also has been recognized in a mare with bilateral granulosa cell tumors and in horses with pheochromocytomas.

Primary diabetes mellitus is rare in horses. Cases have been reported in association with pancreatic disease and one case of type II diabetes. Determination of serum insulin concentrations, as well as a glucose tolerance test and insulin tolerance test, may help in defining the condition. There are no reports of long-term management of equine patients with diabetes mellitus.

Johnson PJ, Goetz TE, Foreman JH, Zachary JF: Pheochromocytoma in two horses. J Am Vet Med Assoc 206:837–841, 1995.

McCoy DJ: Diabetes mellitus associated with bilateral granulosa cell tumors in a mare. J Am Vet Med Assoc 188:733–735, 1986.

Ruoff WW, Baker DC, Morgan SJ: Type II diabetes mellitus in a horse. Equine Vet J 18:143–144, 1986.

Taylor FGR, Hillyer MH: The differential diagnosis of hyperglycaemia in horses. Equine Vet Educ 4:135–138, 1992.

72. Are there any cases of hyperinsulinism in horses?

One case has been reported in a 12-year-old pony with documented hyperinsulinism secondary to a pancreatic neoplasm. The pony had intermittent seizures and hypoglycemia. In some cases, administration of exogenous insulin should be considered.

Ross MW, Lowe JE, Cooper BJ, et al: Hypoglycemic seizures in a Shetland pony. Cornell Vet 73:151–169, 1983.

BIBLIOGRAPHY

1. Allen AL, Townsend HGG, Doige CE, Fretz PB: A case-control study of the congenital hypothyroidism and dysmaturity syndrome of foals. Can Vet J 37:349–358, 1996.
2. Beech J, Garcia M: Hormonal response to thyrotropin-releasing hormone in healthy horses and in horses with pituitary adenoma. Am J Vet Res 46:1941–1943, 1985.
3. Breukink HJ, Van Wegen P, Schotman AJH: Idiopathic diabetes insipidus in a Welsh pony. Equine Vet J 15:284–287, 1983.
4. Cohen ND, Carter GK: Steroid hepatopathy in a horse with glucocorticoid-induced hyperadrenocorticism. J Am Vet Med Assoc 200:1682–1684, 1992.
5. Couetil L, Paradis MR, Knoll J: Plasma adrenocorticotropin concentration in healthy horses and in horses with clinical signs of hyperadrenocorticism. J Vet Intern Med 10:1–6, 1996.
6. Couetil L, Sojka JE, Nachreiner RF: Primary hypoparathyroidism in a horse. J Vet Intern Med 12:45–49, 1998.
7. Dybdal N: Pituitary pars intermedia dysfunction (equine Cushing's-like disease). In Robinson E (ed): Current Therapy in Equine Medicine, 4th ed. Philadelphia, W.B. Saunders, 1997, pp 499–501.
8. Dybdal NO: Endocrine disorders. In Smith BP (ed): Large Animal Internal Medicine, 2nd ed. St. Louis, Mosby, 1996, pp 1444–1454.
9. Dybdal NO, Hargreaves KM, Madigan JE, et al: Diagnostic testing for pituitary pars intermedia dysfunction in horses. J Am Vet Med Assoc 204:627–632, 1994.
10. Dybdal NO, Levy M: Pituitary pars intermedia dysfunction in the horse. Part II: Diagnosis and Treatment. Proceedings ACVIM, Lake Buena Vista, FL, 1997, pp 470–471.
11. Duckett WM: Thyroid gland. In Reed SM, Bayly WM (eds): Equine Internal Medicine. Philadelphia, W.B. Saunders, 1998, pp 916–925.
12. Garcia MC, Beech J: Equine intravenous glucose tolerance tests: Glucose and insulin responses of healthy horses fed grain or hay and of horses with pituitary adenoma. Am J Vet Res 47:570–572, 1986.
13. Hines MT, Gay C, Talcott T: Congenital hypothyroidism and dysmaturity syndrome of foals: Diagnosis and possible risk factors. Proceedings ACVIM, Lake Buena Vista, FL, 1997, pp 363–364.
14. Johnson PJ, Goetz TE, Foreman JH, Zachary JF: Pheochromocytoma in two horses. J Am Vet Med Assoc 206:837–841, 1995.
15. Levy M, Dybdal NO: Pituitary pars intermedia dysfunction in the horse. Part I: Clinical signs and pathophysiology. Proceedings ACVIM, Lake Buena Vista, FL, 1997, pp 468–469.
16. McCoy DJ: Diabetes mellitus associated with bilateral granulosa cell tumors in a mare. J Am Vet Med Assoc 188:733–735, 1986.
17. Messer NT: Thyroid dysfunction in horses. Proc Am Assoc Equine Pract 153–154, 1994.
18. Millington WR, Dybdal NO, Dawson R Jr, et al: Equine Cushing's disease: Differential regulation of β-endorphin processing in tumors of the intermediate pituitary. Endocrinology 123:1598–1604, 1988.
19. Moore JN, Steiss J, Nicholson WE, Orth DN: A case of pituitary adrenocorticotropin-dependent Cushing's syndrome in the horse. Endocrinology 104:576–582, 1979.
20. Orth DN, Holscher MA, Wilson MG, et al: Equine Cushing's disease: Plasma immunoreactive proopiolipomelanocortin peptide and cortisol levels basally and in response to diagnostic tests. Endocrinology 110:1430–1441, 1982.
21. Rivas L: Diseases of the adrenal glands. In Reed SM, Bayly WM (eds): Equine Internal Medicine. Philadelphia, W.B. Saunders, 1998, pp 934–936.

22. Ross MW, Lowe JE, Cooper BJ, et al: Hypoglycemic seizures in a Shetland pony. Cornell Vet 73:151–169, 1983.
23. Ruoff WW, Baker DC, Morgan SJ: Type II diabetes mellitus in a horse. Equine Vet J 18:143–144, 1986.
24. Schott HC: Diabetes insipidus. In Reed SM, Bayly WM (ed): Equine Internal Medicine. Philadelphia, W.B. Saunders, 1998, pp 898–899.
25. Schott HC, Bayly WM, Reed SM, Brobst DF: Nephrogenic diabetes insipidus in sibling colts. J Vet Intern Med 7:68–72, 1993.
26. Taylor FGR, Hillyer MH: The differential diagnosis of hyperglycaemia in horses. Equine Vet Educ 4:135–138, 1992.
27. van der Kolk JH: Equine Cushing's disease. Equine Vet Educ 9:209–214, 1997.
28. van der Kolk JH, Kalsbeek HC, van Garderen E, et al: Equine pituitary neoplasia: A clinical report of 21 cases (1990–1992). Vet Rec 133:594–597, 1993.
29. Wilson MG, Nicholson WE, Holscher MA, et al: Proopiolipomelanocortin peptides in normal pituitary, pituitary tumor, and plasma of normal and Cushing's horses. Endocrinology 110:941–954, 1982.
30. Yovich JV, Ducharme NG: Ruptured pheochromocytoma in a mare with colic. J Am Vet Med Assoc 183:462–464, 1983.

6. THE IMMUNE SYSTEM

Virginia Buechner-Maxwell, D.V.M., M.S., Dip. ACVIM, and
Mark V. Crisman, D.V.M., M.S., Dip. ACVIM

1. Define immunity, immune system, and immune response.
Immunity: protection from disease.
Immune system: cells and molecules responsible for immunity.
Immune response: the collective and coordinated response of the immune system to the introduction of foreign substances (antigens) into the body.

2. List the general ways in which natural and acquired immunity differ.
Characteristics of natural immunity
- The ability to mount a maximal response, which should be present before exposure to the foreign agent.
- The response is not enhanced by repeated exposure.
- The response does not discriminate among most foreign substances.

Characteristics of acquired immunity
- The response is induced by prior exposure.
- The response is specific for distinct foreign substances.
- The response increases in magnitude and effectiveness with successive exposures.

3. Name the mechanisms used by animals to protect themselves from foreign substances (especially infectious agents).
The mechanisms of natural immunity and acquired immunity are (1) physiochemical barriers, (2) circulating molecules, (3) cells, and (4) soluble mediators that act on other cells.

4. Describe the components that contribute to the mechanisms of natural and acquired immunity.

MECHANISMS	NATURAL IMMUNITY	ACQUIRED IMMUNITY
Physiochemical barriers	Skin, mucous membranes	Cutaneous and mucosal immune systems, antibodies in secretions
Circulating molecules	Complement	Antibodies
Cells	Phagocytic cells (macrophages, neutrophils, natural killer cells)	Lymphocytes
Soluble mediators that act on other cells	Macrophage-derived cytokines (e.g., tumor necrosis factor, α and β interferon)	Lymphocyte-derived cytokines (e.g., γ interferon)

5. List the cells that are capable of phagocytosis. Describe the process of phagocytosis.
Neutrophils and macrophages are the primary phagocytic cells of the body. Phagocytic cells are initially drawn to foreign particles by chemical signals emitted by the particle itself or nearby host tissues. This process of moving in the direction of chemical signals is called **chemotaxis**. Once the phagocytic cell arrives at the site where the foreign particle is located, the cell adheres to the particle by extending a portion of the cell membrane around it. The phagocytic cell eventually engulfs or ingests the particle in a structure called a **phagosome**. The ingested particle is then exposed to enzymes and other intracellular substances that serve to digest it into small pieces.

6. What is opsonization? How does it influence phagocytosis?

Opsonization is the process of coating a foreign particle with antibodies or other molecules that facilitate phagocytosis of the particle. Opsonins, the substances that coat the particle, improve recognition and ingestion by phagocytic cells.

7. Discuss the steps required by circulating neutrophils to exit the blood and move toward a site of infection.

In areas of inflammation, signals expressed by the nearby vascular endothelial cells help to direct neutrophils out of the blood and into the affected tissue. Initially, molecules of the selectin family are expressed on the endothelial surface of capillaries near the site of inflammation. These receptors interact with neutrophils to slow the cells and cause them to roll across the vessel surface. Integrins, a second group of molecules expressed by neutrophils, serve to adhere neutrophils to the vessel wall so that the cells can emigrate from the blood into the tissue. Once the neutrophils exit the blood, they respond to chemotactic stimuli that direct cell migration toward the inflamed tissue.

8. What is leukocyte adhesion deficiency (LAD)? What are the predominant clinical signs associated with LAD in domestics animals?

To date, a form of LAD has been recognized in humans, dogs, and cattle; it has not been recognized in horses. LAD develops from an inability to express adhesion molecules on the surface of inflammatory cells. Most often LAD-affected animals are identified by the inability of neutrophils to express some or all integrins (surface antigens). Integrins play an important role in neutrophil adhesion reactions; in the absence of appropriate integrin expression, neutrophils cannot adhere to the capillary wall and emigrate into the tissue. Because neutrophils cannot gain entry into the tissue, infectious organisms cannot be eliminated. In the presence of an infection, appropriate signals are also sent to the bone marrow to increase neutrophil release. As a result, the most common signs associated with LAD include significantly elevated neutrophil concentration in the blood and recurring, persistent infections (e.g., fever, weight loss, lymphadenopathy, gingivitis, pneumonia, diarrhea). Bovine leukocyte adherence deficiency (BLAD), which affects Holstein cattle, is inherited in a simple autosomal mode. Identification of affected calves is based on the presence of clinical signs as described above, the pedigree of the calf, and DNA evaluation via polymerase chain reaction (PCR). PCR has allowed implementation of a control program whereby carriers can be identified.

9. What is the appropriate name for monocytes found in each of the following tissues: blood, brain, lung, liver, connective tissue, kidney, lymph nodes, spleen, bone, and bone marrow?

Blood: monocyte

Brain: microglial cells

Lung: dendritic cells (interstitial),
    alveolar macrophages (airway)

Liver: Kupffer cells

Connective tissue: histiocytes

Lymph nodes: macrophages

Bone marrow: macrophages

Bone: osteoclasts

10. List four major functions of macrophages.

(1) Phagocytosis, (2) cytokine production, (3) antigen presentation, and (4) synthesis of nitric oxide.

11. How is the complement system activated? What is the outcome of activation?

The complement system is activated by two pathways:

1. The **classical pathway** is activated by antigen-antibody complexes.

2. The **alternative pathway** is activated by components on the microbial surface.

Activation of the alternative or classical pathways results in subsequent activation of the **terminal pathway** and formation of the membrane attack complex (MAC). The MAC is a combination of molecules that bind together to form a tubular structure. This structure inserts into the cell membrane, forming a transmembrane channel. When sufficient numbers of MACs penetrate the membrane, the cell is lysed by osmosis.

12. What are the acute-phase proteins and the acute-phase response?

Acute-phase proteins are synthesized mainly by the liver in an acute response to infection or inflammation. The acute-phase proteins include C-reactive protein, amyloid A, fibrinogen, haptoglobin, and transferrin. An **acute-phase reaction** is a nonspecific response to infection or inflammation characterized by the appearance of acute-phase proteins in the blood.

13. Describe the cell type, mechanism, and main immune function of cell-mediated and humoral immunity.

T-lymphocytes direct cell-mediated immunity, which is important in elimination of intracellular organisms (such as viruses and some bacteria) that are inaccessible to circulating antibodies. Cells that contain infectious agents or abnormal cells (e.g., cancer cells) are eliminated by cell-mediated immunity, which causes intracellular destruction and/or lysis of affected cells.

B-lymphocytes produce antibodies required for humoral immunity. Humoral immunity mediates defense against extracellular microbes or toxins, which is achieved through the production of antibodies that recognize and bind foreign substances (called antigens) and assist in their destruction.

14. Define antibody, antigen, and isotype.

An **antibody** (also called immunoglobulin) is a molecule produced by B- and plasma cells. Antibodies have the ability to recognize and bind to specific foreign particles called antigens. An **antigen** is a foreign particle that promotes the synthesis of antibodies and/or a T-cell–mediated response. Antigens stimulate these responses by binding to specific receptors on the lymphocyte surface. **Isotype** (or class) refers to a classification of immunoglobulins (for example, IgG, IgA, IgM, and IgE) based on the constant region of the heavy chain. Isotypes do not vary among members of the same species and are similar across species. Different isotypes perform different functions.

15. Describe the general molecular structure of an antibody.

The basic antibody unit is composed of four peptide chains; two larger "heavy" chains and two smaller "light" chains. Each peptide chain can be divided into a constant, variable, and hypervariable region. Variability depends on the amount of difference in the amino acid sequence in a region of the peptide compared with other antibodies of the same class. The constant regions are highly similar across individuals within the same species, whereas the variable and hypervariable regions differ to permit specificity of antigen recognition. The amino acid sequence in the constant region determines the isotype or class of antibody, whereas antigens interact with small regions in the variable or hypervariable region. The four peptides bind together to form a Y-shaped structure, with the base of the Y representing the Fc (constant) end of the molecule and the two top arms representing the Fab (variable or antigen-binding) fragment.

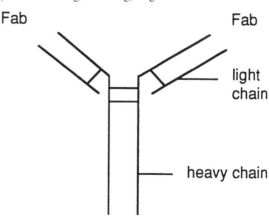

Immunoglobulin G molecule, showing the two antigen-binding fractions (Fab) and the crystallizable (or constant) fraction (Fc), which makes up the base. The structures of light chains, heavy chains, and disulfide bonds (——) are also represented.

16. Describe the origin and function of the common isotypes of antibodies.

Immunoglobulin A (IgA) is synthesized by plasma cells located near a mucosal surface and secreted as a dimer. IgA provides protection from pathogen entry through the gastrointestinal, respiratory, and urogenital tracts, mammary glands, and eyes.

Immunoglobulin G (IgG) is secreted by plasma cells. It is the immunoglobulin found in the highest concentration in the blood. IgG circulates as a monomer and escapes from the blood into interstitial sites, especially near inflamed tissues where vascular permeability is increased. IgG serves to agglutinate and opsonize antigens and may activate complement under specific conditions.

Immunoglobulin M (IgM) is synthesized by plasma cells and found in high concentrations (second to IgG) in serum as a polymer (5 or 6 subunits). IgM is the major immunoglobulin class produced during a primary immune response and mediates complement activation, opsonization, viral neutralization, and agglutination. IgM is mainly confined to blood because of its large size.

Immunoglobulin E (IgE) is produced by plasma cells and found in extremely low concentrations in serum. More commonly IgE is bound to the surface of mast cells or basophils, where it participates in signal transduction. Antigen binding to the Fab portion of the bound IgE results in rapid release of inflammatory molecules from the cells. The resulting inflammation enhances local defenses. IgE also mediates type I hypersensitivity.

17. How do the concentration and isotype of antigen-specific antibodies change over time during primary and secondary immune response to the antigen?

After initial exposure to a new antigen, measurable amounts of antigen-specific antibody can first be detected at 5–7 days and peak at around 10–14 days. The predominant antibody isotype during the primary response is IgM. With subsequent exposures, the response occurs more rapidly, and the peak concentration of antigen-specific antibody is greater. The response also persists longer, and the predominant antibody isotype is IgG.

18. Define active and passive immunity. Give an example of each that is important in veterinary medicine.

Active immunity is induced by exposure to a foreign substance. Vaccination and prior exposure to a pathogen are important examples in veterinary medicine. **Passive immunity** is transferred in the form or cells and/or serum derived from an immunized individual to a nonimmunized (or immunologically naive) individual. The process permits the recipient to develop immediate resistance in the absence of an immune response. Important examples in veterinary medicine are the colostral transfer of antibodies from the dam to the neonate and administration of tetanus antitoxin.

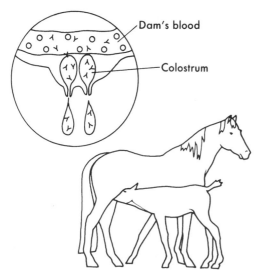

Through passive transfer the neonate receives antibodies concentrated in colostrum. (From Smith BP: Large Animal Internal Medicine. St. Louis, Mosby, 1990, with permission.)

19. What cytokines stimulate a B-cell response?

IL2, IL4, and IL5 promote B-cell response. IL2 is secreted by T-helper cells, and B-cells respond by dividing and differentiating. IL4 is secreted by Th2 cells and stimulates growth and differentiation of activated B-cells. IL5 is also secreted by Th2 cells and acts on activated B-cells to enhance differentiation into plasma cells.

20. What are CD4+ and CD8+ T-cells?

CD4 and CD8 are two glycoproteins expressed on the surface of T-lymphocytes. Both molecules assist in T-cell receptor (TCR) interaction with the major histocompatibility complex (MHC) receptor on the antigen-presenting cell. CD4 is expressed on the surface of T-helper cells and interacts exclusively with MHC class II molecules to promote cytokine secretion. CD8 is found on cytotoxic cells and binds to MHC class I molecules to promote a cytotoxic T-cell response.

21. What are Th1 and Th2 cells?

Th1 and Th2 cells are subpopulations of CD4+ cells. Development of Th1 and Th2 depends on the types of cytokines that cells encounter in their environment. For example, interleukin 12 (IL-12) stimulates cells to become Th1 types and suppresses Th2 differentiation. Th1 cells mediate cellular immunity and delayed-type hypersensitivity reactions and are characterized by synthesis of IL2 and interferon gamma. Th2 cells mediate antibody production and stimulate eosinophil and mast cell response. They are characterized by production of interleukins 4, 5, 6, and 10.

22. What cells express MHC-I and MHC-II? What is the role of these molecules?

MHC molecules are located on the surface of many cells in the body and play a role in defining tissue that is recognized by an individual's immune system as "self."

MHC-I molecules, also called class I antigens, are glycoproteins expressed to varying degrees on the surface of most cells in the body. They play a critical role in tissue allograft (transplant) rejection, because the type of MHC-I expressed on cell surfaces helps to define what the body considers its own tissue. MHC-I molecules also play an important role in presentation of endogenous antigen to cytotoxic T-cells. Endogenous antigens are manufactured within the cell through the guidance of viral or neoplastic genes and are not normally expressed on the cell surface.

MHC-II molecules, also called class II antigens, are expressed on antigen-presenting cells (APCs), including macrophages, monocytes, dendritic cells, B-lymphocytes, and, in horses, activated T-lymphocytes. MHC-II molecules serve as a platform on which processed exogenous antigens are presented to T-helper cells. Exogenous antigens are molecules produced without the use of the host cell's protein synthetic machinery. These antigens are phagocytized, processed within the cell, and presented in small recognizable fragments by APCs to the T-cell.

23. How do T-lymphocytes interact with APCs?

APCs digest antigens into small fragments. These fragments are then processed and moved to the cell's surface, where they become attached to MHC. A complex molecule, called the T-cell receptor (TCR), is located on the surface of the T-lymphocyte. The TCR recognizes and binds to specific combinations of processed antigen and MHC on the APC. In most cases, this binding results in activation of the T-cell. The activated T-cell then responds by proliferating and/or manufacturing cytokines that direct the influx of additional cells into the area. The cytokines produced by activated T-cells also promote the proliferation of additional B- and T-cells.

24. What are natural killer (NK) cells? What is their function?

NK cells are a subpopulation of lymphocytes that recognize and kill virus-infected cells. They differ from CD4+ and CD8+ T-cells because they do not require previous exposure to foreign antigens to be effective. NK cells also may be important in eliminating cancer cells.

25. What is the difference between T-dependent and T-independent antibody response?

Although B-cells recognize antigen directly, the optimal response is achieved when antigen binding occurs in the presence of the correct stimuli from T-helper cells. T-cells promote B-cell division and differentiation as well as isotype switching. As a result, B-cells produce antibodies of different classes, resulting in more specific and effective humoral protection against pathogens. Because T cells play a critical role in activation and isotype switching of B-cells, the response is termed **T-dependent**. Some antigens, however, bind directly to B-cells and stimulate maximal antibody production without assistance from T-helper cells. *Escherichia coli* lipopolysaccharide is an example. Although antibody production can be stimulated, isotype switching does not occur, and subsequent exposure to the antigen results in continued synthesis of IgM class antibodies. This type of humoral response is called **T-independent**.

26. What is the relationship among B-cells, plasma cells, and memory cells?

B-cells are found in the cortex of lymph nodes, the marginal zone of the spleen, bone marrow, Peyers' patches, and, to a small extent, in blood (< 5%). Each B-cell carries a large number of identical receptors on its surface, and when the cell encounters an antigen that is recognized by these receptors, the B-cell becomes activated to proliferate, to differentiate into plasma cells, and to make antibodies. **Plasma cells** are B-cells that have terminally differentiated into cells that can make substantial amounts of antibody. Plasma cells contain extensive endoplasmic reticulum to facilitate increased protein (immunoglobulin) synthesis. Their life span is short (i.e., 3 days to 4 weeks). Most activated B-cells also die as exposure to antigen diminishes. However, a subset of these cells is reserved and becomes antigen-sensitive or **memory cells**. Memory cells can be called on to mount a more rapid and efficient response if subsequent exposure should occur.

27. Based on serum protein electrophoretic results, what is the significance of polyclonal vs. monoclonal gammopathies?

Monoclonal gammopathies are associated with the presence of myeloma. They appear as a single large peak on electrophoresis and represent the expansion of a single clonal line of antibodies. **Polyclonal gammopathies** are more commonly associated with inflammation or infection. They appear as a broad, nonspecific peak on electrophoresis and represent the expansion of multiple clonal lines of antibodies, as expected with infection or inflammation.

28. What are the four basic types of hypersensitivities?

Type I (immediate) hypersensitivity is an acute inflammatory reaction mediated by IgE bound to mast cells and basophils. The reaction results from a release of pharmacologically active molecules from associated mast cells and basophils.

Type II (antibody-mediated) hypersensitivity results from cell or tissue destruction mediated by antibodies that recognize antigens on the tissue surface. For example, antibodies that recognize surface antigens on red blood cells attach and coat the cells. The antibody coating signals the removal of cells by antibody-complement–mediated intravascular hemolysis and/or extravascular elimination.

Type III (immune complex-mediated) hypersensitivity occurs when antigen-antibody complexes deposit in tissues, where they generate chemotactic peptides that attract neutrophils. Neutrophils release free radicals and enzymes that cause tissue destruction and inflammation.

Type IV (T-cell–mediated) hypersensitivity requires a cellular immune response, such as the tuberculin test in cattle. These reactions are slow and considered to be delayed hypersensitivities, because antigen processing, presentation, and T-cell response must occur before the immune response is mounted.

29. What classes and subclasses of immunoglobulins have been identified in horses?

IgG [subclasses: Ga; Gb; Gc; G(B); G(T)a; and G(T)b], IgA, IgM, and IgE.

30. Describe the time table of immune development in the equine fetus.

- Lymphocytes present in thymus   60–80 days of gestation
- Lymphocytes present in blood   80 days of gestation

- Lymphocytes present in mesenteric lymph node   90 days of gestation
- Lymphocytes present in spleen   240 days of gestation
- Graft vs. host response   80 days of gestation
- Antibody response to pathogen   200–230 days of gestation
- IgM, IgG   Birth

31. Are foals immunocompetent at birth?

Foals are immunocompetent (able to mount an immune response) at birth. However, their immune system has had little previous exposure to pathogens and other foreign antigens. As a result, the foal's immune system is considered naive, and most initial responses to pathogens are slow, primary responses.

32. What is the most common immunologic disease recognized in horses?

Failure of passive transfer of colostral immunoglobulins from the mare to the foal is the most common immunologic disease of the horse.

33. What are the concentrations of the different classes of immunoglobulins in equine colostrum and milk?

Immunoglobulin Concentration (mg/dl)

	IgA	IgM	IgG	IgG(T)	IgG(B)
Colostrum	500–1500	100–350	1500–5000	500–2500	500–150
Milk	50–100	5–10	20–50	5–20	—

34. What is considered evidence of failure of passive transfer in the equine neonate?

A serum immunoglobulin concentration greater than 800 mg/dl is considered representative of good passive transfer of colostral antibodies. A concentration of 400–800 mg/dl may be considered adequate if the foal and mare are in good health and there is little chance of exposure to pathogens during the first 6 weeks of the foal's life (i.e., appropriate environment and management). Less than 400 mg/dl is evidence of failure of passive transfer.

35. What methods are used to detect failure of passive transfer in foals?

Serum immunoglobulin concentration is usually not measured until the foal is 18–24 hours of age to permit adequate time for absorption of colostral antibodies. Serum immunoglobulin concentration can be measured by several different techniques. The **zinc sulfate turbidity test** is rapid and cheap, but it is difficult to obtain exact values if a spectrophotometer and appropriate standards are not available. **Single radial immunodiffusion** is more accurate but also more expensive and requires 18–24 hours before it can be read. The **latex agglutination test** uses beads coated with antiequine IgG. The equine IgG in the serum binds with the beads, causing them to agglutinate. The test is reliable, fast, and accurate. A semiquantitative membrane filter test (**enzyme-linked immunosorbent assay [ELISA]**) is also commercially available. This test measures the IgG concentration in the foal's serum or whole blood. The color intensity of the reaction from the foal's serum is compared with membrane-ELISA results obtained with standardized immunoglobulin preparations. This test is also quick and reliable.

36. How is failure of passive transfer treated?

Failure of passive transfer can be predicted in foals, such as orphans, that do not have access to good-quality colostrum. If the problem is identified before the foal is 12 hours old, immunoglobulins can be supplied by providing 2 liters (for 50-kg foals) of good-quality colostrum, divided into 4 feedings given at 2–3-hour intervals. Colostral quality can be determined by measuring colostral specific gravity with a hydrometer. Good colostrum should have a specific gravity greater than 1.060 (indicating about 3000 mg/dl IgG). If the foal is older than 12 hours or unable to be fed enterally or if colostrum is not available, a plasma transfusion can be administered to provide immunoglobulins. One liter of plasma increases a foal's IgG concentration from 200 to 400 mg, and it is best to reevaluate immunoglobulin concentration after the transfusion is complete. Foals with preexisting infections may need substantially more plasma to achieve acceptable serum levels of IgG. Colostrum from other species (e.g., cow) does not provide equine-specific pathogen antibodies. The half-life of bovine antibodies is shorter in foals; however, some veterinarians think that the IgA may be useful in decreasing enteric disease.

37. What is the time course of maternal antibody concentration in foals?
Most colostral immunoglobulins are absorbed in the foal within the first 24 hours of life, at which time the serum concentration peaks. Colostral antibody concentration gradually declines over 3–6 months. The foal initiates greater immunoglobulin production 2–4 weeks after birth. Therefore, as colostral antibody concentration declines, immunoglobulins are replaced by those synthesized by the foal.

38. What is severe combined immunodeficiency (SCID)? What breeds of horses are affected?
SCID is a lethal primary immune disease of Arabian and Arabian-Cross horses and is inherited as an autosomal recessive trait. Affected foals fail to produce T- or B-lymphocytes, whereas heterozygous horses show no abnormalities. The frequency of the disease among Arabian foals is 2–3%, and affected animals die of overwhelming infections within the first few months of life

39. What clinical signs are associated with SCID? How is a definitive antemortem diagnosis made?
Affected Arabian foals appear normal at birth, but if blood is sampled before the foal is allowed to suckle, an absence of serum IgM is detected. Foals develop signs of recurring infections (especially pneumonia) within the first weeks to months of life. A consistent hematologic finding of lymphopenia (< 1000 cells/μl of blood) is also suggestive of SCID. At necropsy, affected foals have small or absent lymph nodes and thymus. Histopathologic examination of tissue reveals severe cellular hypoplasia. Definitive antemortem diagnosis is made by detecting the aberrant gene in cells obtained from blood samples of affected or carrier horses, using PCR technology.

40. List and describe at least three additional immunologic disorders of foals.
1. **Selective IgM deficiency** has been reported predominantly in Arabian and Quarter Horse breeds. Three clinical syndromes have been described. Most affected animals develop severe recurring infections and die within the first year of life. A smaller proportion of animals have recurring infections that improve with therapy but return when treatment is stopped. Such horses have decreased average daily gain and often die within 2 years. The third syndrome is an acquired selective IgM deficiency, which generally affects horses between 2 and 5 years old and is associated with the concurrent or subsequent development of lymphoma. IgM deficiency is diagnosed by measuring serum immunoglobulins. Horses with selective IgM deficiency have concentrations that are two standard deviations below the mean, with normal concentrations of IgG and normal peripheral blood lymphocyte count. Treatment is usually unrewarding, although spontaneous recovery has been noted in rare cases.

2. **Transient hypogammaglobulinemia** is a rare disease characterized by a transient delay in the onset of immunoglobulin synthesis. Transient hypogammaglobulinemia has been reported in the Arabian breed. Affected foals present with infections around the time that colostral immunity begins to wane. Diagnosis is based on low serum immunoglobulin concentrations with normal lymphocyte counts, a finding that helps to distinguish this disease from SCID. Foals usually begin to produce immunoglobulins around 3 months of age, and will survive if they receive adequate medical support until this time.

3. **Agammaglobulinemia** is a rare immunodeficiency characterized by absence of B-lymphocytes in the blood and failure to produce immunoglobulins. Cell-mediated immunity is normal. Cases have been identified in colts of the Thoroughbred, Standardbred, and Quarter

Horse breeds. Affected animals do not develop clinical signs of disease until colostral immunity begins to wane. Colts present with recurring infections and low serum protein concentrations due to the lack of immunoglobulins in blood and tissue. Diagnosis is based on low serum immunoglobulin concentrations, poor response to vaccination, and/or absence of B-lymphocytes as determined by immunofluorescence. Most animals die of infection by 2 years of age.

41. Describe the pathogenesis of equine neonatal isoerythrolysis.
    Neonatal isoerythrolysis (NI) is a disease that affects foals during the first few days of life. The disease is noted in 0.5–2% of Standardbreds and Thoroughbreds. Offspring of mares that have had previous foals are at greatest risk. The mare is rarely exposed to fetal blood during pregnancy, but some exposure may occur at parturition. If the foal's red blood cells express paternal antigens that are not expressed on the mare's red cells, the mare mounts an immune response and titer to these antigens. If exposure occurs at parturition, maternal immunoglobulins are not synthesized in time to enter the colostrum of the foal produced by this pregnancy. In future pregnancies, however, it is likely that antibodies against the paternal red cell antigens will be included in the colostrum that the mare produces. Subsequent foals will ingest these antibodies, along with all of the immunoglobulins in colostrum. If the foal's red blood cells express these antigens, the ingested antibodies attach themselves to the red cells and cause hemolysis.

42. What factors contribute to the severity of NI?
    The severity of NI depends on the antigen that the colostral antibody recognizes and the amount of colostrum that the foal is allowed to ingest. The most severe form of the disease occurs when the colostral antibodies are directed against the blood group Aa. Antibodies that recognize the Qa group also cause severe disease, but the onset tends to be slower. Foals that develop severe NI often require blood transfusions and intense supportive care but will recover if appropriate therapy can be delivered.

43. If a brood mare has one foal that is diagnosed with NI, how can the disease be avoided in future foals from the same mare?
    Recurring problems can be prevented by identifying incompatibilities between the dam and sire before parturition and preventing the foal from ingesting colostrum from its dam. When subsequent pregnancies are by a different stallion, the mare and stallion blood should still be examined for incompatibilities (i.e., in case the subsequent stallion is Aa- or Qa-positive) before birth of the anticipated foal.

44. What is the best source of red blood cells to transfuse foals with NI?
    The anti-red blood cell antibodies found in the dam's colostrum recognize red cell antigens that are not present on the mare's cells. Therefore, the colostral antibodies do not react with red blood cells from the mare. As a result, the dam is a good potential source for red blood cells for the foal with NI. However, whole blood also contains plasma, and the dam's plasma will contain antibodies that continue to destroy the foal's red blood cells. Therefore, red blood cells from the dam must be washed free of plasma before the cells are delivered to the foal. The equipment required to wash red blood cells is often available at a local hospital, but the procedure may be too costly and time-consuming. A gelding that has never had a blood transfusion may serve as an alternative source of red blood cells for the foal. The antibodies produced by the dam of a foal with NI probably recognize red cell antigens that are common to most horses, and the donor's cells undergo some hemolysis because of interaction with these antibodies. Although this situation is not ideal, the hemolysis is limited by the amount of antibody that the foal received in colostrum, and the process should eventually cease.

45. What is autoimmunity?
    Autoimmunity is the process of mounting an immune response against a normal tissue or organ within the body.

46. What is the proposed cause of equine polyneuritis?

Equine polyneuritis (neuritis of the cauda equina) is thought to occur secondary to an autoimmune reaction against the myelin sheath of the affected peripheral nerves. Histologic evaluation of affected nerves reveals a loss of myelinated axons and an infiltration of macrophages, lymphocytes, giant cells, and plasma cells, suggestive of an immune-mediated etiology.

47. What is an anaphylactic reaction? What dose of epinephrine should be used to treat anaphylaxis in horses?

An anaphylactic reaction is an immediate hypersensitivity reaction (type I, IgE-mediated) that results in severe systemic shock. The dose of epinephrine prescribed for use in cardiac collapse, secondary to anaphylactic shock, is 10–20 µg/kg or 5–10 ml total of 1:1000 IU concentration (i.e., 0.1% solution) for a 450-kg horse. Epinephrine should be administered intravenously or intramuscularly. Subcutaneous administration is not recommended in horses because epinephrine may cause profound vasoconstriction, resulting in poor absorption and tissue necrosis. In emergency situations with a grave prognosis, in which venous administration is difficult, the epinephrine may be delivered via intracardiac injection or intratracheal administration.

48. Describe the pathogenesis of purpura hemorrhagica associated with *Streptococcus equi* respiratory infections.

The clinical syndrome of purpura hemorrhagica most commonly occurs 2–4 weeks after exposure to *S. equi* or other *Streptococcus* species antigens and results in the development of an immune-mediated vasculitis. Circulating immune complexes composed of IgA and *S. equi* M protein become deposited in vessel walls and other tissue. It is predicted that these immune complexes initiate an immediate-type hypersensitivity reaction, resulting in vasculitis. Similar injuries may occur to other tissues, such as the kidneys, in which immune complexes also have accumulated.

49. What is a Coggin's test?

A Coggin's test is a serologic test that uses immunodiffusion. Two round wells are cut in a gel layer, about 1 cm apart. Soluble antigen is placed in one well and soluble antibody in the other. The two solutions diffuse through the gel. When the antibody and antigen meet, they form a precipitate that appears as a white line. The Coggin's test is a gel-diffusion method used to detect antibodies against equine infectious anemia (EIA) virus in the horse's serum. An extract of infected horse spleen or an EIA antigen derived from cell culture is placed in one well, and serum from the test horse is placed in a second well. If the test horse has equine infectious anemia, antibodies in its serum react with the spleen or cell culture antigen and form a white line of precipitate in the gel.

50. What factors in the horse's environment or circumstances have a negative effect on the immune system?

1. **Malnutrition**, which includes starvation as well as nutrient imbalances.

2. **Toxin exposure**, which includes exposure to industrial toxins, such as polychlorinated biphenyls, and mycotoxins.

3. **Strenuous exercise**, which in unfit animals results in increased susceptibility to infection.

4. **Age**, which is associated with decreased cellular and humoral immune response in most animals.

5. **Parasitic infection**, especially with organisms such as *Toxoplasma* species or trypanosomes, results in immunosuppression.

51. Give a general description of how each of the following drugs affects immune function: (1) corticosteroids, (2) cytotoxic drugs, and (3) cyclosporine.

1. The effects of **corticosteroids** on immune function vary significantly among species. In general, corticosteroids decrease the number of circulating lymphocytes in blood, depressing the ability of T-lymphocytes and other cells to make cytokines. They also inhibit the increase in

vascular permeability and vasodilatation associated with inflammation. Corticosteroids are potent inhibitors of arachidonic acid metabolism.

  2. **Cytotoxic drugs** inhibit cell division. Because cells of the immune system are short-lived, cytotoxic drugs have a profound effect on immune function. Some cytotoxin drugs are beneficial in the treatment of immune-mediated diseases. However, when used for other purposes (such as chemotherapy in patients with cancer), the effect on immune cell proliferation is considered an undesirable side effect.

  3. **Cyclosporine** is derived from two species of fungi and serves to inhibit specifically the synthesis of IL-2 and interferon gamma by T-cells. As a result, cyclosporine therapy blocks Th1 differentiation of T-cells.

52. Describe the proposed mechanism by which the following drugs improve immune function: (1) bacterial products, (2) levamisole, (3) vitamins C and E, and (4) exogenous cytokines.

  1. Several **bacterial products** have been developed for use in horses. These products are phagocytized by macrophages and thus stimulate the synthesis of a wide variety of cytokines. Two popular bacterial products are bacille Calmette-Guérin (BCG), the live, attenuated vaccine strain of *Mycobacterium bovis*, and an anaerobic coryneform, *Propionibacterium acnes*. The exact mechanism by which these products work has not been well defined.

  2. **Levamisole** is an anthelmintic that has been used as an immune modulator in the treatment of several equine diseases. At lower doses, it is thought to stimulate immune response; at higher doses, the immune response is attenuated. The mechanisms by which these products modulate the immune system are not well defined.

  3. **Vitamins C and E** have been shown either directly or indirectly to improve immune function. Vitamin E supplementation improves cellular immunity. Vitamin C has been shown to have beneficial effects in the treatment of respiratory disease outbreaks in some species.

  4. **Cytokines**
  • *Interferons* are generally thought to promote immune response against viral infection.
  • *IL2* improves cellular and humoral immune response and has been used to promote response to certain vaccines. IL2 therapy results in a number of undesirable side effects, however, and it is unlikely that the drug will be used routinely in its present form.
  • *Others*, such as granulocyte-macrophage colony-stimulating factor (GM-CSF), have been used to stimulate immune cell proliferation and response.

53. What is the difference in composition between live and killed vaccine? What is the advantage of each?

Live vaccine: a vaccine containing a living but avirulent strain of pathogen. Its advantages include the following:
  • Fewer doses are required to achieve good response.
  • Adjuvants are not required.
  • The risk of hypersensitivity is decreased.
  • They are usually inexpensive.

Killed vaccine: a vaccine containing an inactivated (dead) strain of the pathogen. Its advantages include the following:
  • Longer half-life in storage.
  • Unlikely to cause disease through residual virulence.
  • Unlikely to become contaminated with other organisms.

54. What is an adjuvant?

When given with an antigen, an adjuvant enhances the immune response. Adjuvants are often added to dead vaccine to enhance the response to pathogenic antigens.

55. List ten reasons why vaccines may fail.

  1. Inappropriate storage of vaccine (e.g., incorrect temperature)
  2. Inappropriate route of administration

3. Inappropriate dose
4. Death of organism in a live vaccine
5. Administration of vaccine to animal protected by passive immunity
6. Administration of vaccine after the animal was infected
7. Vaccine with wrong strain of organism
8. Vaccine with an antigen that did not produce a protective response
9. Administration to immunosuppressed animal
10. Predicted variation in animal response

BIBLIOGRAPHY

1. Abbas AK, Lichtman AH, Pobe JS (eds): Cellular and Molecular Immunology. Philadelphia, W.B. Saunders, 1994.
2. Clough NC, Roth JA (eds): Understanding Immunology. St. Louis, Mosby, 1998.
3. Reed SM, Bayly WM (eds): Equine Internal Medicine. Philadelphia, W.B.Saunders, 1988.
4. Shinn EK, Perryman LE, Meek K: Evaluation of a test for identification of Arabian horses heterozygous for the severe combined immunodeficiency trait. J Am Vet Med Assoc 211:1268–1270, 1998.
5. Tizard IA (ed): Veterinary Immunology: An Introduction. Philadelphia, W.B. Saunders, 1996.

7. TOXICOLOGY

C. E. Dickinson, D.V.M., M.S., Dip. ACVIM, and
A. P. Knight, B.V.Sc., M.S., M.R.C.V.S., Dip. ACVIM

1. Are horses susceptible to poisoning by high nitrate levels in plants?

Compared with ruminants, horses are rarely affected by high nitrate levels in plants. Nitrates must first be reduced to nitrite to induce poisoning. This process occurs rapidly in ruminants through the action of rumen microorganisms, whereas the horse, a hindgut fermentor, reduces nitrate to nitrite more slowly. Cattle are about 10 times more susceptible to nitrate poisoning than horses. If a horse ingests significant quantities of nitrite, it is as susceptible to poisoning as any other animal. Nitrite converts hemoglobin to methemoglobin, which cannot bind or transport oxygen; thus cells become hypoxic. Clinical signs of nitrate poisoning develop when about 20% of hemoglobin is converted to methemoglobin, and death results when methemoglobin levels exceed 80%.

Fertilizers and agricultural water runoff from fertilized fields are also potential sources of excessive nitrate. Horses that gain access to fertilizer containing nitrates develop signs of poisoning related to the irritant effects of the nitrates on the digestive system. Colic and diarrhea are likely clinical findings.

2. What is the treatment for nitrate poisoning?

Methylene blue (1% solution, 10 mg/ml) at a dose of 1–2 mg/kg body weight injected intravenously is the standard treatment for nitrate or nitrite poisoning. Methylene blue converts reduced nicotinamide adenine dinucleotide phosphate (NADPH) to its unreduced form (NADP). NADP reduces methylene blue to leukomethylene blue, which in turn converts methemoglobin to hemoglobin, thereby restoring oxygen transportation.

3. What plants containing cyanogenic glycosides are most likely to be hazardous to horses?

Over 2,000 species of plants are known to contain cyanogenic glycosides. The more common plants associated with cyanide poisoning include *Sorghum* species (Johnson and Sudan grass), *Prunus* species (e.g., choke cherry, cherries, peaches), *Linum* species (flax), and *Triglochin* species (arrow grass).

4. What is the mechanism of cyanide poisoning?

When horses eat cyanogenic plants, damage to plant cells enables beta-glycosidases to come in contact with the plant cyanogenic glycosides, thereby releasing free cyanide (hydrocyanic acid [HCN]). The cyanide is rapidly absorbed from the digestive tract into the blood, where it inhibits the enzyme cytochrome oxidase, an essential component of the oxygen transport system in red blood cells. Cyanide has a high affinity for the ferric iron in the cytochrome oxidase, preventing electron transfer; thus hemoglobin becomes saturated with oxygen that cannot be released at the tissues. Acute cellular hypoxia results, leading to death. The blood of animals dying from cyanide is characteristically cherry-red.

5. What are the signs of chronic Sudan grass poisoning in horses?

Sudan grass (*Sorghum vulgare var. Sudanesis*) has been associated with acute cyanide and nitrate poisoning. It also has been associated with a syndrome of posterior ataxia and cystitis that is thought to be due to the presence of a lathyrogen, beta-cyanoalanine. Similar lathyrogens are found in various members of the pea family (*Lathyrus* species). Horses that are fed solely Sudan grass hay over a period of weeks may develop a syndrome of hindquarter ataxia, urinary incontinence, and constipation due to loss of rectal tone. Clinical signs resemble those encountered in equine herpes virus 1 myeloencephalitis (rhinopneumonitis) and cauda equina neuritis.

6. What is the best treatment for cyanide poisoning?

Traditionally cyanide poisoning is treated with intravenous administration of sodium nitrite and sodium thiosulfate. The sodium nitrite causes a low level of methemoglobinemia, which displaces the cyanide molecule from the cytochrome oxidase enzyme to form cyanmethemoglobin. The sodium thiosulfate then reacts with the cyanide under the influence of the enzyme rhodanase to form thiocyanate, which is readily excreted in the urine. A solution containing 1 ml of 20% sodium nitrite and 3 ml of 20% sodium thiosulfate, given intravenously at a dose of 4 ml per 100 lb (45 kg) body weight, is recommended. The animal should be handled carefully to avoid stress and excitement.

7. Heinz bodies in the red blood cells of a horse are indicative of what toxicoses?

Heinz bodies are indicative of oxidative denaturation of hemoglobin. The horse is highly susceptible to oxidants such as those found in red maple leaves, onions, and *Brassica* species (e.g., cabbage, turnip, mustards, kale) and to chemicals such as methylene blue and phenothiazine.

8. Are horses susceptible to hemlock poisoning?

Yes. Horses are susceptible to the toxic effects of both the water hemlock (*Cicuta* species) and poison or spotted hemlock (*Conium maculatum*). Cicutoxin, a highly unsaturated alcohol found in the leaves and tubers of water hemlock, is a potent neurotoxin that causes violent convulsions and death. Poison hemlock contains various piperidine alkaloids that cause neuromuscular blockade, leading to weakness, depression, coma, respiratory paralysis, and death. The teratogenic effects of poison hemlock encountered in other livestock have not been reported in horses.

9. Are all maple trees toxic to horses?

Only the red maple (*Acer rubrum*) has been associated with poisoning in horses (see question 7). More specifically, only the wilted or dried leaves and the bark are toxic. Hybrids of the red maple tree may be toxic.

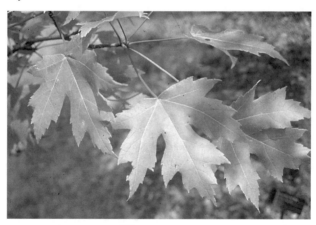

Red maple leaves (*Acer rubrum*).

10. What plants contain toxins that exert their primary effect on myocardial function and pose a threat to horses?

Although cardiac glycosides capable of causing tachyarrhythmias, heart block, and death are found in plants such as foxglove (*Digitalis purpurea*) and lily of the valley (*Convallaria majalis*), horses are more likely to be poisoned by plants such as oleander (*Nerium oleander*) and milkweeds (*Asclepias* species). These plants contain glycosides similar in effect to the digitalis glycosides found in foxglove. The glycosides act on cardiac musculature by inhibiting the cellular sodium-potassium pump (sodium-potassium-adenosine triphosphatase system) with resulting depletion of intracellular potassium. Progressive decrease in electrical conductivity through the heart causes irregular heart activity and eventually complete block of cardiac activity. Oleander leaves administered experimentally via nasogastric tube at 40–80 mg/kg body weight consistently cause cardiac toxicity. Although reduced, toxicity is retained in the dried leaves.

11. What plants are most likely to cause chronic weight loss, icterus, and severe photosensitivity in horses? How is the diagnosis confirmed?

A horse with this combination of signs in all probability has severe chronic liver disease induced by pyrrolizidine alkaloids (PAs),which are found in various plant species. The most common of the PA-containing plants are the senecios or groundsels (*Senecio* species), the best known of which is tansy ragwort (*S. jacobea*). Fiddleneck (*Amsinckia intermedia*) is also a common weed of the southwestern states that contains PA. A noxious weed introduced from Europe that contains high levels of PA is hound's tongue (*Cynoglossum officinalis*). This plant remains toxic in hay and is spreading extensively in the western United States. Rattlepod (*Crotalaria* species) and viper's bugloss (*Echium vulgare*) are PA-containing plants that may be problematic to horses.

PA poisoning is best confirmed by liver biopsy or a postmortem examination of the liver because PAs are cumulative toxins; their effects become evident many weeks after the plant has been consumed and is no longer detectable in the digestive system. The histologic changes in the liver characteristic of PA poisoning include megalocytosis, biliary hyperplasia, and extensive bridging fibrosis. Another common toxin that mimics these changes is aflatoxin.

12. How can yew poisoning be confirmed in horses?

As little as 8 ounces (~230 gm) of yew (*Taxus* species) leaves can fatally poison an adult horse. Yews contain a group of 10 or more toxic alkaloids, collectively referred to as taxine, that inhibit normal sodium and calcium exchange across the myocardial cells, thereby depressing depolarization. All parts of the plant, green or dried, but especially the leaves in winter, are toxic. A diagnosis of yew poisoning is usually based on the history of access to the plant and the finding of leaf parts in the stomach of the horse. Identification of taxine from chewed plant material and stomach contents using mass spectrometry is a precise means of confirming yew poisoning.

13. What is the pathogenesis of locoweed poisoning?

Locoweeds, a large group of plants belonging to the genera *Astragalus* and *Oxytropis* (with similarities to *Swainsonia* species) contain the alkaloid swainsonine, which inhibits the action of two lysosomal enzymes (alpha D-mannosidase and Golgi mannosidase II) that aid in the metabolism of saccharides. The inhibition of alpha D-mannosidase causes cells to accumulate oligosaccharides. Inhibition of Golgi mannosidase II affects the normal structure of oligosaccharide components of glycoproteins, furthering their accumulation. As a result, oligosaccharides accumulate in the cells of the brain and many other organs, interfering with normal cellular function. In effect, swainsonine causes a generalized lysosomal storage disease similar to the the genetically transmitted disease, mannosidosis.

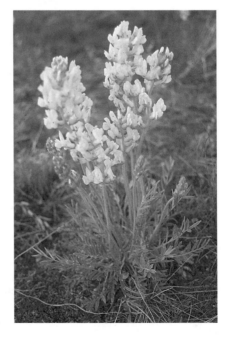

White locoweed.

14. What are the clinical signs of locoweed poisoning in horses?

The sudden onset of abnormal behavior in a horse that otherwise was normal suggests loco-ism, especially if the horse has had prolonged access to locoweeds. Affected horses show depression, circling, incoordination, staggering gait, and unpredictable behavior, especially if stressed or excited. Some horses become totally unpredictable in their response to handling and may fall down when being haltered or ridden. Poor vision, incoordination, and sudden changes in behavior such as rearing and falling over backward make horses dangerous and unsafe to ride. Weight loss despite ample forage and grain is typical. In addition to the neurologic signs of locoism, mares that consume locoweeds during pregnancy may produce foals with congenital deformities of the lower leg.

15. How can locoism be confirmed in horses?

Locoism may be confirmed in horses and other animals by demonstrating the presence of vacuoles in the cytoplasm of neurons in the brain and cells of other tissues, including the liver, thyroid gland, and lymphocytes. Vacuoles in the cytoplasm of lymphocytes in the blood is a useful indicator of locoweed poisoning, especially if the horse demonstrates characteristic neurologic signs and has had access to locoweeds. Swainsonine levels detectable in the blood indicate that the horse has recently consumed locoweed. Blood samples submitted for the detection of swainsonine levels must be collected within 1 day of ingestion of locoweed because the serum half-life is short (17–20 hours). If coupled with decreased serum alpha-mannosidase activity, detectable swainsonine levels in the animal are highly suggestive of locoweed poisoning.

16. What clinical signs are associated with sage poisoning?

The clinical signs of sagebrush (*Artemisia* species) poisoning in horses may closely resemble those associated with locoweed poisoning. *Artemisia* species contain terpene alkaloids that are neurotoxic to horses but not to ruminants. Incoordination, circling, muscle tremors, sudden collapse, and abnormal "drunken" behavior, especially if the horse is stressed or excited, are typical of a "saged" horse. Affected animals have a strong sage smell to the breath and feces. If removed from the sage, the horse usually recovers completely, whereas a locoweed-poisoned horse may never fully recover because of residual brain damage.

Horses usually do not eat toxic amounts of sage unless they are forced to do so when hungry and normal forages are unavailable. Classically horses develop sage poisoning when deep snow covers rangeland grasses and the only accessible vegetation is the sagebrush protruding above the snow.

17. What are the characteristic clinical signs of yellow star thistle and Russian knapweed poisoning in horses?

The neurotoxin in yellow star thistle (*Centaurea solstitialis*) (see figure) and Russian knapweed (*Acroptilon repens*) specifically destroys the dopaminergic nigrostriatal pathways of the cerebral cortex and affects cranial nerves V, VII, and IX, which coordinate the prehension and chewing of food. Affected horses exhibit hypertonicity of the muscles of the muzzle and lips so that the mouth is held open, the incisor teeth are exposed, and the tongue hangs out. Continuous movements of the tongue may cause frothing of saliva as the horse tries to eat. Some horses may wander about with their lips brushing through the grass; to the unobservant, this behavior may be mistaken for normal grazing. If offered hay, the horse attempts to scoop up the hay and hold it in its mouth. Swallowing is unaffected, and some less severely affected horses may learn to submerge their heads far enough into a deep trough of water to allow water to reach the pharyngeal area and be swallowed. Some affected horses appear depressed. If the lesions in the brain affect one side more than the other, the lips may be pulled to one side and the horse may circle in one direction. Other abnormal behavior may include violent head tossing and excessive yawning. Weight loss is severe; if not euthanized, affected horses eventually die from starvation and/or inhalation pneumonia.

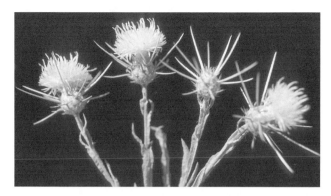

Yellow star thistle (*Centaurea solstitialis*).

18. Are horses likely to develop laminitis from merely standing in black walnut shavings without eating them?

Horses bedded with wood shavings containing 15–20% black walnut (*Juglans nigra*) shavings can develop acute laminitis without eating the shavings. Although juglone, a toxic naphthoquinone found in the black walnut, hickory, pecan, butternut, and English walnut, is involved in the development of laminitis, the precise cause is unknown. Black walnut shavings or sawdust should not be used for horse bedding, and it is not advisable to plant black walnut trees in or surrounding horse pastures.

19. Can plants other than black walnut cause limb edema?

Yes. Hoary alyssum (*Berteroa incana*), a common weed of the north central and eastern United States and Canada, causes limb edema and laminitis in horses that eat the plant. The plant as a contaminant of alfalfa hay has been associated with fever and early parturition in horses.

20. Can horses develop primary photosensitization?

Horses grazing on plants such as buckwheat (*Fagopyrum esculentum*) and St. John's wort (*Hypericum perforatum*) may ingest sufficient amounts of the plant's photoreactive pigments to cause photosensitization. Horses recover once removed from the source of the plant; there is no underlying hepatopathy.

21. Are oak leaves and acorns toxic to horses?

All oaks (*Quercus* species) contain gallotannins that produce the potent phenolic astringents tannic and gallic acid when eaten by animals. Cattle and occasionally horses develop acute gastroenteritis and renal tubular necrosis. Hemorrhagic diarrhea, tenesmus, colic, and hemoglobinuria are likely clinical signs before death. Detection of phenolic acids in the urine is helpful in confirming the diagnosis of oak poisoning.

22. What are the clinical signs of avocado poisoning?

The leaves and fruit of the avocado (*Persea americana var. guatamalensis*) are toxic to horses, causing cardiomyopathy. Horses may develop edematous swelling of the lips, mouth, eyelids, head, and neck that causes upper respiratory distress. Hydrothorax may develop. Colic is seen in some horses.

23. When can horses safely be allowed to graze a pasture recently sprayed with herbicide?

Horses have been reported to show depression, salivation, muscular tremors, icterus, and occasionally death after grazing pastures sprayed with 2,4-D and 2,4,5-T. In addition to the direct toxic effects of some herbicides, plants may increase the levels of toxic compounds such as nitrates, cyanide, and some alkaloids after being sprayed with herbicides. As a general rule, horses and other animals should be held off pastures that have been treated with herbicides until the treated plants have dried.

24. What is orchard disease?

Horses grazing in orchards in southern Florida were found to develop a neurologic disease that was originally attributed to chemical poisoning but subsequently shown to be due to creeping indigo (*Indigofera spicata*). A similar disease occurs in horses in Australia (Birdsville disease) grazing *Indigofera* species. The plant contains the toxic amino acid indospicine, which is similar to arginine and prevents the incorporation of arginine into protein. Affected horses show muscle weakness, ataxia, incoordination, seizures, and collapse. Erosion of the gums and corneal opacity are frequent findings. Pregnant mares may abort. Hepatopathy due to consumption of *Indigofera* species is apparently limited to cattle and sheep.

25. Are castor beans poisonous to horses?

Yes. Castor beans (*Ricinus communis*) contain the lectin ricin, one of the most toxic plant compounds known. Lectins as glycoproteins (toxalbumins) bind to receptor sites on certain cells, causing inhibition of protein synthesis and cell death. Castor oil also contains ricinoleic acid, a potent irritant and cathartic. Horses are reportedly fatally poisoned by as few as 60 seeds if they are well chewed before being swallowed. Unchewed seeds may pass through the intestinal tract without causing poisoning. The signs of castor bean poisoning are primarily associated with severe gastrointestinal irritation. Signs of poisoning usually begin several days after consumption of a toxic dose of lectins. Colic is often severe. Rapid loss of water and electrolytes through diarrhea results in dehydration and hypovolemic shock. Increases in serum liver enzymes, creatinine, urea nitrogen, sodium, and potassium levels and a decrease in serum total protein reflect the loss of fluid, protein, and electrolytes and the effects of the lectins on organ function. Animals left untreated die from hypovolemic shock. The black locust (*Robinia pseudoacacia*) and the rosary pea (*Abrus precatorius*) also contain lectins and are similarly toxic to horses.

26. What clinical signs are associated with bracken fern poisoning in horses?

Bracken fern (*Pteridium aquilinum*) contains thiaminase, an enzyme that destroys thiamin. Thiamin is essential for energy metabolism, specifically the conversion of pyruvate to acetyl-CoA and the oxidation of alpha-ketogluconate to succinyl CoA in the citric acid cycle. Horses are more likely to be poisoned by bracken when it is incorporated in hay. After consuming the dried bracken for several weeks, horses develop a thiamin deficiency that causes anorexia, depression, convulsions, opisthotonus, coma, and death. Blood pyruvate levels are elevated, whereas thiamin is decreased. Large doses of thiamin effectively treat the vitamin deficiency.

27. Is white snake root toxic to horses?

White snake root (*Eupatorium rugosum*) is rarely a problem to horses unless they are forced to eat it in times of drought. Tremetol, an alcohol, induces muscle tremors (especially after exercise), depression, colic, constipation, blood in the feces, and a peculiar acetone-like odor to the breath. Once muscle tremors begin, animals are reluctant to move, showing marked stiffness and eventual recumbency. Mortality is usually high in livestock showing "trembles." Fatty degeneration of the liver and kidney is a prominent necropsy finding. Tremetol is passed in the milk of lactating animals and poses a risk to the nursing foal.

28. Is day blooming jessamine poisonous to horses?

The leaves of day-blooming jessamine (*Cestrum diurnum*) contain substances with activity similar to 1,2-dihydroxycholecalciferol, the active form of vitamin D3. Horses eating the plant therefore absorb from the intestines excessive amounts of calcium, which are deposited in the soft tissues. Affected animals initially show stiffness, lameness, and weight loss with eventual recumbency. Hypercalcemia, hyperphosphatemia, and calcification of the tendons, ligaments, lungs, diaphragm, kidneys, heart, and blood vessels are likely in more chronic cases.

29. What are the signs of chronic selenium poisoning in horses?

Horses that chronically eat plants that accumulate high levels of selenium develop hair loss and lameness due to defective keratin formation; selenium displaces sulfur in the formation of normal keratin. As a result, the keratin molecule is defective, causing the hair to break and the hoof wall to crack at sites where the selenium is incorporated in keratin. The long hairs of the main and tail tend to break off, and the hooves develop circular ridges and cracks that cause severe lameness. Diets high in sulfur or sulfur-containing amino acids (e.g., methionine, cysteine) and with adequate copper help to prevent poisoning in areas where soil, plant, and water selenium levels are high.

30. Is it safe to feed plants containing high levels of oxalates to horses?

Because horses generally do not like oxalate-containing plants, poisoning is uncommon. However, sodium and potassium oxalates found in many plants are toxic and may induce hypocalcemia, oxalate nephrosis, and renal failure. Horses should not be fed oxalate-containing plants such as rhubarb leaves, sorrel (*Oxalis* species), curly leafed dock (*Rumex* species), greasewood (*Sarcobatus vermiculatus*), or halogeton (*Halogeton glomeratus*). Many plants containing oxalates may be recognized by the red color of their stems.

31. Are onions poisonous to horses?

Yes. Although less susceptible to onion poisoning than cattle, horses develop Heinz body anemia due to the oxidant effects of n-propyl disulfide and other sulfides. These sulfides are liberated from thiosulfinates formed when the methyl and propylcysteine sulfoxides in the onion are hydrolyzed in the chewing and digestive process.

32. Are larkspurs poisonous to horses?

Larkspurs (*Delphinium* species) contain various alkaloids that act on the neuromuscular junction to block the action of nicotinic acetylcholine receptors. Paralysis and death may result, depending on the dose of alkaloid and the species involved. Cattle are highly susceptible to larkspur poisoning, whereas horses are less susceptible and sheep are quite resistant. Both wild and cultivated varieties of larkspur should be considered toxic until proved otherwise. The effects of larkspur poisoning can be reversed by the timely use of physostigmine.

33. What effect is water with a "bloom" of blue-green algae likely to have on horses that drink it?

Although horses have not been reported to be affected by blue-green algae poisoning, they are more than likely susceptible to the potent neurotoxins and hepatotoxins produced by some species of algae (*Microcystis, Anabaena*, and *Nodularia* species). Algae blooms often occur in ponds contaminated with large amounts of organic matter or fertilizer runoff. Acute death may follow severe hepatic necrosis or neuromuscular blockade that results in respiratory paralysis.

34. What are aflatoxins? How do they affect horses?

Aflatoxins are mutagenic, hepatotoxic mycotoxins produced by various fungi. Aflatoxins are produced primarily by *Aspergillus* species but also by *Penicillium, Rhizopus, Mucor,* and *Streptomyces* species, which commonly grow on soybeans, corn, peanuts, cottonseed, and other grains. Compared with other species, reports of aflatoxicosis in horses are relatively rare. Aflatoxins are mutagenic, carcinogenic, teratogenic, and immunosuppressive because they alkylate nucleic acids and nucleoproteins. Acute toxicity generally reflects severe hepatocellular necrosis that results in acute hepatic failure. Chronic exposure may present as anorexia, weight loss, and hepatopathy.

35. What epidemiologic factors are associated with fescue toxicosis in horses?

Fescue toxicosis occurs when mares in late pregnancy consume tall fescue (*Festuca arundinacea*) that is infected with the fungus *Acremonium coenophialum*. The grass and fungus have a symbiotic relationship; infected fescue is much hardier than noninfected grass. Thus endophyte-infected fescue is the predominant variety. The grass grows commonly in the southern United States and has been distributed throughout the U.S. because of its many agricultural and commercial uses. Toxicity is apparently due to fungal ergopeptine alkaloids, which inhibit prolactin secretion, thereby seriously disturbing hormonal activity associated with udder development, lactation, placentation, and parturition. The alkaloids also may cause embryonic loss during the first 21 days of pregnancy.

Prevention involves reducing or eliminating exposure of mares to infected fescue during the first 21 days and last 30 days of pregnancy. Pasture management practices include eradication of fescue and reseeding with endophyte-free fescue or other forage (not always practical); increasing the legume content of fescue pastures; and/or reducing the endophyte load by cutting or grazing infected pastures before the grass flowers and seeds. Mares in late pregnancy should be removed from infected pastures. If infected hay must be fed, dilution of the ration with good-quality legume hay is advised.

36. What are the clinical manifestations of fescue toxicosis in mares?

Mares consuming endophyte-infected fescue during late pregnancy can develop various abnormalities associated with placentation, lactation, and parturition, including poor udder development, hypogalactia, agalactia, prolonged gestation, placental edema, premature placental separation, abortion, dystocia, stillbirths, weak foals, and retained fetal membranes. Pregnant mares exposed to infested fescue that exhibit poor udder development in late pregnancy should be treated with domperidone (1 mg/kg orally once daily), a dopamine agonist that promotes prolactin production.

37. What is slaframine?

Slaframine is the so-called slobber factor, a mycotoxin produced by the black patch mold (*Rhizoctonia leguminicola*) that infests legume forage, classically red clover (*Trifolium repens*). Intoxication is characterized by signs of excessive parasympathetic stimulation, including hypersalivation, diarrhea, pollakyuria, and lacrimation.

38. Tremorogenic mycotoxins are involved with which forage-associated diseases?

Paspalum staggers may occur when horses and other livestock consume paspalum grasses infested with the fungus *Claviceps paspali*. The fungus produces neurotoxic metabolites called paspaletrems, which cause a reversible syndrome of incoordination and tremors. The disease occurs in the southern U.S. and New Zealand.

Perennial ryegrass staggers is a similar but more severe syndrome caused by the tremorogen lolitrem B, which is produced by the fungus *Acremonium loliae*. The disease occurs in North America, Australia, and New Zealand when horses are kept on drought-stressed, overgrazed perennial ryegrass pastures. Horses exhibit muscle tremors, head bobbing, and incoordination. When stimulated, affected horses may show severe incoordination, collapse, and tetanic spasms. Clinical signs generally subside 1–2 weeks after horses are removed from toxic ryegrass.

Annual ryegrass staggers is a severe, often fatal syndrome of tremors and incoordination that occurs in horses and livestock in Australia and South Africa. In contrast to paspalum staggers and perennial ryegrass staggers, annual ryegrass staggers is due to glycolipid corynetoxins produced by bacteria of the *Clavibacter* species.

39. What is leukoencephalomalacia (LEM) in horses?

Otherwise known as moldy corn poisoning, LEM is a liquefactive necrosis of the cerebral white matter caused by fumonisin-B1, a mycotoxin produced by the fungus *Fusarium moniliforme*. Clinical signs include sudden death, depression, blindness, ataxia, hyperexcitability, and head pressing. The mold tends to grow on corn that is harvested after a dry growing season, has been altered by insects or processing, and is subsequently exposed to moist conditions. Therefore, the disease generally occurs during the cooler months of the year. Fumonisin-B also may cause hepatopathy. Not all moldy corn contains the toxin, and affected corn may not appear grossly moldy. Therefore, definitive diagnosis requires identification of toxic concentrations of fumonisin-B1 in the feed. Presumptive diagnosis is made through history, clinical signs, and necropsy findings. Treatment is supportive, and the mortality rate is high.

40. What is cantharidin? How does it affect horses? What can be done to avoid poisoning?

Cantharidin is a vesicant toxin contained in the hemolymph of *Epicauta* species beetles and is the cause of blister beetle poisoning in horses and other livestock. The toxin damages mucous membranes and other epithelial tissues. Poisoning in horses is characterized by colic, acute renal dysfunction, cystitis, hypocalcemia, and shock. The toxicosis may be severe and fatal. Treatment is supportive. The beetles swarm in alfalfa in mid-to-late summer when the legume is blooming. If the alfalfa is harvested during the swarm, particularly if the harvesting technique includes crimping of the forage, dead beetles will be present in the hay. Blister beetle toxicosis can be prevented by avoiding harvesting alfalfa during the bloom when grasshoppers and beetles are swarming and by moving alfalfa without crimping. Since movement of alfalfa hay around the United States has increased, cantharidin toxicosis may occur in states not typically affected.

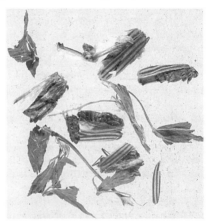

Blister beetles (*Epicauta* species) produce cantharidin toxin.

41. What is the mechanism of toxicity of ionophore antimicrobials? What is the clinical course of events after accidental exposure of horses to feeds containing ionophores?

Carboxylic ionophore antimicrobials, which are used in poultry, swine, and cattle rations as coccidiostats and growth promotants, are highly toxic to horses. Ionophores include monensin, salinomycin, narisin, and lasalocid. They form lipid-soluble complexes with cations (sodium and potassium) that readily cross biologic membranes and disrupt transmembrane electrochemical gradients, causing cell death. Tissues with high metabolic demand are most susceptible, and clinical signs in horses reflect damage to the myocardium, skeletal muscle, and renal tissues. Poisoned horses initially go off feed, often show signs of colic, and may sweat profusely. As the poisoning progresses, the clinical picture includes acute cardiac failure, hypovolemic shock, and renal failure. Laboratory abnormalities reflect the effects of shock, renal failure, and myonecrosis and may include hemoconcentration, electrolyte disturbances, elevations in serum muscle enzyme activities, hematuria, and myoglobinuria. Treatment is supportive and should include large volumes of intravenous fluids to support cardiovascular and renal function. Administration of mineral oil, activated charcoal, and/or saline cathartics is indicated to reduce absorption of the toxin. Severe poisonings often result in death due to acute myocardial failure. Horses that survive the acute poisoning may succumb later or become incapacitated by myocardial fibrosis.

42. How does vitamin K antagonism occur? How is the diagnosis confirmed? How is it corrected?

Vitamin K antagonism results from exposure to anticoagulant rodenticides and also occurs naturally when horses are exposed to moldy sweet clover containing toxic levels of dicumeral, a fungal metabolite of Coumarin. Vitamin K is required in the synthesis of coagulation factors I (fibrinogen), II (prothrombin), VII (prothrombinogen), IX (Christmas factor, hemophilic factor B), and X (Stuart factor). Inhibition of vitamin K results in deficiency of these factors; ultimately the system is unable to generate thrombin, and coagulopathy ensues. Since both intrinsic and extrinsic arms of the coagulation cascade are affected, prothrombin time (PT), activated partial thromboplastin time (aPTT), and thrombin time (TT) are prolonged. However, because factor VII has a short half-life relative to clotting factors associated with the intrinsic and common pathways, the PT (extrinsic pathway) becomes prolonged before signs of coagulopathy are evident. Therefore, in patients with a history of possible exposure to an anticoagulant, PT is useful in confirming or ruling out poisoning. When clinical signs are apparent, they reflect the consequences of hemorrhage and may include depression, weakness, tachypnea, tachycardia, anemia, epistaxis, hematoma formation, hemarthrosis, hemothorax, and hemoperitoneum.

Vitamin K1 given by subcutaneous injection is the treatment of choice. Dosage, frequency of administration, and length of treatment depend on the specific anticoagulant involved. Anticoagulants may be classifed as short-acting (warfarin), intermediate-acting (diphacinone, chlorophacinone), and long-acting (brodifacoum, bromadialone). Poisoning with short-acting anticoagulants generally requires 1 week of vitamin K1 treatment, whereas horses poisoned with intermediate- and long-acting anticoagulant rodenticides may require a treatment period exceeding 30 days. Clotting times can be used to monitor therapy and to identify the therapeutic endpoint. Vitamin K3 (menadione sodium bisulfite) must not be used; it may cause acute renal tubular necrosis and renal failure in horses.

43. What are the clinical signs of lead poisoning in horses? How is the diagnosis confirmed? What is the treatment?

Classically, lead poisoning in horses is a neurologic syndrome accompanied by weight loss and depression after chronic exposure. The neuropathy is characterized by cranial nerve dysfunction. Dysphagia, dysphonia, and "roaring" result from pharyngeal and laryngeal paresis or paralysis, and aspiration pneumonia may be a complication. Additional clinical signs may include facial paralysis, poor anal tone, proprioceptive deficits, incoordination, stiffness, muscle tremors, colic, diarrhea, and anemia. Since the disease results from chronic exposure, blood lead levels are often normal, although high levels are present in bone. The diagnosis may be confirmed by measuring urine lead levels after chelation. Measurement of free erythrocyte porphyrins, erythrocyte concentrations of alpha-aminolevulinic acid, and/or blood gamma-aminolevulinic acid hydratase also may substantiate the diagnosis. Treatment is based on chelation with calcium disodium ethylenediamine tetraacetic acid (EDTA) and should include fluid and nutritional support.

44. What types of venomous snakes are indigenous to the United States?

Pit vipers (family Crotalidae) are by far the predominant type of venomous snake in North America and therefore account for the vast majority of venomous snakebites. North American pit vipers include the rattlesnakes (genus *Crotalus*), pigmy and massasauga rattlesnakes (genus *Sistrurus*), and cottonmouths and moccasins (genus *Agkistrodon*). Rattlesnakes are the most widely distributed and are probably involved in the majority of envenomations in livestock in the U.S. The venoms of all North American pit vipers are quite similar in overall composition, although specific composition varies among species, subspecies, and individual snakes. The venoms have potent necrotizing and hemorrhagic properties and variable neurotoxicity, which takes the form of somatic motor paralysis when present. Corral snakes (family Elapidae, genus *Micrurus*) produce a less complex but highly lethal neurotoxic venom. Because of their limited geographic distribution (coastal Florida and Texas, extreme southern New Mexico and Arizona), reclusive nature, and rear-fanged anatomy, envenomation of livestock by corral snakes is quite rare.

45. What are the clinical manifestations of pit viper venom poisoning in horses?

Envenomation by pit vipers is a complex poisoning characterized by local swelling, tissue damage, hypotension, hemorrhage, and hematologic disorders, including hemolysis, thrombocytopenia, and coagulopathy. Because horses are most often bitten on or near the muzzle while grazing, head swelling is often the most obvious clinical sign. Mild epistaxis is typically present, and swelling in the nasal passages and pharynx results in upper airway obstruction. When horses are bitten on an extremity, swelling and lameness are apparent. Acute signs may include mild fever, tachycardia, tachypnea, pain, and excitement. Various laboratory abnormalities may be present, including anemia, thrombocytopenia, prolonged clotting times, stress leukogram, azotemia, acidosis, hypocalcemia, hyperglycemia, elevations in serum hepatic and muscle enzyme activities, and pigmenturia. Complications may include acute airway obstruction, severe hemolytic anemia, colic, colitis, acute renal dysfunction, pharyngeal paralysis, paralysis of the muscles of mastication, and necrosis and/or chronic inflammation at the envenomation site. In addition, severe myocarditis may occur, resulting in acute or chronic myocardial failure. Envenomations by the Mojave rattlesnake in the southwest U.S. may result in somatic motor paralysis, leading to recumbency and death by asphyxiation due to paralysis of the diaphragm.

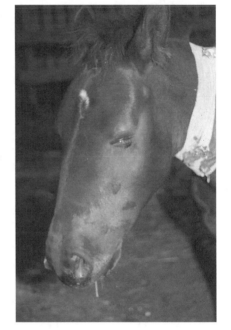

Swollen head with syringes in nares following rattlesnake envenomation.

46. How should pit viper bites in horses be treated?

The definitive treatment for pit viper venom poisoning in the U.S. is intravenous administration of specific antivenom, marketed as antivenin (Crotalidae) polyvalent by Wyeth (human label) and as antivenin by Fort Dodge (veterinary label). Moderately-to-severely envenomated horses should receive at least 1 or 2 vials within 24 hours of the poisoning, preferably sooner. Acute placement of nasal tubes (e.g., modified syringe cases) is useful in maintaining a patent airway. Tracheotomy may be necessary in certain cases but is often troublesome because of severe ventral cervical swelling and inflammation and persistent bleeding at the surgical site. Hematocrit should be monitored frequently to assess the degree of hemolysis. Fluid therapy is beneficial. Horses should be treated with broad-spectrum antimicrobials and receive tetanus prophylaxis. Administration of NSAIDs at analgesic dosages is appropriate. Administration of short-acting corticosteroids may temporarily inhibit swelling, but repeated dosing may be contraindicated. Affected limbs should be treated with hydrotherapy daily and wrapped appropriately. Nursing care is important, because the horse may not be able to eat and drink adequately.

Appropriate first aid procedures in the field include nasal intubation for horses bitten on the muzzle and application of light pressure wraps (with cotton padding) to affected distal limbs, which help to slow venom absorption by impeding lymphatic flow. For horses bitten on the head, halters should be applied loosely and removed when not needed for handling. Physical activity should be kept to a minimum, and horses with severe upper airway obstruction should be handled with care to avoid acute respiratory embarrassment and collapse. Incision and suction of the bite site may be beneficial in reducing the venom load if performed within 30 minutes of envenomation, but this procedure may exacerbate tissue damage and introduce infection if not done properly. It should not be attempted by laymen. Application of tourniquets or cryotherapy (ice baths) is strictly contraindicated.

BIBLIOGRAPHY

1. Cheeke PR: Natural Toxicants in Feeds, Forages, and Poisonous Plants, 2nd ed. Interstate Publishers, 1997.
2. Colegate SM, Dorling PR: Plant-associated Toxins. Wallingford, U.K., CAB International, 1994.
3. Fraser CM (ed): The Merck Veterinary Manual, 7th ed. Rahway, NJ, Merck & Co., 1991.
4. Plumlee KH, Galey FO: Neurotoxic mycotoxins: A review of fungal toxins that cause neurological disease in large animals. J Vet Intern Med 8:49–54, 1994.
5. Robinson NE (ed): Current Therapy in Equine Medicine, 4th ed. Philadelphia, W.B. Saunders, 1997.
6. Smith BP (ed): Large Animal Medicine, 2nd ed. St. Louis, Mosby, 1996.

8. CARDIOLOGY

Melinda A. Edwards, D.V.M., and
Catherine J. Savage, B.V.Sc., M.S., Ph.D., Dip. ACVIM

1. What are the elements of a thorough evaluation of the equine cardiovascular system?

1. Obtain a detailed history, including any duration of poor performance.

2. Observe the horse from a distance (e.g., 3–12 meters) to note general disposition, presence of edema, and other relevant characteristics.

3. Palpate the left hemithorax (generally in the fifth intercostal space for the maximal impulse), obtain the pulse, palpate the limbs and ventrum for edema, and evaluate the temperature of the limbs.

4. Percuss both hemithoraces to see whether pleural or pericardial effusion is present.

5. Auscultate the heart and lungs thoroughly, beginning on the left side and then listening to the right chest.

6. Perform echocardiography, if needed.

7. Perform electrocardiography (EKG), if needed.

2. What are the normal cardiac physical examination findings in horses?

As with any system assessment, one should begin the examination by observing the animal at a distance. The patient should be bright, alert, and willing to move about freely. The head, ventrum, and extremities are normally without edema. Once should assess the respiratory system by observing the patient for abdominal and/or intercostal muscle use, tachypnea, or coughing, because pulmonary pathology can arise from primary cardiac dysfunction. Mucous membranes should be light pink and have a capillary refill time of less than 2 seconds. With the patient's head in a neutral position, it is normal for a jugular pulse to extend from the level of the thoracic inlet to a point approximately one-third of the way up the neck. A normal jugular vein should fill within 2–3 seconds after occlusion and immediately disappear once pressure is relieved. A nondistended jugular vein is normally not palpable.

The heart rate or pulse rate in adult horses should be 26–48 beats per minute. Because of the great variability among different classes of horses, it is wise for owners to learn what is normal for their horse. Arterial pulse can be assessed by palpating the digital, facial, transverse facial, or median arteries digitally. The strength of the pulse is related to the difference between systolic and diastolic pressures and thus is decreased in cases of cardiac tamponade and cardiomyopathy. The appreciable arterial pulse may be altered with heart rate and excitement; in addition, it is often weak in cases of hypovolemic shock (e.g., severe colitis or colic) because strength of pulsations reflects changes in stroke volume. A palpable pulse should be associated with each heart beat. It is often useful to auscultate the heart while palpating the facial artery to ensure that no pulse deficits are present. Pulse deficits are associated with premature beats or short R-R intervals, as may occur in atrial fibrillation.

Both left and right hemithoraces should be auscultated thoroughly, with the left chest receiving attention first. It is normal to hear up to four heart sounds in equine patients (e.g., du-LUBB-DUPP-boo). The rhythm of these four sounds is S4-S1-S2-S3. However, most commonly one auscultates only the first (S1) and second (S2) heart sounds (i.e., LUBB-DUPP).

Physiologic murmurs may vary in intensity with changing heart rates (e.g., exercise), generally occur sporadically, are often subtle, and may tend to have a focal point of maximal intensity (PMI). Conversely, persistent or prominent murmurs are often pathologic and may be auscultated over a more diffuse field.

Patteson M: Equine Cardiology. Oxford, Blackwell Science, 1996.

3. Which main cardiac functions are associated with each of the four heart sounds?

The first heart sound (S1) represents the onset of systole and occurs when the mitral and tricuspid valves close. The second heart sound (S2) occurs at the onset of diastole and represents closure of the aortic and pulmonic valves. The third heart sound (S3) is associated with rapid ventricular filling. The fourth heart sound (S4) signifies atrial contraction. At heart rates less than 48 beats per minute, it is possible to hear all four heart sounds. The four heart sounds should be distinguished from split heart sounds, which can be appreciated in some normal equine hearts. This phenomenon represents asynchronous valve closure. A split S1 may occur when the mitral and tricuspid valves do not close simultaneously, whereas a split S2 represents asynchronous aortic and pulmonic valve closure. A split S2 may be pathologic when it represents pulmonary hypertension.

4. In what locations on the equine thorax are the sounds associated with each valve best auscultated?

The pulmonic, aortic, and mitral valves are best auscultated on the left side of the equine thorax, whereas the tricuspid valve is best appreciated on the right hemithorax. Specifically, activity associated with the **pulmonic valve** is best appreciated over the third intercostal space, slightly ventral to the point of the shoulder on the left hemithorax. Sounds associated with the **aortic valve** are best heard in the fourth intercostal space just ventral to the level of the point of the shoulder on the left side of the thorax. The **mitral valve** is best auscultated in the area of the left fifth intercostal space just dorsal to the level of the olecranon. The **tricuspid valve** is best auscultated on the right side of the thorax at the level just above the olecranon over the fourth intercostal space but also may be heard on the left hemithorax cranial and slightly dorsal to the olecranon. It is useful to remember that the caudal edge of the triceps muscle overlies the fifth intercostal space.

Since anatomic landmarks may be difficult to appreciate and since points of maximal impulse do not correlate with anatomic location of valvular structures, it is beneficial to know how to identify the valves based on characteristic sounds heard in various locations on the thorax. S1, representing closure of the atrioventricular valves, is most prominent over the mitral area on the left side of the chest and the tricuspid area on the right side of the chest. Likewise, S2 is best appreciated at the heart base, where aortic and pulmonic valvular activity occurs.

Patteson M: Equine Cardiology. Oxford, Blackwell Science, 1996.

5. Describe the four characteristics by which cardiac murmurs are classified.

A consistent, universally accepted means of identifying various characteristics of cardiac murmurs is helpful in monitoring change in a patient's condition over time and also helps to define a murmur as either physiologic or pathologic. Murmurs are classified according to (1) timing/duration, (2) character, (3) intensity, and (4) location (point of maximal intensity).

1. **Timing** of the murmur refers to the point in the cardiac cycle in which the murmur occurs. *Pan-* means that the murmur obscures the heart sounds, *holo-* means that the murmur begins/ends immediately after/before the heart sounds, *systolic* means between S1 and S2, and *diastolic* means between S2 and S1. Thus, a pansystolic murmur obscures S1 and S2. A holosystolic murmur is present from the end of S1 to the beginning of S2. Likewise, a holodiastolic murmur is auscultated from the ends of S2 to the beginning of S1. Murmurs also may be described as occurring early, midway through, or late in systole or diastole.

2. **Character** of the murmur refers to intensity and pitch. Changes in *intensity* result from various pressure gradients and velocity of flow. If the pressure gradient remains constant during the time that the murmur occurs, it is termed a *plateau murmur*. This type of sound is appreciated in the case of atrioventricular (e.g., mitral and tricuspid) valve regurgitation, because the pressure difference between ventricles and atria (i.e., across the valve) remains consistent throughout systole. In contrast, a murmur associated with aortic regurgitation is described as a *decrescendo murmur* because the pressure across the valve during diastole gradually decreases as the blood flows distally through the aorta. *Crescendo-decrescendo murmurs* also have been described in cases in which intensity increases, peaks, then decreases. Pulmonary valve insufficiency is rarely associated with a murmur, because the pressure gradient across the pulmonary valve is low. *Pitch*

ranges from musical to harsh and sonorous. Both intensity and pitch may vary from beat to beat or change with varying heart rates.

3. Murmur **intensity** is divided into six grades:
- *Grade I:* barely audible murmur; discernible only after careful auscultation over a focal area.
- *Grade II:* low-intensity murmur; heard immediately to a few seconds after the stethoscope is placed over the point of maximal impulse of the murmur; softer than S1.
- *Grade III:* loud murmur that is immediately audible; may be heard over a wide area of the chest; equally as loud as S1.
- *Grade IV:* a prominent, widespread murmur that is louder than S1 and may be heard over a wide area of the chest.
- *Grade V:* a prominent murmur (the loudest that becomes inaudible when the stethoscope is removed) with a palpable thrill.
- *Grade VI:* a loud murmur with accompanying precordial thrill that can be auscultated with the stethoscope off the chest wall.

4. **Location of the point of maximal intensity** (PMI) of the murmur is helpful in associating the sound with a particular valve (see question 4 for the positions of valves in the chest). The extent of radiation of sound helps to determine whether the sound is physiologic or pathologic. Physiologic murmurs are usually focal and do not radiate. Pathologic murmurs may be local or auscultated over a wide area on the thorax. Often the degree of valvular incompetence is directly proportional to the degree of radiation of the murmur. In addition, in rare cases one can ascertain the direction of the jet creating the murmur by determining the extent and direction of sound radiation.

Patteson M: Equine Cardiology. Oxford, Blackwell Science, 1996.

6. How does the electrical and mechanical activity of the heart correlate with the EKG tracing?

The P-wave of the normal EKG tracing represents depolarization and subsequent contraction of the atria. The length of the PR interval indicates velocity of conduction through the atria, atrioventricular (AV) node, and bundle of His. The QRS complex represents depolarization of the ventricles. Auscultation of S1, the heart sound associated with systole, occurs during the S-wave of the EKG. S2, the diastolic heart sound, occurs at the peak of the T-wave. S3, representing ventricular filling, occurs between the T-wave and the subsequent P-wave. Atrial contraction, coinciding with S4, is associated with the Q-wave of the EKG.

7. What basic components of the EKG should be evaluated in each tracing?

One should begin by assessing quality of the tracing for artifact and determining paper speed. Then the heart rate should be determined by counting over a 60-second interval. A normal rate should be differentiated from a slow rate (bradycardia) or an accelerated rate (tachycardia); an arrhythmia may affect the calculation of heart rate substantially. Next the rhythm should be determined, checking whether changes in rate are regular or irregular and whether the variability is continuous or intermittent. Finally, the EKG complexes should be evaluated. A QRS complex should follow every P-wave, and every QRS should be preceded by a P-wave. Duration and amplitude of the P-wave and QRS complex should be evaluated, and the duration of the PR interval should be determined. Many normal alterations of the P-wave (split or biphasic) and T-wave are found in horses; occurrence of the Q and R portions of a QRS complex is also variable. Little significance can be ascribed to these variations; however, the P-QRS-T complex should be consistent in shape and deflection throughout a 2-minute tracing.

Patteson M: Equine Cardiology. Oxford, Blackwell Science, 1996.

8. Give normal durations and amplitudes of the P-wave, PR interval, QRS complex, ST segment, and T-wave. What alterations commonly occur? What pathology is represented by each?

The **P-wave** is usually positive (i.e., has an upward deflection) with an amplitude of 0.1–0.3 millivolts and a duration of < 0.16 seconds. A normal P-wave may be notched.

Enlargement of the right atrium is characterized by increased amplitude of the P-wave, whereas left atrial enlargement is represented by a prolonged P-wave that is often notched. Variability in the shape of the P-wave represents variability in the focus of the electrical impulse. A P-wave arising from the atria has a different shape from a P-wave arising from the sinoatrial node. A P-wave may be superimposed on the preceding T-wave in cases of tachycardia and thus difficult to identify.

The average **PR interval** is < 0.5 (0.22–0.50) seconds. Prolonged or inconsistent PR intervals may occur with atrioventricular block. Prolongation of the PR interval also may occur with atrial myocarditis and treatment with cardiac glycosides.

The **QRS complex** normally has a duration of < 0.14 (0.08–0.14) seconds. In a normal equine EKG the amplitude of the Q-wave is > 0.18–0.28 millivolts; of the R-wave, 0.8–1.2 millivolts; and of the S-wave, 0.2–0.38 millivolts. Right ventricular hypertrophy is characterized by increased S-wave amplitude, whereas exaggerated R-wave amplitude is present in cases of left ventricular enlargement. Low QRS amplitude is characteristic of pericardial effusion.

The **ST segment** should form a straight baseline with the PR segment. Elevation or depression of the ST segment may occur with myocarditis, infarction, endotoxic shock, hypoxia, or hypokalemia.

The normal equine **T-wave** has an amplitude of 0.2–0.6 millivolts and many possible variations in appearance. Hyperkalemia, hypoxia, and a number of medications can alter the shape and amplitude of the T-wave. Changes in T-wave morphology are not a reliable indicator for any particular pathology.

Patterson M: Equine Cardiology. Oxford, Blackwell Science, 1996.

9. EKG leads are chosen to minimize error attributable to movement, to improve the size and clarity of waveforms, and thus to increase the likelihood of evaluating structures accurately. Which lead is used most commonly for producing the equine EKG?

When limb leads are used in the horse, a strong panniculus reflex and shifting movements often result in artifact that interferes with interpretation of the tracing. Placing the leads over the trunk and neck helps to alleviate this problem. Since the direction of ventricular depolarization is cranial and dorsal, a bipolar lead placed on the thorax/neck in a cranial-caudal or dorsal-ventral plane is most likely to yield tracings with large complexes and minimal artifact.

The base-apex lead (i.e., Y-lead or base-to-apex lead) incorporates these principles. The positive electrode (e.g., LA lead) can be placed on the left thorax in the region overlying the apex of the heart—at the level of, and just caudal to, the olecranon on the left thorax. Alternatively, the positive electrode can be placed on the ventral midline in the area of the xiphoid of the sternum. The negative electrode (e.g., RA lead) is placed on the region overlying the heart base. The left jugular furrow or the area just cranial to the scapula are appropriate sites. The ground electrode can be placed at any distant site away from the base-apex circuit, usually over the withers or at the thoracic inlet. Since the vector of depolarization is directed away from the positive electrode, the QRS complex has a predominantly negative deflection.

10. In what disease states is the P-wave likely to be absent or hidden?

Absence of P-waves may indicate atrial fibrillation (multiple, variable F-waves occur in sequence without associated QRS complexes); hyperkalemia (serum potassium > 6 mEq/L); junctional rhythm (i.e., when a rhythm originates in the atrioventricular node and P-waves become hidden in the QRS complexes by incorporation); or, in rare cases, sinus arrest. In third-degree (complete) heart block and supraventricular tachycardia, some P-waves may be obscured occasionally in the QRS complex or T-waves.

11. Describe the best approach to performing echocardiography in horses.

The horse should be positioned in stocks if they are available. Generally no chemical restraint is used. A region from the right third-to-seventh intercostal spaces and left fourth-to-seventh intercostal spaces from several inches above the olecranon to several inches below should be clipped if the horse's coat is thick. Some horses with thin hair coats (e.g., horses that are blanketed and stabled) may be examined after application of alcohol and ultrasonic transmission gel. The leg should be pulled forward and slightly abducted so that the transducer can be pushed in front of the olecranon if necessary. The right side is examined first for the standard long- and short-axis views. Then the left side is imaged to complete any portions of the study that could not be imaged on the right side. The left side is also useful if Doppler is to be used.

The normal equine heart just fits onto the sector image of ultrasonographic equipment with a depth of 24 cm. It is rare to be able to image the entire left atrium in either transverse or long-axis planes. However, the best images of the left atrium and left ventricular wall can be obtained from imaging the left side.

In imaging an equine heart on either the left or right side, it is best to think in terms of a clock face with 12 o'clock pointing to the dorsum and 3 o'clock pointing to the leg (on the right) and the tail (on the left). Then one uses the **long-axis left ventricular outflow view** as a reference plane; all movements occur around the clock away from this plane. Some ultrasonographers may choose other reference points; thus, it is essential to know the location of the transducer reference mark at all times. To obtain the long-axis left ventricular outflow view, one should place the transducer in the third-to-fifth intercostal space approximately 2–3 inches above the point of the olecranon on the right side, while keeping the transducer perpendicular to the chest wall. The reference mark is directed toward 1 o'clock (i.e., the sound beam should be aligned along the imaginary line joining 1 o'clock and 7 o'clock). The cable end of the transducer (i.e., not the crystal head/end) should be pushed into the right leg of the horse so that the crystal head points slightly caudal. This maneuver lengthens the left ventricle view. To obtain a better view of the aorta, it may be necessary to rotate the transducer so that the reference mark (i.e., on top of the transducer crystal head) moves toward the leg.

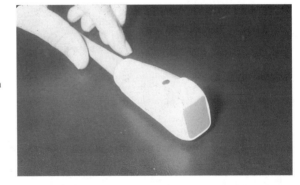

2.5-mHz ultrasound transducer with black reference mark.

To obtain the **right parasternal long-axis view** with left ventricular outflow, rotate the transducer back to the 12 o'clock mark. Continue to rotate until the aorta disappears from view and the interatrial septum is seen. To keep the full length of the left ventricle in view, the transducer should be pointed caudal (i.e., the transducer cable end should be pushed into the leg). Pointing the transducer crystal face dorsally produces a tipped (i.e., apex at top) four-chamber view.

To obtain **transverse views** of the heart, the transducer should be rotated clockwise until the reference mark is at approximately 4 o'clock and a circular aorta or left ventricle is seen. Then pivot the transducer ventrally (i.e., face toward the sternum) for an image of the left ventricle and dorsally to the neck for the heart base.

The **four-chambered view** of the heart is obtained from a cranial location (i.e., fourth-to-fifth intercostal space), approximately 2–3 inches above the olecranon on the left side. The reference mark should be at 12 o'clock, and the transducer should be kept almost perpendicular to the thoracic wall. Then one can point the transducer in a dorsal and cranial direction until the largest view of the left ventricle is obtained. To obtain the **five-chambered view** with the aorta, the transducer should be rotated counterclockwise to approximately 10–11 o'clock. These four- and five-chambered views are examples of the **left parasternal long-axis images**.

To obtain the left ventricle and heart base (i.e., right ventricle and pulmonary artery), one may use **left parasternal short-axis imaging**. Start with the left parasternal long-axis four-chambered view, and then rotate the transducer so that the reference mark is at 3–4 o'clock and a circular left ventricle is seen. One may then pivot the transducer crystal to find the view in which the left ventricle is largest and symmetric. To obtain a heart base view, the transducer must be moved to the level of the olecranon and as far cranial as possible. The reference mark is 12–2 o'-clock, and the crystal head should be pointed caudally and slightly dorsally until both the pulmonic and tricuspid valves can be seen.

The **left parasternal apical view** is not a true apical view because the left ventricle is foreshortened to a great degree. However, it is useful because it allows the aorta to be visualized in the long axis. The transducer should be moved to a point just above the level of the olecranon and caudally by 2–3 intercostal spaces (to the point where the left parasternal four- and five-chambered views were obtained). The reference mark should be located in a 1–2 o'clock position (i.e., left side so that the direction toward the tail is 3 o'clock) with the face of the transducer directing cranially and dorsally. Then pivot the transducer toward and away from the body to obtain the clearest images.

Long KJ, Bonagura JD, Darke PGG: Standardized imaging technique for guided M-mode and Doppler echocardiography in the horse. Equine Vet J 24:226–235, 1992.

Boon JA: The echocardiographic examination. In Boon JA (ed): Manual of Veterinary Echocardiography. Baltimore, Williams & Wilkins, 1998, pp 35–150.

12. What are the five goals of treatment of congestive heart failure (CHF) in horses?

1. **Positive inotropy** (i.e., increasing stroke volume through increasing contractility). Digoxin is the drug most often used for this purpose.

2. **Negative chronotropy** (i.e., decreasing heart rate). In addition to being a positive inotrope, digoxin is also a negative chronotrope.

3. **Reduced preload.** Use of venodilators and arteriodilators has been poorly evaluated in horses. Diuretics (e.g., furosemide) are most commonly chosen for this purpose; however, great care must be taken when furosemide is used because tissue perfusion may be compromised further.

4. **Reduced afterload.** The angiotensin-converting enzyme (ACE) inhibitor, lisinopril (Zenaca Pharmaceuticals, Wilmington, DE, 19850), has been shown anecdotally to be beneficial in decreasing vasoconstriction of both veins (thereby reducing preload) and arteries (thereby reducing afterload). ACE inhibitors also minimize fluid retention via a decrease in aldosterone, which also decreases preload.

5. **Control of atrial and ventricular dysrhythmias.** Quinidine and lidocaine are treatment options. Specific therapy is dictated by the type of dysrhythmia.

13. What is the most common equine congenital cardiac effect? How may one differentiate this anomaly from other congenital abnormalities?

Ventricular septal defect (VSD) is the most frequently diagnosed congenital cardiac abnormality in horses. The malformation is usually an opening high in the membranous portion of the septum. The murmur auscultated in cases of VSD is best appreciated on the right side of the thorax because of the left-to-right direction of flow in the majority of cases. As opposed to the continuous murmur associated with patent ductus arteriosus, the murmur resulting from VSD is harsh, plateau-shaped, and holosystolic; it may be accompanied by a palpable thrill. A second component of the murmur may be auscultated on the left side of the thorax during diastole if concomitant aortic insufficiency is present. Definitive diagnosis may be made by echocardiography.

14. What recommendations should a veterinarian make to the owner of a foal with VSD?

It is prudent to advise that the affected horse not be bred, because the hereditary component of the disease has not been fully elucidated. There is no practical treatment for VSD, although open heart surgery with septal repair may be attempted in a valuable foal. It is also prudent to advise caution regarding exercise, especially riding. However, some horses can race or otherwise perform well even with the defect, although predicting the consistency and frequency of performance is difficult.

15. When does a patent ductus arteriosus (PDA) occur?

PDA occurs when the ductus arteriosus, a vessel connecting the aorta to the pulmonary artery in the fetus, remains patent for an uncommon length of time after birth.

16. How may one verify the presence of PDA in an 8-day-old foal with a persistent murmur that has a PMI over the left third-to-fourth intercostal space?

In cases of PDA, one often can auscultate a continuous murmur over the left and right hemithoraces at the third-to-fourth intercostal spaces at the level of the shoulder. In some cases, only a holosystolic murmur can be appreciated because the diastolic component may be quite subtle as pulmonary hypertension increases. An augmentation in murmur intensity often occurs with elevations in heart rate secondary to excitement, exercise, or pain. The arterial pulse is often bounding because blood leaves the left side via the shunt, thus decreasing the diastolic pressure rapidly. Tests to assist in verifying the diagnosis, although not very useful, include the following:

1. Radiographic changes associated with PDA are seen with any left-to-right shunt and are therefore not pathognomonic for the syndrome. Foals with uncomplicated PDA may have an enlarged cardiac silhouette and pulmonary overcirculation. In cases of secondary right heart failure, one may note changes consistent with pulmonary venous congestion, interstitial pulmonary edema, and alveolar edema.

2. There are no specific EKG changes. The amplitude of the S-wave may be heightened in cases of right ventricular hypertrophy.

3. Echocardiography may demonstrate increased left atrial-to-aortic root dimension, decreased velocity of circumferential fiber shortening, and increased left ventricular end-diastolic dimension. Unfortunately it is rare to be able to see the PDA because the lung often obscures the descending aorta.

4. Oximetry may be used to demonstrate an increase in pulmonary artery oxygen saturation.

5. Although rarely performed in horses, angiography and cardiac catheterization may reveal increased pulmonary artery and right ventricular pressures.

17. How should you counsel the owner of a 12-hour-old term foal with suspected PDA vs. the owner of a 12-day-old foal with the same condition?

Normal foals may have PDA for up to 96 hours. Rarely, a foal may exhibit signs for up to 8 days without suffering long-term sequelae as an adult. A foal under 96 hours of age with suspected PDA should simply be monitored for circulatory and respiratory compromise. Location and intensity of the murmur should be noted and assessed for changes. A 12-day-old foal with persistent signs of PDA should be further evaluated and possibly treated. Echocardiography and radiography should be incorporated into the work-up so that the degree of heart failure may be observed.

18. Is there any way to close a PDA?

Treatment attempting closure of a PDA may include the use of prostaglandin inhibitors such as the nonsteroidal antiinflammatory drugs (NSAIDs). Flunixin meglumine has been used at a dose rate of 0.5–1.0 mg/kg IV every 24 hours for 3 days. Alternatively, ketoprofen has been used at a dose rate of 1.0 mg/kg IV every 24 hours. The putative mechanism of action in reducing PDA is alteration of eicosanoid balance in favor of the vasoconstrictor thromboxane at this site. Undesirable side effects include renal papillary necrosis, platelet dysfunction, and gastrointestinal ulceration. Since even normal foals are susceptible to gastric ulceration, it is wise to reserve NSAID therapy for foals over 7–8 days old and to provide concomitant ulcer prophylaxis. Recommended therapy includes the use of H2 receptor antagonists such as cimetidine, 8–18 mg/kg orally every 4–6 hours or ranitidine, 6.6 mg/kg orally every 8 hours, and mucosal protectants, such as sucralfate, 20 mg/kg orally every 6 hours.

19. How is aortic valvular insufficiency differentiated from mitral insufficiency?

Of the four heart valves, the aortic and mitral valves are most commonly affected by bacterial endocarditis, which may lead to valvular insufficiency. Differentiating which structure is affected may be facilitated by various means. Cardiac auscultation is a simple and straightforward method of assessing the nature of the dysfunction. Murmurs associated with aortic valvular insufficiency are best auscultated on the left side of the thorax at the fourth intercostal space just ventral to the level of the point of the shoulder. The murmur is usually diastolic and decrescendo in nature and may radiate ventrally. An insufficient mitral valve is associated with a holosystolic plateau murmur that may radiate dorsally, cranially, and caudally (see question 5). The murmur in this case is best heard over the left thorax at the fourth-to-fifth intercostal spaces just dorsal to the olecranon.

If valvular insufficiency has progressed to the point of inducing heart failure, one may appreciate EKG changes consistent with right atrial enlargement in the case of mitral regurgitation or right ventricular enlargement when the aortic valve is affected. Echocardiography, preferably with color flow Doppler, helps greatly in verifying presence and degree of valvular insufficiency.

Patteson M: Equine Cardiology. Oxford, Blackwell Science, 1996.

20. Which is more common in horses—congenital or acquired valvular heart disease?

Acquired valvular heart disease is more common than congenital valvular disease in horses. Congenital valvular heart disease is rarely observed in horses. In contrast, one study of horses at a slaughter house demonstrated that approximately 23% (356 of 1557) had acquired valvular heart disease.

Else RW, Holmes JR: Cardiac pathology in the horse. I: Gross pathology. Equine Vet J 4:1–8, 1972.

21. Which valves are more commonly involved in acquired valvular heart disease in horses?

The aortic valve is most commonly affected, closely followed by the mitral valve. Lesions also have been described affecting the tricuspid and pulmonary valves.

22. Which factors may contribute to the pathogenesis of acquired valvular heart disease?

Bacterial endocarditis is one form of acquired disease; the structures most commonly affected include the aortic and mitral valves. The tricuspid valve is less commonly affected, and the pulmonic valve is rarely affected. Degenerative changes also may occur, although such cases do not always result in valvular incompetence. Viral infections, inflammation, trauma, rupture of valve leaflets or chordae tendinae, neoplasia, and cardiac dilation may contribute to valvular damage and insufficiency.

23. A 10-year-old Quarter Horse gelding with a history of endotoxemia has a holosystolic, grade IV murmur, best appreciated over the aortic to mitral region of the thorax. What other findings support a diagnosis of bacterial endocarditis?

1. **Other signs and symptoms** supporting a diagnosis of bacterial endocarditis include recurrent fever, tachypnea, tachycardia, anorexia, and weight loss. Signs of disseminated sepsis include lameness (although it does not appear to be as common in horses with bacterial endocarditis as in cattle), joint distention, coughing, pneumonia, hematuria, pyuria, mastitis (rare), and occasionally neurologic signs. Embolic or metastatic disease may occur secondarily to the initial valvular nidus.

2. **Positive growth on blood cultures** may provide information about the causative organism as well as antimicrobials to which it is susceptible. The cultures are ideally drawn before antimicrobial therapy is initiated. A sample that is free from contamination is essential. Multiple (e.g., 3–5) cultures should be obtained over a 48-hour period. Both aerobic and anaerobic cultures should be requested. If fevers are cyclic, the likelihood of isolating an organism is optimized by collecting the sample 1 hour before predicted febrile episodes.

3. **Clinicopathologic changes** include anemia of chronic inflammation, leukocytosis, and hyperglobulinemia. Azotemia may be present in cases of septic emboli to the kidneys. EKG changes may include arrhythmias such as atrial fibrillation and premature ventricular contractions.

4. A **valvular mass** may be determined by echocardiographic evaluation. Echocardiography is invaluable in demonstrating valvular lesions, disturbances in flow, and heart failure. The B-mode sector scanner is usually superior to M-mode for detection and measurement of valvular masses. M-mode is superior for documentation of chamber enlargement. Doppler echocardiography is useful in assessing the severity of valvular regurgitation.

24. Which infectious agents contribute most often to the pathogenesis of bacterial endocarditis? Which antimicrobials are most efficacious for treatment?

Streptococcus species are the most commonly isolated agent in equine bacterial endocarditis. However, *Actinobacillus* species, *Serratia marcescens*, *Escherichia coli*, and *Pseudomonas* species has been less commonly identified. The best way to determine which antimicrobials are useful in individual cases of bacterial endocarditis is to perform blood cultures and then determine sensitivity patterns. While you are awaiting culture and sensitivity results or if bacteria do not grow but bacterial endocarditis is still suspected, broad-spectrum antimicrobial combinations may be used:

    1. Penicillin and ceftiofur (broad-spectrum coverage with strong gram-positive coverage). Some veterinarians prefer two beta-lactams.

    2. Penicillin and gentamicin (broad-spectrum coverage). Gentamicin may be nephrotoxic.

    3. Ceftiofur and gentamicin (broad-spectrum coverage with strong gram-negative coverage).

Penicillin is an appropriate antimicrobial selection in cases of suspected gram-positive involvement. Problems may occur with client compliance because of the difficulty of long-term (e.g., 4–15 weeks) intramuscular (IM) administration of procaine penicillin or ampicillin. If the client is able to maintain a long-term intravenous (IV) catheter, potassium penicillin or ampicillin may be used. (**Note:** Ampicillin may be given by the IM or IV routes). Another option is ceftiofur (Naxcel, Smith-Kline-Beecham, Philadelphia), a cephalosporin that is effective against many gram-negative bacteria and maintains a good level of activity against anaerobes and gram-positive bacteria. Disadvantages of Naxcel therapy include expense, anecdotal associations with diarrhea, and resistance by some *Streptococcus* species. A combination of penicillin and gentamicin provides broad-spectrum antimicrobial coverage, but gentamicin may cause renal tubular damage.

25. Myocarditis may result from a variety of insults. Name the five broad categories of etiologic agents, and give examples of each.

    1. **Bacteria:** *Streptococcus* species, especially *S. equi*, and *Staphylococcus aureus*

    2. **Viruses:** equine infectious anemia, equine viral arteritis, equine influenza, African horse sickness

    3. **Parasites:** *Strongylus vulgaris, Onchocerca* species

    4. **Toxins:** ionophores and cantharidin from the blister beetle (*Epicauta* species)

    5. **Deficiencies:** vitamin E, selenium

McGuirk SM, Shaftoe S, Lunn DP: Diseases of the cardiovascular system. In Smith BP (ed): Large Animal Internal Medicine. St. Louis, Mosby, 1990, pp 454–488.

26. A 15-year-old Thoroughbred mare with a history of strangles *(S. equi var. equi)* is febrile, tachycardic, and myalgic. Her complete blood count reveals leukocytosis with neutrophilia. Myocarditis is suspected. What clinical signs and pathologic findings should be expected if the mare does not respond to treatment and develops congestive heart failure?

Signs of congestive heart failure vary depending on which side of the heart is affected. When the right side of the heart is dysfunctional, the clinician may note ventral edema, edema of the extremities, and jugular distention with or without appreciable pulsation of the vein. If the left side of the heart is failing, one may note the presence of inspiratory crackles on lung auscultation, and the horse may have respiratory distress and a cough.

As a result of congestive liver failure, the biochemical profile may reveal a mild-to-moderate increase in hepatic enzymes (aspartate aminotransferase [AST], gamma glutamyl transferase [GGT], L-iditol dehydrogenase [L-iDH], alkaline phosphatase [AP]) as well as bilirubin. A decrease in blood urea nitrogen, glucose, and albumin may be present and represents the inability of the congested liver to carry out its functions (e.g., conversion of ammonia to urea, gluconeogenesis, and production of albumin).

Cardiac isoenzymes of creatinine kinase (CK-MB) and lactate dehydrogenase (LDH-1) are usually elevated in horses with acute myocarditis with or without concomitant heart failure. However, in horses with chronic myocardial damage these isoenzymes may be normal and thus not helpful in diagnosis. Arterial blood gas analysis may reveal a subnormal partial pressure of oxygen in arterial blood (PaO_2).

27. Which neoplasms are most likely to be involved in the rare cases of equine cardiac neoplasia?

The most common neoplasia involving the heart and pericardium is lymphoma. Other neoplasms that have been described include fibrosarcoma, adenocarcinoma, squamous cell carcinoma, mesothelioma, hemangiosarcoma, and an infiltrative cardiac lipoma.

28. How can the practitioner differentiate pleural from pericardial fluid accumulation solely on the basis of physical examination findings?

The key to distinguishing pleural from pericardial fluid accumulation lies in thoracic auscultation, especially if the horse can tolerate a rebreathing system (e.g., a plastic bag placed over the muzzle). In cases of pericardial effusion, heart sounds are muffled. When pleural effusion is present, the heart sounds are of normal intensity but radiate over a wider-than-normal region of the thorax. Lung auscultation also assists in differentiating the two conditions. A horse with pleural effusion has decreased or absent breath sound ventrally, whereas dorsal sounds are of normal intensity. Pericardial effusion may emulate this condition in that dorsal breath sounds may appear louder; however, ventral sounds are present in many cases. In some cases, pericarditis and pleuritis may occur concomitantly. The "washing machine murmur" characteristic of bovine pericarditis is not typical of equine pericarditis.

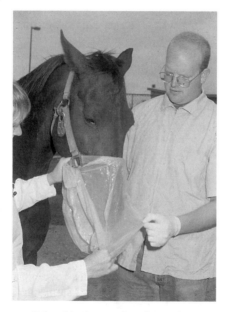

Rebreathing bag over horse's muzzle.

29. A 19-year-old Arabian gelding presents with fever, anorexia, depression, and weight loss. What findings on cardiac examination may lead to the suspicion of infective pericarditis? What EKG findings and clinicopathologic data support this diagnosis?

Cardiac auscultation is likely to reveal the presence of muffled heart sounds. A pericardial friction rub occasionally may be auscultated in the presence of small amounts of fluid and significant pericardial inflammation. When fluid accumulation restricts ventricular filling, stroke volume is decreased and signs of decompensation may become apparent. Such signs include congestion and cyanosis of the mucous membranes, prolongation of the capillary refill time, and jugular venous distention/pulsation. The peripheral arterial pulses are diminished in strength and amplitude because the difference between systolic and diastolic pressures is less than normal. The degree of cardiac decompensation and therefore clinical signs depend on the acuity of the pericardial effusion. Since the pericardium is somewhat elastic, it stretches in response to slow accumulation of pericardial fluid. In cases of rapid accumulation, the pericardial sac is not able to alleviate increasing pressures through compensatory stretching; therefore, clinical signs may be more apparent.

Although cases of pericarditis are not necessarily accompanied by EKG changes, characteristic findings often include a decrease in the QRS amplitude and ST-segment elevation. Electrical alternans, an altered configuration of P-, QRS-, and T-waves occurring consistently throughout the tracing, also may be observed.

Clinicopathologic data may support clinical findings. Examples include an inflammatory leukogram, hyperfibrinoginemia, and hyperglobulinemia.

Patteson M: Equine Cardiology. Oxford, Blackwell Science, 1996.

30. What are the six broad categories of potential causes of pericarditis?

1. Hematogenous infection
2. Extension of infection from pleura or lung
3. Viral infection (equine viral arteritis, equine influenza)
4. Neoplasia (rare)
5. Idiopathic disease (aseptic inflammation, frequently diagnosed in horses)
6. External wounds (especially penetrating)

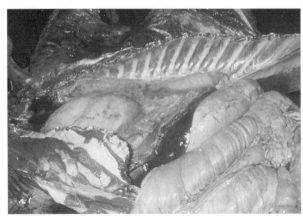

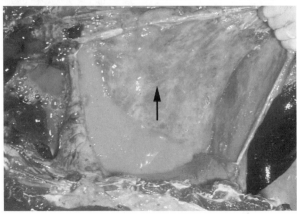

Thoracic cavity *(top)* and heart *(bottom)* from a horse with traumatic pericarditis after suspected penetration of a foreign body into the thorax via a wound in the left pectoral region. Note thickened pericardium *(arrow)*.

31. Why is pericardiocentesis useful in horses with pericarditis? How is it performed? How can one minimize the associated risks?

Pericardiocentesis helps to evaluate pericardial fluid, thus providing a better estimation of etiology and prognosis. A region in the left fifth intercostal space, approximately 5 cm above the olecranon, should be prepared in a sterile fashion. The skin and intercostal muscle are infiltrated with local anesthetic. The catheter (e.g., Argyle catheter or Abbocath) should be advanced along the cranial portion of the rib to avoid the intercostal vessels and nerves coursing along the caudal rib border. Ideally and commonly, pericardiocentesis is performed under ultrasonographic guidance so that the risk of penetrating the myocardium is decreased. In addition, this modality helps to identify and target specific structures. Risk also can be minimized by running a continuous EKG during the procedure so that arrhythmias can be detected and quickly addressed.

32. How is infectious pericarditis differentiated from other causes of pericarditis?

If echogenic fluid or fibrin is visualized on echocardiography, an infectious or inflammatory process is assumed. Highly echogenic regions with shadowing suggestive of gas accumulation should arouse the suspicion of anaerobic bacteria. Pericardiocentesis aids in both diagnosis and treatment. Cytologic examination as well as culture and sensitivity testing should be performed on the pericardial fluid. Horses with congestive heart failure may have a small amount of clear (e.g., hypoechoic) fluid that does not inhibit ventricular filling; attempts at drainage are contraindicated in such cases. Clinicopathologic data also help to determine the cause. Presence of an inflammatory leukogram, hyperfibrinoginemia, and hyperglobulinemia is consistent with an infectious process.

33. How is infectious pericarditis treated?

Antimicrobial selection is ideally based on culture and sensitivity testing of the pericardial fluid; however, broad-spectrum coverage is commonly used when pericardiocentesis was not performed. If the presence of anaerobic bacteria is suspected, metronidazole is often one of the drugs of choice. It is important to define the therapeutic regimen and prognosis to the owner before initiation of treatment. Antimicrobial therapy often must be carried out for 3–15 weeks, resulting in significant expense and effort. Anecdotal evidence suggests that pericardiocentesis with lavage (0.9% sterile saline) and subsequent instillation of antimicrobials may be helpful. No controlled data support this approach. If lavage is performed, it is prudent to have continuous EKG evaluation of the heart.

Patteson M: Equine Cardiology. Oxford, Blackwell Science, 1996.

34. What are the two major causes of acute hemorrhage into the pericardial sac? How do they differ in clinical signs and prognosis?

Acute hemorrhage into the pericardial space may occur with aortic ring rupture and pulmonary artery rupture. (**Note:** A coagulopathy also may cause pericardial hemorrhage.) Aortic ring rupture is invariably fatal and usually occurs in a stallion during the act of breeding at the beginning of the breeding season. There is no known association with copper deficiency in affected stallions (vs. pigs with copper deficiency and elastin deterioration). Pulmonary artery rupture has occurred rarely in stallions in the early breeding season, with signs of cardiac tamponade immediately after breeding. Affected horses may present with a history of acute colic. Patients with rupture of the pulmonary artery can survive, although they require stabilization and subsequent removal of the serous fluid via pericardiocentesis once the hemorrhage has subsided (e.g., 12 hours later if possible). Echocardiography is not likely to demonstrate the area of rupture, although it is certainly helpful in defining the extent and nature of the existing fluid as well as guiding the performance of pericardiocentesis.

35. Are equine patients more or less likely to have cardiac dysrhythmias than other domestic species? Why?

Horses are more prone to cardiac dysrhythmias than other domestic species. The reason is thought to be related to the larger heart size and therefore more extensive myocardial circuit, which allows a higher rate of reentry phenomena. High vagal tone in equine patients predisposes them to benign arrhythmias, primarily atrioventricular blocks, that disappear with exercise, excitement, or administration of a parasympatholytic agent (e.g., atropine, 0.02 mg/kg subcutaneously).

36. Identify the arrhythmias in the EKG tracings shown below.

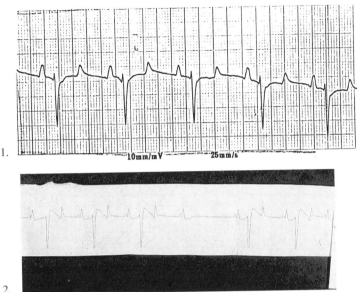

Answers: 1. Normal sinus rhythm; there is no arrhythmia. 2. Second-degree atrioventricular block, Mobitz type II. This tracing shows a consistent, normal PR interval with regularly dropped QRS complexes. Like the Mobitz type I (which is characterized by a progressively longer PR interval until a QRS complex is completely dropped [e.g., no QRS follows the P-wave]), this arrhythmia is usually benign; however, if the condition persists with a heart rate > 50 or if syncope occurs concomitantly, atrioventricular nodal disease should be considered.

Patteson M: Equine Cardiology. Oxford, Blackwell Science, 1996.

Reimer JM: Cardiac arrhythmias. In Robinson NE (ed): Current Therapy in Equine Medicine, 3rd ed. Philadelphia, W.B. Saunders, 1992, pp 383–393.

37. What is the most common pathologic dysrhythmia is horses? What auscultatory findings support the diagnosis?

Atrial fibrillation is the most common, clinically significant (and pathologic) arrhythmia in horses. It usually occurs without evidence of underlying cardiac disease, especially in racehorses. The many putative causes include heat, sweating losses, electrolyte imbalances, and possible predisposition in the Standardbred breed. Atrial fibrillation also may result from atrial disease, as in horses with atrial dilation in congestive heart failure.

Diagnosis can be established fairly reliably with auscultation alone, although EKG confirmation is ideal. The heart sounds are often of variable intensity, and the rhythm is irregularly irregular. S4 is not auscultable. In cases of atrial fibrillation with no underlying cardiac disease, the resting heart rate is usually normal. Tachycardia with rates > 60 beats per minute and murmurs (> grade III–V mitral or tricuspid insufficiency) are poor prognosticators, because they indicate primary cardiac disease. Such horses are notoriously difficult to convert to normal sinus rhythm.

38. What are the most prominent features of the EKG in cases of atrial fibrillation?

The EKG tracing is characterized by many fibrillation waves (f-waves) between QRS complexes. The f-waves are not associated with subsequent QRS complexes, as are P-waves in normal sinus rhythm. P-waves are absent because of the lack of coordinated atrial contraction. R-R intervals are irregular. QRS complexes usually appear normal; in horses with underlying cardiac disease, however, chamber enlargement due to congestive heart failure may be represented as a variation in normal QRS complex morphology. The resting ventricular rate is typically normal in the absence of underlying cardiac pathology.

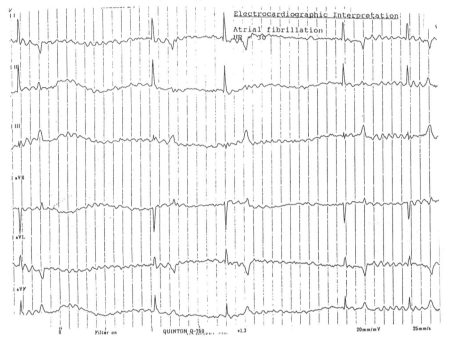

EKG from a horse with atrial fibrillation.

39. Outline a treatment plan for the three following equine patients diagnosed with atrial fibrillation.

1. A 1000-lb (450-kg) 15-year-old Quarter Horse broodmare with no evidence of cardiac disease or poor performance and a heart rate of 40 bpm.

The horse is not asked to perform athletically and is not symptomatic. The normal resting heart rate suggests that cardiac output is probably sufficient (whereas with a heart rate of 80 bpm, for example, the time between beats is probably insufficient to allow adequate ventricular filling). The owner may elect not to treat the mare, because the atrial fibrillation does not prevent her from carrying a foal to term and is unaccompanied by syncope or signs of congestive heart failure. If decompensation occurs or the mare becomes symptomatic, quinidine conversion may be indicated.

2. An 1100-lb (500-kg) 2-year-old Standardbred gelding that raced poorly 3 days ago.

Factors such as heat, electrolyte imbalances, and breed (Standardbred) are thought to be contributors to the development of atrial fibrillation. Since the gelding is unable to maximize his athletic capabilities and since the dysrhythmia is probably acute in onset and therefore more responsive to attempts at conversion, it is prudent to attempt conversion with quinidine.

3. An 1100-lb (500-kg) Saddlebred stallion in early congestive heart failure.

The practitioner must address both atrial fibrillation and congestive heart failure. Digoxin is the drug of choice for treating heart failure in horses. Quinidine reduces renal excretion of digoxin, thus enhancing the likelihood of toxicity. It is possible to monitor both medications by ensuring that blood levels are within therapeutic range. Horses in atrial fibrillation with concomitant congestive heart failure ideally should be digitalized first, although this regimen is not without risk of digoxin toxicity. One should initiate digoxin therapy at a dose of 0.01 mg/kg orally 2 times/day for 3 days, then start the quinidine conversion regimen. The EKG should be monitored carefully for QRS prolongation, supraventricular dysrhythmias (> 100 bpm), and ventricular rhythms. Some equine patients require digoxin therapy for the remainder of their lives.

40. What type of drug is quinidine? Describe two different treatment regimens.

Quinidine is a sodium channel blocker that is a positive chronotrope (i.e., increases heart rate) and a negative inotrope (i.e., decreases contractility of the heart and therefore stroke volume). EKG monitoring should be in place during administration. Quinidine sulfate (oral formulation) may be given as a test dose (4 mg/kg; e.g., 2.0 gm per 500-kg horse) via the nasogastric tube approximately 12–24 hours before the conversion attempt to test for allergic reaction to quinidine. The nasogastric tube should be placed (e.g., indwelling) before commencement of conversion. The quinidine sulfate then is given at a dose rate of 20–22 mg/kg (e.g., 10–11 gm per dose for a 500-kg horse). Additional 10–11-gm boluses are given every 1–2 hours until (1) conversion occurs, (2) a maximal total dosage of 60–66 gm is achieved, or (3) signs of toxicity are noted. An alternative is an intravenous protocol using quinidine gluconate. Bolus injections of 1.0–1.5 mg/kg are administered every 10–15 minutes until a total dose of 1.8–5.8 mg/kg is achieved.

41. It is important to educate owners about potential side effects of quinidine before attempting conversion of a horse in atrial fibrillation. What are they?

Administration of quinidine is associated with numerous idiosyncratic and toxic side effects, including urticaria, laminitis, nasal edema with or without respiratory distress, ataxia, soft feces/diarrhea, depression, nervousness, anorexia, atrioventricular block, and severe hypotension. The idiosyncratic reactions such as urticaria, nasal mucosal edema, and ataxia can be minimized by administering a test dose (4 mg/kg quinidine sulfate) before initiation of therapy. However, sudden death may occur even after the administration of a test dose. The toxic effects of quinidine can be decreased by clinical vigilance as well as EKG monitoring for QRS prolongation (> 25% of the original [preconversion] QRS width). Frequent and thorough physical examinations during therapy are prudent, and therapeutic monitoring of plasma quinidine concentrations is recommended (therapeutic: 0.5–3.0 μg/ml of plasma).

42. By what mode of action does digoxin exert its effect? What are the indications for its use?

Digoxin, a cardiac glycoside, inhibits membrane-bound sodium-potassium-adenosine triphosphatase, which acts to increase intracellular sodium, thus inhibiting calcium transport out of the cell via the sodium-calcium exchange. The increased calcium concentration enhances sarcomere contractility, thereby exerting a positive inotropic effect. Digoxin exerts both direct and indirect effects on the electrical conduction system of the heart. Digoxin works directly by shortening the duration of the action potential. In the atria, this effect is manifested by a shortened refractory period and inhibition of sinoatrial node automaticity. In the atrioventricular node, the refractory period is increased and conduction velocity is inhibited. Effects on the ventricles and Purkinje system include inhibition of conduction velocity and promotion of abnormal automaticity. Indirect effects on the cardiac conduction system include a parasympathomimetic influence on the autonomic nervous system. As a result, the atrial refractory period is reduced, and the atrioventricular refractory period is increased. Atrioventricular node conduction velocity is suppressed.

Digoxin enhances cardiac output in cases of congestive heart failure. The net electrical effect of digoxin is to slow the ventricular response in cases of supraventricular arrhythmias. Atrial fibrillation does not convert to sinus rhythm with digoxin, but the reduced ventricular rate and increased myocardial contractility may result in a diminution of clinical signs due to congestive heart failure.

Katzung BG, Parmley WW: Cardiac glycosides and other drugs used in congestive heart failure. In Basic and Clinical Pharmacology, 5th ed. Norwalk, CT, Appleton & Lange, 1992, pp 176–189.

43. Why must the practitioner be especially alert to the development of digoxin toxicity when it is administered with quinidine?

Quinidine decreases renal excretion of digoxin. Simultaneous administration of both drugs greatly increases the risk of digoxin toxicity.

44. What are signs of digoxin toxicity? What level of digoxin is acceptable in the plasma?

Signs of digoxin intoxication include an increase in the P-R interval, atrioventricular block, and prolongation of the QRS complex. Digoxin toxicity also may be manifested by various arrhythmias; the most common include sinus bradycardia, ventricular premature depolarizations, ventricular tachycardia, and ventricular fibrillation. Other manifestations of digoxin toxicity include obtunded mentation, inappetance, and diarrhea.

To minimize the unpleasant and potentially fatal effects of digoxin, regular monitoring of serum digoxin levels should be included in the therapeutic regimen. The dosage should be altered as needed to maintain levels between 0.5–2.0 ng/ml of plasma.

Katzung BG, Parmley WW: Cardiac glycosides and other drugs used in congestive heart failure. In Basic and Clinical Pharmacology, 5th ed. Norwalk, CT, Appleton & Lange, 1992, pp 176–189.

45. How can beats originating from the ventricles be differentiated from beats arising from a supraventricular focus?

Premature supraventricular beats, whether of atrial, sinoatrial, or junctional origin, are generally similar in QRS configuration to the normal sinus rhythm complexes, although they may appear tall and narrow. In contrast, QRS complexes originating from a ventricular focus are often tall and wide. Supraventricular foci produce a complex of normal duration (< 0.14 seconds). Beats with a ventricular focus often produce T-waves that are wider and of higher amplitude than normal; these T-waves are often of opposite polarity to the preceding QRS complex.

When a beat originating in the ventricles is conducted, the subsequent P-wave does not elicit a QRS because the ventricles are still refractory from the premature ventricular complex (PVC). The R-R interval from the PVC to the next normally conducted sinus beat is subsequently prolonged; this phenomenon is termed a compensatory pause. A premature atrial contraction is rarely followed by a compensatory pause. Although an EKG should be incorporated into the work-up to ensure an accurate diagnosis, the compensatory pause is a useful method by which to estimate focus by auscultation alone.

Patteson M: Equine Cardiology. Oxford, Blackwell Science, 1996.

46. How can one recognize whether the ventricular ectopic beat originates from the right or left side of the heart?

In general, ventricular ectopic beats originating from the right side go upward first, whereas those originating from the left go downward first.

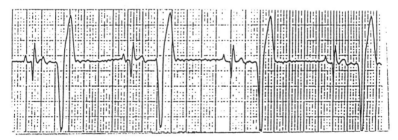

Ventricular ectopic beat originating from the left side.

47. What risk factors are associated with increased incidence of jugular venous thrombosis and thrombophlebitis?

Whenever the tunica intima is compromised, risk for thrombosis and thrombophlebitis is augmented. Insertion of intravenous catheters and administration of intravenous medications are the most clinically relevant procedures associated with increased risk for thrombosis and throm-bophlebitis. Multiple venous punctures and stiffer catheters (e.g., Teflon) are also contributory factors as well as long-term maintenance of any intravenous catheter. Etiologic factors contribut-ing to thrombophlebitis include catheter and injection contamination, movement of skin flora from the catheter through the puncture site, and hematogenous spread of microbes from a distant site of origin. Without concomitant intimal disruption, coagulopathies (e.g., disseminated in-travascular coagulopathy [DIC]) may cause thrombosis. Endotoxemia, vasculitis, and sepsis are conditions that may favor this process. Certain drugs promote jugular venous thrombosis when injected intravenously. One study demonstrated that 10% guaifenesin was thrombogenic in 100% of the 7 horses tested.

Bayly WM, Reed SM: Equine Internal Medicine. Philadelphia, W.B. Saunders, 1998.

Donawick WJ, Gardner SY: Jugular vein thrombosis. In Robinson NE (ed): Current Therapy in Equine Medicine, 3rd ed. Philadelphia, W.B. Saunders, 1992, pp 406–408.

Herschl MA, Mahaffey EA, Trim CM: Effects of 5% and 10% guaifenesin infusion on equine vascular endothelium. Vet Surg 21:494–497, 1992.

48. How are catheter materials ranked according to thrombogenicity?

Polypropylene (most thrombogenic), Teflon (polytetrafluoroethylene), silicon, rubber, nylon, polyvinylchloride, and polyurethane (least thrombogenic). Polyurethane catheters should be used if the catheter is to remain in the horse for longer than 12–48 hours. Examples of polyurethane catheters used in horses are Mila catheter (Mila International, Covington, KY 41011), Arrow catheter (Arrow International, Reading, PA 19610), and Jorgansen catheter (Jorvet, Loveland, CO 80538).

49. What clinical signs and pathologic data are associated with septic thrombophlebitis?

Horses with septic thrombophlebitis display heat, swelling, and tenderness over the affected area. There also may be a palpable corded vein with slow fill when the vein is held off. If jugular venous thrombosis is present, facial venous distention is sometimes seen. If sepsis is present, the patient may demonstrate signs of inappetance, fever, and depression as well as injected mucous membranes and prolonged capillary refill time.

A complete blood count, especially in cases of sepsis, often reveals neutrophilic leukocytosis with hyperfibrinoginemia. If septic thrombi have migrated to other organs, such as the liver or kidneys, elevations in organ-specific parameters may be noted.

Donawick WJ, Gardner SY: Jugular vein thrombosis. In Robinson NE (ed): Current Therapy in Equine Medicine, 3rd ed. Philadelphia, W.B. Saunders, 1992, pp 406–408.

50. What are the current treatments for jugular venous thrombosis?

Intravenous catheters should be removed from the affected jugular vein, and alternative sites used for venipuncture. The contralateral jugular vein should not be used. Local treatment of the affected vein may include topical application of a thin layer of dimethyl sulfoxide (DMSO) with subsequent application of hot packs.

NSAIDs also may be used. Such a strategy may include flunixin meglumine (0.5 mg/kg orally every 12 hours) or phenylbutazone (2 mg/kg orally every 12–24 hours). It is prudent to limit treatment to the acute inflammatory phase so that adverse effects are minimized. Compromised, septic animals should be evaluated carefully before treatment, because dehydra-tion may exacerbate the renal papillary necrosis potentially associated with NSAIDs.

Selection of antimicrobial therapy is best based on culture and sensitivity results, of either a catheter tip or blood. If this information is unavailable when treatment is deemed necessary, a broad-spectrum antimicrobial regimen should be instituted. If the practitioner suspects that anaer-obes are causative, as when hyperechoic gas pockets are visualized with ultrasonographic eval-uation, metronidazole (15 mg/kg orally every 6 hours) should be part of the therapeutic regimen.

When the affected portion of vein acts as a nidus and promotes persistent sepsis or toxemia, surgical resection of the vein should be considered.

Bayly WM, Reed SM: Equine Internal Medicine. Philadelphia, W.B. Saunders, 1998.

51. What should you tell an owner about the long-term implications of jugular venous thrombosis?

A simple thrombosis without phlebitis is likely to recanalize without long-term deleterious effects. In cases of septic thrombophlebitis, prolonged antimicrobial therapy may be indicated. Whereas some markedly affected veins may resume patency, others may exhibit stenosis secondary to fibrosis. However, collateral circulation develops over time, often alleviating clinical signs.

Donawick WJ, Gardner SY: Jugular vein thrombosis. In Robinson NE (ed): Current Therapy in Equine Medicine, 3rd ed. Philadelphia, W.B. Saunders, 1992, pp 406–408.

Patteson M: Equine Cardiology. Oxford, Blackwell Science, 1996.

52. A 2-year-old Quarter Horse colt presents with hindlimb lameness and stiffness that are exacerbated by work. What historical and physical findings support a diagnosis of aortic-iliac thrombosis? What methods can be used to define the presence and extent of the lesion?

Young male horses in work are most commonly presented for this problem. They may be asymptomatic with rest or minimal exertion, but signs recur during strenuous exercise. Affected animals exhibit stiffness in the hindlimbs and, in cases of increased severity, may knuckle over onto the dorsal surface of the fetlock. If the animal has been in work, physical signs may have abated with development of collateral circulation. The signs of aortic-iliac thrombosis are most prominent after the animal has been rested, when collateral circulation is likely to regress. Animals suffering from aortic-iliac thrombosis may kick out or stamp their hindleg(s).

On palpation of the extremities, one should note that the affected leg or legs are cool and devoid of distal peripheral pulses. The saphenous veins may have a prolonged fill time. Occasionally, one may note atrophy of the muscles of the hindquarters. On palpation of the distal aorta and branches of the iliac arteries by rectal examination, one may note an exceptionally prominent aortic pulse cranial to the obstruction with transfer of waves along the walls of the obstructed vessel, as opposed to abrupt cessation of palpable pulses caudal to the obstruction. Other supportive findings on rectal examination include indurated, enlarged iliac arteries and/or iliac arteries that are asymmetric in size and pulse quality. Two stallions with aortic-iliac thrombosis have been described with ejaculatory failure.

If the practitioner wishes to confirm the presence or define the extent of an aortic-iliac thrombosis, ultrasonography per rectum or angiography may be helpful.

Maxie MG, Physick-Sheard PW: Peripheral vascular disease. In Robinson NE (ed): Current Therapy in Equine Medicine, 2nd ed. Philadelphia, W.B. Saunders, 1987, pp 173–176.

McDonnell SM, Love CC, Martin BB, et al: Ejaculatory failure associated with aortic-iliac thrombosis in two stallions. J Am Vet Med Assoc 7:954–957, 1992.

Reef VB, Roby KAW, Richardson DW, et al: Use of ultrasonography for the detection of aortic-iliac thrombosis in horses. J Am Vet Med Assoc 190:286–288, 1987.

53. How does the cardiovascular system of a normal horse respond to exercise?

Changes associated with exercise are a direct result of enhanced sympathetic output and diminished parasympathetic effects as well as species-specific adaptations of the equine cardiovascular system. Horses have a tremendous cardiac reserve; they are able to increase cardiac output significantly as physiologic needs dictate. This capacity explains the low resting heart rate of the equine patient compared with other species of similar size.

Exercise stimulates the sympathetic nervous system. Red blood cells are mobilized from the spleen and liver, thus enhancing oxygen-carrying capacity of the blood. In addition, organs such as the liver, spleen, gastrointestinal tract, and urogenital system experience a decrease in blood flow due to local vasoconstrictive effects, whereas the musculoskeletal system, nervous system, skin, and thoracic organs have enhanced flow through local vasodilatory effects.

Stroke volume and therefore cardiac output are also enhanced by increased myocardial contractility. The average horse in work enhances contractility by 20–30% of resting performance, whereas the equine athlete may reach a degree of contractility that is 50% of resting levels. Exercise-induced increases in heart rate also contribute to an overall increase in cardiac output. Rates of 7 times the normal resting heart rate have been noted during maximal physical exertion.

The practitioner must realize, however, that maximal heart rates do not allow ideal ventricular filling times; thus, exercise-induced tachycardia may be detrimental to cardiac output.

Patteson M: Equine Cardiology. Oxford, Blackwell Science, 1996.

Littlejohn A: Exercise-related cardiovascular problems. In Robinson NE (ed): Current Therapy in Equine Medicine, vol. 2. Philadelphia, W.B. Saunders, 1987, pp 176–180.

54. What factors contribute to the development of exercise-induced cardiac arrhythmias?

Supraventricular tachycardia, atrial tachycardia, atrial fibrillation, premature ventricular complexes, ventricular tachycardia, and ventricular fibrillation may occur with exercise. Substantial evidence suggests that myocardial hypoxia is the underlying cause of exercise-induced cardiac arrhythmias. Altered myocardial microvasculature and fibrotic degeneration have been identified in tissues from horses suffering from exercise-induced arrhythmias. Since these lesions were not present in normal horses, myocardial hypoxia may contribute to the development of such changes. Any preexisting pathology that inhibits oxygenation of tissues also may contribute to exercise-induced arrhythmias. Anemia and pulmonary disease are two examples.

Littlejohn A: Exercise-related cardiovascular problems. In Robinson NE (ed): Current Therapy in Equine Medicine, vol. 2. Philadelphia, W.B. Saunders, 1987, pp 176–180.

55. Ionophores are antimicrobial compounds used as coccidiostats and growth promotants in cattle. Horses are highly sensitive to the toxic effects of these compounds, even in small doses. Describe the pathogenesis, clinical signs, pathologic data, postmortem findings, and treatment of ionophore toxicity in horses.

Ionophores such as monensin, lasalocid, and salinomycin exert their toxic effect by incorporating cations (e.g., sodium and potassium ions) into the lipid-soluble complexes that they form. These cation-containing structures are carried across cell membranes, and physiologic ionic gradients of microbial cell units are subsequently disturbed. The resulting disruption in cellular function also may occur in host (e.g., mammalian) cells but usually at higher concentrations. However, ionophores are extremely toxic to horses; therefore, concentrations that are safe in poultry, pigs, and cattle are markedly toxic to horses.

Clinical signs of ionophore toxicity include inappetance, abdominal pain, sweating, tetraparesis, tetraplegia, ataxia, conscious propioceptive deficits, myopathy, myocarditis, and cardiac dysrhythmias. Sudden death may be the only pertinent historical finding and warrants questions about the nutritional history of the horse. For example, were any feeds for food animals fed to the horse, or did a new shipment of feed arrive? The second question is pertinent because an equine feed may have been manufactured directly after a food animal feed containing high levels of ionophores.

Signs consistent with hemolysis may be present, including hemoglobinuria and hyperbilirubinemia. Azotemia, diminished urine concentrating ability, and hematuria reflect renal compromise. Muscle damage may result in myoglobinuria as well as elevations in creatinine kinase (CK), lactate dehydrogenase (LDH), and aspartate aminotransferase (AST). Liver enzymes also may be increased. Serum concentrations of potassium and calcium may be low, especially acutely. However, if renal failure occurs, the potassium concentration may increase.

Gross lesions are often not appreciated on postmortem examination. The ventricular myocardium may have visible areas of pallor. Pericardial and epicardial hemorrhages may be present. Occasionally necrotic foci may be seen in the renal cortex and skeletal muscle.

Histologic examination of tissues from affected animals may reveal tubular nephritis and hepatitis. Microscopic lesions consistent with diffuse myocarditis are the primary cardiac abnormalities. Mitochondrial swelling and vacuolar degeneration may be noted on histologic examination of myocardial cells.

Treatment is supportive; no antidote currently exists. If the practitioner knows or suspects that ingestion was recent, gastric lavage and/or administration of mineral oil or activated charcoal via nasogastric tube may be undertaken in hope of removing feed containing ionophores or inhibiting ionophore absorption, respectively. Intravenous fluid therapy assists in reversal of dehydration and maintenance of perfusion of vital organs as well as correction of any electrolyte abnormalities. If the horse survives the acute period after intoxication, rest and appropriate supportive care should be continued for several months. It may be wise to suggest an echocardiographic evaluation before a person rides the horse.

George L: Localization and differentiation of neurologic disease. In Smith BP (ed): Large Animal Internal Medicine. St. Louis, Mosby, 1990, p 167.

Hodgson DR: Diseases of muscle. In Smith BP (ed): Large Animal Internal Medicine. St. Louis, Mosby, 1990, p 1351.

BIBLIOGRAPHY

1. Bayly WM, Reed SM: Equine Internal Medicine. Philadelphia, W.B. Saunders, 1998.
2. Boon JA: The echocardiographic examination. In Boon JA (ed): Manual of Veterinary Echocardiography. Baltimore, Williams & Wilkins, 1998, pp 35–150.
3. Donawick WJ, Gardner SY: Jugular vein thrombosis. In Robinson NE (ed): Current Therapy in Equine Medicine, 3rd ed. Philadelphia, W.B. Saunders, 1992, pp 406–408.
4. Else RW, Holmes JR: Cardiac pathology in the horse. I: Gross pathology. Equine Vet J 4:1–8, 1972.
5. George L: Localization and differentiation of neurologic disease. In Smith BP (ed): Large Animal Internal Medicine. St. Louis, Mosby, 1990, p 167.
6. Herschl MA, Mahaffey EA, Trim CM: Effects of 5% and 10% guaifenesin infusion on equine vascular endothelium. Vet Surg 21:494–497, 1992.
7. Hodgson DR: Diseases of muscle. In Smith BP (ed): Large Animal Internal Medicine. St. Louis, Mosby, 1990, p 1351.
8. Katzung BG, Parmley WW: Cardiac glycosides and other drugs used in congestive heart failure. In Basic and Clinical Pharmacology, 5th ed. Norwalk, CT, Appleton & Lange, 1992, pp 176–189.
9. Littlejohn A: Exercise-related cardiovascular problems. In Robinson NE (ed): Current Therapy in Equine Medicine, vol. 2. Philadelphia, W.B. Saunders, 1987, pp 176–180.
10. Long KJ, Bonagura JD, Darke PGG: Standardized imaging technique for guided M-mode and Doppler echocardiography in the horse. Equine Vet J 24:226–235, 1992.
11. Maxie MG, Physick-Sheard PW: Peripheral vascular disease. In Robinson NE (ed): Current Therapy in Equine Medicine, 2nd ed. Philadelphia, W.B. Saunders, 1987, pp 173–176.
12. McDonnell SM, Love CC, Martin BB, et al: Ejaculatory failure associated with aortic-iliac thrombosis in two stallions. J Am Vet Med Assoc 7:954–957, 1992.
13. McGuirk SM, Shaftoe S, Lunn DP: Diseases of the cardiovascular system. In Smith BP (ed): Large Animal Internal Medicine. St. Louis, Mosby, 1990, pp 454–488.
14. Patteson M: Equine Cardiology. Oxford, Blackwell Science, 1996.
15. Reef VB, Roby KAW, Richardson DW, et al: Use of ultrasonography for the detection of aortic-iliac thrombosis in horses. J Am Vet Med Assoc 190:286–288, 1987.
16. Reimer JM: Cardiac arrhythmias. In Robinson NE (ed): Current Therapy in Equine Medicine, 3rd ed. Philadelphia, W.B. Saunders, 1992, pp 383–393.

9. RESPIRATORY SYSTEM

Corinne R. Sweeney, D.V.M., Dip. ACVIM,
and Laura K. Reilly, V.M.D., Dip. ACVIM

1. Why is the horse considered an obligate nasal breather?

The caudal free edge of the soft palate forms a tight seal around the base of the larynx. This seal is broken only during swallowing and coughing and in certain disease conditions. Since the horse does not have the ability to breathe through the mouth, obstructions of the upper airway have the potential to reduce airflow significantly.

2. What is the cause of laryngeal hemiplegia?

Most cases of laryngeal hemiplegia involve damage to the left recurrent laryngeal nerve (RLN) and are idiopathic. In idiopathic laryngeal hemiplegia (ILH), a distal axonopathy of the RLN results in neurogenic atrophy of all intrinsic muscles of the larynx except the cricothyroideus muscle. ILH is most common in large-breed horses, and some evidence suggests that it is a heritable condition. Sporadic cases of left- or right-sided laryngeal hemiplegia may result from trauma or iatrogenic perivascular irritation (the RLN courses with the carotid artery and vagosympathetic trunk in the ventral neck), guttural pouch mycosis, retropharyngeal abscess, neoplasia, and organophosphate and lead toxicity. When right-sided laryngeal hemiplegia is detected in young horses, it is most commonly due to a congenital developmental abnormality of the arytenoid and/or thyroid cartilages.

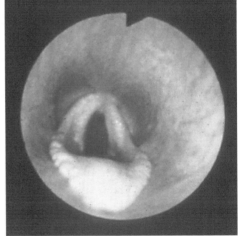

Endoscopic view of idiopathic laryngeal hemiplegia.

3. How does ILH cause respiratory dysfunction?

A normal horse accommodates increased negative inspiratory pressure during exercise by dilation of the larynx. The RLN innervates the major abductor of the arytenoid cartilages, the cricoarytenoideus dorsalis muscle, as well as the adductors—the arytenoideus transversus, cricoarytenoideus lateralis, ventricularis, and vocalis muscles. Damage to the RLN results in neurogenic atrophy of these muscles and reduced abduction of the arytenoid cartilage during inspiration. Consequently, the horse cannot dilate the rima glottis appropriately, and the arytenoid obstructs the airway during inhalation. Inadequate abduction results in an increased resistance to airflow during exercise.

4. How is ILH diagnosed?

ILH should be suspected in horses with a history of an abnormal inspiratory noise during exercise, possibly accompanied by exercise intolerance. The noise is usually characterized as "whistling" or "roaring." Palpation of the dorsal larynx reveals a prominent muscular process of the arytenoid cartilage due to atrophy of the cricoarytenoideus dorsalis muscle. The diagnosis is confirmed with endoscopic examination and visualization of the asymmetric position of the arytenoid cartilages during inspiration or after swallowing. A grading system is frequently used to assess the severity of the disease:

Grade I	Synchronous symmetric full abduction and adduction of both arytenoid cartilages.
Grade II	Asynchronous movement of the left arytenoid cartilage, but full abduction can be induced by swallowing or nasal occlusion.
Grade III	Asynchronous movement of the left arytenoid; full abduction of the left arytenoid cartilage cannot be induced by swallowing or nasal occlusion.
Grade IV	Marked asymmetry of the arytenoid cartilages at rest and lack of substantial movement of the left arytenoid during any phase of respiration.

5. Which horses are candidates for surgical correction of ILH? What surgical options are available?

Since horses with ILH almost never improve spontaneously, surgical correction is indicated when exercise intolerance or abnormal inspiratory noise can be attributed to laryngeal dysfunction. Exercising endoscopy (i.e., treadmill endoscopy) is useful in determining the degree of compromise, but as a rule grade IV horses and grade III horses that are unable to abduct fully the arytenoid cartilages during exercise are most likely to benefit from surgery. Grade I and grade II horses are able to abduct fully the arytenoid cartilages during exercise.

The most commonly performed surgery is the laryngoplasty, in which a prosthesis ("tieback") is placed to maintain abduction of the affected arytenoid cartilage. Ventriculectomy may be performed in conjunction with a laryngoplasty; when performed alone, it is ineffective at maintaining arytenoid abduction.

6. What is the cause of sinusitis?

Sinusitis is classified as primary or secondary. Primary sinusitis is a result of bacterial infection of the upper respiratory tract. *Streptococcus* species are the most common bacterial isolates. Secondary sinusitis is usually the result of dental disease; the upper first molar is most commonly involved. It also may be due to sinus masses and trauma. Secondary sinusitis is uncommon in horses less than 5 years old.

7. What are the clinical signs of sinusitis?

Unilateral, mucopurulent nasal discharge is the most common clinical sign because the nasomaxillary opening is rostral to the end of the nasal septum. In sinusitis secondary to dental disease or with involvement of anaerobic bacteria for any reason, the discharge may have a foul odor. In chronic cases, deformation of the bone overlying the sinuses or exophthalmos may be observed. Airflow from the nares may be asymmetric when bone deformation is present. Percussion of the affected sinus may produce discomfort or a dull sound.

8. How is sinusitis diagnosed?

The presence of typical clinical signs should arouse suspicion of sinusitis. Sinus percussion with the tongue of the horse held in the hand (to enhance resonance) should be performed to ascertain whether a dull sound can be heard or discomfort is elicited. Endoscopy is used to rule out other abnormalities (including abnormalities of the guttural pouches) and to evaluate whether discharge can be observed in the middle meatus near the nasomaxillary opening. Skull radiographs may show an increased opacity and/or fluid lines in the affected sinus and also may assist in the diagnosis of dental disease.

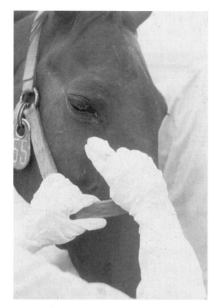

Right, Percussion of maxillary sinus.
Bottom Left, Outline of frontal sinus.
Bottom Right, Outline of frontal (◇) and maxillary sinuses (⊟).

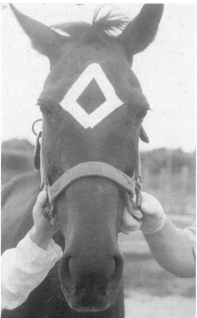

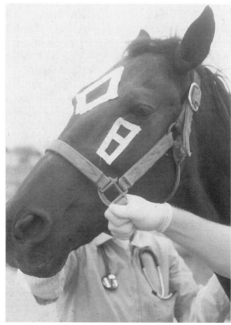

9. What are the indications and landmarks for sinus paracentesis?

Sinus centesis can be used for both diagnosis and treatment of sinusitis. Culture and cytology of a sinus aspirate aid in confirmation of the cause (whether there is primary or secondary bacterial infection). Sinoscopy may be performed for further characterization of sinus abnormalities. If infectious sinusitis is present, repeated lavage of the sinus is therapeutic.

Sinus centesis is performed using a Steinmann pin after aseptic preparation of the site and local block. The rostral maxillary sinus is entered at a site 2–3 cm dorsal to the facial crest and

2–3 cm caudal to the infraorbital foramen. The site for the caudal maxillary sinus is 2–3 cm dorsal to the facial crest and 2–3 cm rostral to the medial canthus. The frontal sinus, which communicates with the caudal maxillary sinus, is entered either at a site midway between the dorsal midline and medial canthus of the eye or on a dorsal midline 1–3 cm caudal to the medial canthus of the eye.

10. Describe the endoscopic anatomy of the guttural pouches.

The guttural pouches are diverticula of the auditory tubes of domestic animals; their function has not been determined. The pharyngeal orifice of the guttural pouch may be entered with the aid of a stylet passed through the endoscope. Each pouch is divided into a large medial compartment and a smaller lateral compartment by the stylohyoid bone. The external carotid artery (maxillary artery) and external maxillary vein course through the lateral compartment along with the pharyngeal branch of the vagus nerve, cranial laryngeal nerve, CN VII, and the mandibular branch of CN V. The internal carotid artery and cranial nerves IX (glossopharyngeal) and XII (hypoglossal) can be seen clearly in the medial compartment. Cranial nerves X (vagus) and XI (accessory) and the pharyngeal branch of cranial nerve X also course under the medial compartment and sometimes can be visualized endoscopically.

11. What are the clinical signs of guttural pouch mycosis (GPM)?

The clinical signs vary according to the structures affected by the fungal plaque. Fungal plaques are most commonly observed in the dorsal wall of the medial compartment of the guttural pouch, overlying the internal carotid artery. They also may be observed in the lateral compartment associated with the external carotid artery. Before the onset of frank hemorrhage, some owners have noted a unilateral mucopurulent discharge that sometimes becomes serosanguinous or sanguinopurulent. Erosion of major vessels causes intermittent severe epistaxis, which ultimately may be fatal. If nervous structures are involved, corneal ulceration secondary to keratoconjunctivitis sicca, dysphagia, facial nerve paresis, laryngeal paresis, or Horner's syndrome may be observed. GPM is usually unilateral. Its pathogenesis is not known, although *Aspergillus* species are most commonly cultured. Bilateral epistaxis can be seen if (1) the septum has been eroded and blood from one side can enter the other guttural pouch; (2) the hemorrhage is profuse; or (3) both left and right guttural pouches have mycotic lesions. (**Note:** The editor has seen one horse with true bilateral GPM.)

12. What is the recommended treatment for GPM?

Aspergillus species are the fungi isolated most frequently from fungal plaques in the guttural pouch. Topical or systemic antifungal treatment, although potentially effective, generally requires several weeks for resolution of the lesions, and the risk for fatal hemorrhage during this time is great. A recent approach involves instillation of 50–100 ml of enilconazole (diluted to a 1% solution) into the affected pouch once or twice daily; however, no controlled data prove regression of fungus. Therefore, surgical treatment is preferred before high-volume lavage. The recommended procedure is to occlude the affected artery (identified by endoscopy) both proximal and distal to the lesion. This technique prevents hemorrhage and also usually leads to resolution of the fungal lesions. Horses with neurologic deficits have a guarded prognosis for recovery of function.

13. Describe the cause and treatment of guttural pouch empyema.

Guttural pouch empyema is either an extension of a bacterial upper respiratory infection or the result of rupture and drainage of an infected retropharyngeal lymph node directly into the pouch. The most common clinical sign, unilateral nasal discharge, is similar to sinusitis; thus endoscopy or radiographs are necessary to confirm the diagnosis. Treatment involves lavage of the affected pouch(es), occasionally aided by systemic antimicrobials. In chronic cases, inspissated materials known as chondroids accumulate in the pouches and may require removal via endoscopic snare and lavage or surgery.

14. What is the cause of dorsal displacement of the soft palate (DDSP)?

Intermittent DDSP is an exercise-induced elevation of the soft palate. The cause has not been defined, but theories include inflammation of the larynx and/ or pharynx, inflammation of the pharyngeal branch of the vagus nerve, excessive flexion of the head, swallowing during exercise, hypoplastic epiglottis, caudal retraction of the larynx, and retraction of the tongue. Persistent DDSP is usually neurogenic and associated with GPM, equine protozoal myeloencephalitis (EPM), or botulism. Affected animals are usually dysphagic.

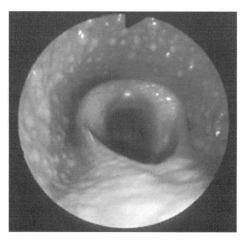

Endoscopic view of dorsal displacement of the soft palate.

15. What are the clinical signs of DDSP?

The elevation of the soft palate reduces the size of the airway and results in exercise intolerance and a gurgling or choking noise, which is usually louder during expiration. Most horses are normal at rest unless DDSP is neurogenic and accompanied by other nerve dysfunction such as dysphagia. DDSP should be suspected with a history of exercise intolerance and a gurgling noise and can be confirmed by endoscopy. To increase the chances of visualization of significant DDSP, endoscopy should be performed (1) at rest with 60 seconds of nasal occlusion, (2) during exercise (i.e., treadmill endoscopy), or (3) immediately after exercise.

16. How does the endoscopic appearance of DDSP differ from epiglottic entrapment?

With epiglottic entrapment, the outline of the epiglottis is visible but the normal distinct margins and vascular pattern are not visible because of elevation of the aryepiglottic fold over the epiglottis. In cases of DDSP, the epiglottis is completely obscured from view and the caudal margin of the soft palate is easily visualized.

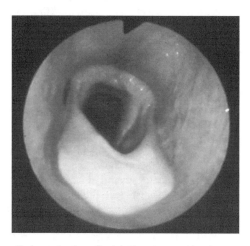

Endoscopic view of epiglottic entrapment in a horse.

17. What is an ethmoid hematoma?

Ethmoid hematoma is a progressively enlarging vascular mass that originates from the ethmoid turbinates. It may be unilateral or bilateral and in some cases extends caudally into the frontal sinus; therefore, it is not readily apparent on endoscopic evaluation. It is seen most frequently in mature horses. The main clinical sign is intermittent unilateral mild epistaxis, although mucopurulent discharge also may be seen. The mass behaves like a tumor but is not neoplastic, and the cause is unknown. In most cases the disease may be diagnosed by endoscopy.

18. What are the treatment and prognosis for ethmoid hematoma?

Traditionally the treatment has been surgical excision. Severe hemorrhage frequently accompanies this procedure, and blood transfusion may be necessary. Recently, however, 4% formaldehyde has been injected into ethmoid hematomas, using a guarded endoscopy needle and the endoscope, with some success. About 20–50% of ethmoid hematomas recur.

19. What are the most common equine respiratory viral diseases? How may they be differentiated?

Influenza and equine herpes virus (EHV) are the most important respiratory viruses in horses. The most important strains of influenza are A/equine 1 and A/equine 2. Two herpes viruses, EHV1 and EHV4, cause significant respiratory disease. The clinical signs of influenza, EHV1, and EHV4 are similar and do not generally provide a means to diagnose the specific virus. Usually affected horses have fever, depression, anorexia, cough, and serous nasal discharge. The diagnosis can be confirmed by virus isolation or an enzyme-linked immunosorbent assay (Directogen) for influenza antigen performed on nasopharyngeal swabs or by serology. Horses infected with equine arteritis virus (EAV) may show similar respiratory symptoms accompanied by conjunctivitis and vasculitis. Virus isolation and serology should be performed to confirm the diagnosis.

20. What clinical syndromes are associated with equine herpes viruses?

Both EHV1 and EHV4 cause similar respiratory disease; however, EHV1 also may cause abortions, neurologic disease (equine herpes myeloencephalitis), and fatal infections in neonatal foals. EHV4 has been associated only with respiratory disease and is considered a more important respiratory pathogen than EHV1. EHV2 and EHV5 are found in normal horses and described as equine cytomegaloviruses. Their role as pathogens has not been determined. EHV3 causes equine coital exanthema.

21. How does a viral respiratory infection predispose to bacterial pneumonia?

Viruses invade and replicate in the ciliated endothelial cells that line the upper airways. Necrosis of the endothelial cells leads to impairment of mucociliary clearance and reduced clearance of bacteria and debris from the lower respiratory tract.

22. Define "strangles."

Strangles is a bacterial infection caused by *Streptococcus equi* subspecies *equi*. Infection is achieved by contact with purulent material from infected horses. *S. equi* is not a normal resident of the equine respiratory tract. Clinical signs include fever, anorexia, depression, mucopurulent nasal discharge, submandibular and retropharyngeal lymph node enlargement, and in some cases dysphagia. Lymph node suppuration develops, and typically the horse recovers uneventfully after rupture of the abscessed lymph nodes. The entire course of disease in an uncomplicated case is about 3 weeks. Diagnosis is based on the clinical signs and culture of the nasopharynx, draining lymph nodes, or sometimes guttural pouches. The name "strangles" refers to the respiratory obstruction due to severe lymph node enlargement that occurs in some cases.

23. What is the recommended treatment for strangles?

The treatment regimen is controversial and depends on the stage and severity of the infection. First, all affected horses should be isolated from other horses, because *S. equi* subspecies *equi* is contagious. If the horse has early clinical signs but no lymph node abscessation, procaine penicillin G may be administered at a dose of 22,000 IU/kg intramuscularly twice daily for 3–10 days. On the other hand, if a lymph node abscess is present, the recommendation is to withhold antimicrobials and to encourage maturation of the abscess by hot packing. If antimicrobials are used in such cases, they may actually prolong the course of the disease. Horses that are severely ill or have developed complications should be treated with antimicrobials even if abscesses are present.

24. What complications may be seen with strangles?

Most horses recover uneventfully from strangles, but numerous complications have been reported. Internal abscessation (metastatic or "bastard" strangles) may involve any lymph node and can be particularly difficult to diagnose and treat. Purpura hemorrhagica, an immune complex reaction to the streptococcal antigen, results in fever, depression, marked edema of the limbs and ventrum, and, in some cases, petechiae. Corticosteroids are used in addition to penicillin to treat purpura hemorrhagica. Guttural pouch empyema is seen relatively frequently. Other reported complications include septicemia, dyspnea secondary to retropharyngeal abscessation, laryngeal hemiplegia, endocarditis, myocarditis, and suppurative bronchopneumonia.

25. What is the significance of pharyngeal lymphoid hyperplasia (PLH)?

PLH is a common endoscopic finding in horses less than 5 years of age. Numerous small follicles are observed in the dorsal and lateral walls of the pharynx. PLH is believed to represent the response of lymphoid tissue to antigens of viruses, bacteria, and allergens. The role of PLH in poor performance has been debated, but it is generally believed to have no effect on performance.

26. What are the most common causes of pleural effusion in horses?

Most pleural effusions reported in horses are secondary to bacterial pleuropneumonia or thoracic neoplasia. Pleural effusion may occur in any horse with pleuropneumonia; it is not restricted to severe cases. Lymphoma is the most common neoplasia of the thorax in horses. Pleural effusion has been reported with many thoracic neoplasms including lymphoma, adenocarcinoma, squamous cell carcinoma, hemangiosarcoma, and pleural mesothelioma.

27. What does thoracic ultrasound detect in abnormal horses?

Pleural fluid can be seen as a separation of the lung from parietal pleura by an anechoic space (black). Fibrin strands can be seen frequently in horses with pleuropneumonia. They appear as "fronds" (relatively echogenic) waving in the anechoic pleural fluid. Lung consolidation in cases of pneumonia presents as hyperechoic lung with multifocal areas of aeration. Atelectasis, which is compression of the ventral lung margins, is frequently seen with marked pleural effusions. Abscessation, pleural thickening, and pleural adhesions also may be seen. Thoracic ultrasound also allows characterization of a pleural effusion. Pneumothorax can be diagnosed ultrasonographically but requires an experienced examiner.

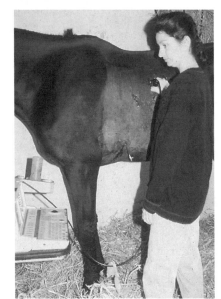

Ultrasound examination of the equine chest.

28. Describe the difference between a tracheal aspirate and a bronchoalveolar lavage. How are they collected?

A **tracheal aspirate** collects cells in the distal trachea. A tracheal aspirate is collected by infusing a small volume (< 50 cc) of saline into the trachea, allowing it to mix with tracheal secretions, and then retrieving it by aspiration. A tracheal aspirate can be collected via percutaneous puncture of the trachea or endoscopically.

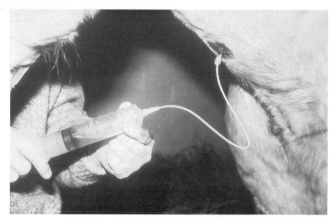

Percutaneouos tracheal aspirate.

A **bronchoalveolar lavage** (BAL) collects cells located in the segmental and subsegmental bronchi. A BAL is collected by infusing a large volume (> 200 ml) of saline into a segmental bronchus and then aspirating to collect the infused saline mixed with the epithelial lining fluid. A BAL can be collected by wedging a long cuffed tube or endoscope into a segmental bronchus.

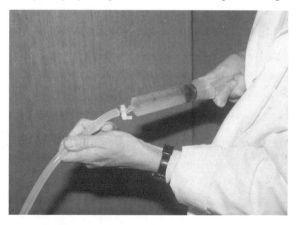

Aspiration of fluid from a BAL tube.

29. How does one collect pleural fluid for examination?

Thoracocentesis is the technique for removal of pleural fluid for analyses. This procedure is performed in the standing position after local anesthetic infiltration and possible chemical sedation. Thoracic ultrasound may help to detect a specific area for thoracocentesis. Without ultrasound guidance, the preferred site for thoracocentesis is the right seventh intercostal space just dorsal to the palpable costochrondral junction or the left eighth intercostal space approximately 5 cm above the point of the elbow. Thoracocentesis may have both diagnostic and therapeutic value.

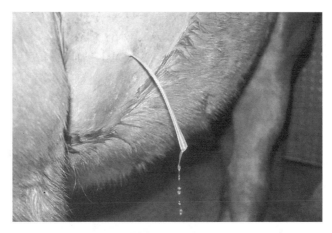

Thoracocentesis.

30. What are the normal cellular contents of pleural fluid?

Pleural fluid from healthy horses may contain up to 10,000 enucleated cells/μl and 3.5 gm/dl of protein. Most horses have less than 5000 enucleated cells/μl and less than 2.5 gm/dl of protein.

31. What are the two basic types of pleural effusions?

A pleural effusion represents an increase in fluid in the pleural space. The two basic categories are transudative and exudative. A transudative effusion is classically associated with volume overload states, such as congestive heart failure. An exudative effusion is a protein-rich effusion secondary to inflammation or failure of lymphatic protein removal. Exudative effusion occurs with infection and neoplasms.

32. What findings on physical examination are suggestive of pleural effusion?

Small effusions frequently elicit minimal clinical findings. Larger effusions, however, demonstrate dullness to percussion and diminished breath sounds of the ventral lung field. As the effusion increases with concomitant atelectasis, physical examination findings reveal either a complete absence of sounds in the ventral lung fields or loud bronchial breath sounds. With chronicity, substernal edema develops. Cardiac sounds are not muffled (unless pericardial effusion is also present) but may radiate over a larger region than normal.

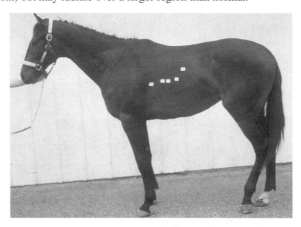

Horse with taped marking of boundaries of pleural effusion.

33. In what group of horses is pleuropneumonia most commonly seen?

Although pleuropneumonia may occur in any horse at any age, the young racehorse or competitive horse that is transported a long distance is at greatest risk. Pleuropneumonia is an extension of the infectious process from the lung into the pleural cavity. Any condition predisposing a horse to develop pneumonia predisposes the horse to develop pleuropneumonia.

34. What are the most likely etiologic agents in horses with pleuropneumonia?

Since pleuropneumonia is an extension of primary pneumonia, the common pathogens for pneumonia are most often responsible for pleuropneumonia, including gram-positive organisms such as *Streptococcus* species and gram-negative organisms such as *Pasteurella* species and *E. coli*. Anaerobic organisms frequently identified in horses with pleuropneumonia include *Bacteroides* and *Clostridium* species.

35. How is pleuropneumonia diagnosed?

Pleuropneumonia should be suspected from the physical examination findings in a horse with respiratory signs, including increased respiratory rate, decreased lung sounds ventrally, pleuritic pain (pleurodynia, which is only sometimes present), substernal edema (if chronic), and abducted elbows (usually if pleurodynia is present). Breath sounds may be absent or decreased in the ventral thorax. Only large airway sounds with no normal bronchovesicular sounds may be heard. Normal-to-loud airway sounds may be heard dorsally. Pleural friction rubs may be present. Thoracic percussion may indicate the presence of pleural fluid by dullness of the ventral aspect of the thorax. Thoracic ultrasound determines the presence and approximate volume of the pleural effusion and helps to characterize it (i.e., cellular, acellular, fibrin tags/adhesions, "gas echoes"). Thoracic ultrasound also allows examination of the underlying lung that is the source of the infection. Thoracocentesis allows collection of pleural fluid for further cytologic and microbiologic examination. As described earlier, however, most cases of pleuropneumonia originate in the pulmonary parenchyma; thus, tracheal aspirate cytology with culture and sensitivity testing is usually rewarding.

36. What is the treatment of pleuropneumonia?

Four major modalities need to be considered in treatment: antimicrobial therapy, pleural fluid drainage, analgesics, and nursing care. The most important aspect of treatment is antimicrobial therapy. The antibiotic may be selected on the basis of culture of bacteria from the tracheal aspirate and pleural fluid. Frequently both gram-positive and gram-negative aerobic and anaerobic bacteria are present. A typical treatment may include a penicillin, an aminoglycoside, and metronidazole to broaden coverage for anaerobes. Pleural fluid can be drained using intermittent thoracocentesis or by placing indwelling chest tubes with a one-way valve attached. Pleural lavage may be used in selective cases to help remove fibrin. Thoracotomy with or without rib resection permits removal of organized fibrin from the pleural space. Pain relief and efforts to address the horse's comfort and long-term nutritional needs are important because of the chronic nature of the disease.

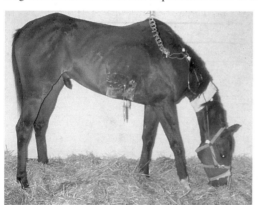

Horse with pleuropneumonia (indwelling argyle catheters with Heimlich valves).

37. What are the common clinical signs of chronic obstructive pulmonary disease (COPD)?
COPD is a complex syndrome with clinical signs ranging from exercise intolerance in the performance horse to expiratory dyspnea, chronic purulent nasal discharge, cough, and weight loss in chronic cases. Other clinical signs include increased respiratory rate, flared nostrils, exaggerated abdominal expiration, heave line, and wheezes and crackles heard on thoracic auscultation. Expiratory wheezes are the most characteristic abnormal sound. If emphysema is present, the field of auscultation may appear larger.

38. What are the common pathologic findings in a horse with COPD?
The main lesion of COPD is bronchiolitis characterized by diffuse epithelial hyperplasia, mucus plugging of airways, and neutrophilic, lymphocytic, and plasmacytic infiltrates. Lesions commonly extend into the peribronchial tissues, and peribronchial fibrosis is also present. Chronic bronchiolitis is the most consistent histologic abnormality in COPD.

39. What are the pathophysiologic changes in a horse with COPD?
Horses affected with COPD generally have increased airway resistance and decreased dynamic compliance. These changes are compatible with diffuse lower airway obstruction. Plugging of the airways with mucus cellular debris and exudate contributes to the airway obstruction. Airway obstruction is also caused by airway smooth muscle contraction. Airway hyperresponsiveness also may contribute to obstruction and clinical signs.

40. Describe the treatment of COPD.
1. Reduce the horse's exposure to the offending agent, most often air-borne dust and molds. Management and change of the environment (i.e., bedding, feed, ventilation) are paramount to successful therapy.
2. Pharmacologic intervention may be necessary, including antiinflammatory agents, bronchodilators, and mucolytics. Antiinflammatory drugs primarily affect the delayed response in bronchial hyperactivity. Systemically administered corticosteroids most commonly used are prednisolone and dexamethasone. Bronchodilators may include drugs from three groups: (1) muscarinic receptor antagonists (i.e., parasympatholytics); (2) β_2-adrenoceptor agonists (i.e., sympathomimetics); and (3) methylxanthine derivatives. Mucokinetic drugs increase the transport of airway secretions by differing mechanisms; agents to consider in horses include clenbuterol, albuterol, bromhexine, dembrexine, and theophylline. Corticosteroids (e.g., beclomethasone) and bronchodilators (e.g., albuterol, ipratropium bromide) also may be administered by metered-dose inhalation using the Aeromask (Canadian Monaghan, London, Ontario, Canada).

41. What is the most common tumor in the thorax of horses?
Thoracic lymphoma is the most common neoplasm of the thorax. Equine lymphoma occurs in mediastinal, alimentary, generalized, and cutaneous forms. Combinations of one or more of these presentations are not infrequent.

42. What are the most common clinical features among horses with thoracic lymphoma?
Weight loss, ventral edema, dyspnea, pleural effusion, and distention of jugular veins often are seen in horses with thoracic lymphoma.

43. What are the most common primary pulmonary tumors reported in horses?
Granular cell tumor (myoblastoma), a neoplasm of mesenchymal origin, is the most frequently reported primary pulmonary tumor in horses. The granular cell tumor may invade from the pulmonary parenchyma into the bronchi and sometimes can be visualized endoscopically as a tracheal (bronchial) mass. Other primary pulmonary tumors reported in horses include lymphoma, bronchial myxoma, pulmonary carcinoma, pulmonary chondrosarcoma, pleural mesothelioma, and thymoma.

44. What are other frequently reported metastatic thoracic neoplasia?

Lymphoma, adenocarcinoma, squamous cell carcinoma, and hemangiosarcoma have been frequently reported to metastasize to the thorax. The primary neoplasia site, although often unknown, may include organs such as kidney, uterus, ovary, stomach, and muscle.

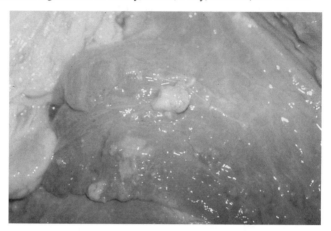

Metastatic squamous cell carcinoma.

45. What is the incidence of exercise-induced pulmonary hemorrhage (EIPH) in race-horses?

Data from large surveys performed in a number of areas around the world indicate that EIPH occurs in virtually all horses racing at speed, although the degree of hemorrhage may vary. In most cases, horses do not demonstrate epistaxis; instead, blood may be present in the trachea. If it is present in sufficient volume, it moves into the pharynx and is swallowed.

46. How is EIPH diagnosed?

Blood at the nares, seen during or after strenuous exercise, is highly suggestive of EIPH. Documentation that the blood originated from the lungs requires endoscopic examination. In most horses without gross evidence of hemorrhage at the nares, endoscopic examination carried out 30–60 minutes after exercise reveals blood in the trachea and large bronchi. Cytologic examination of tracheal aspirates or bronchoalveolar lavage samples reveals hemosiderophages (macrophages containing hemosiderin). These cells can be identified in samples obtained for many weeks after the incident of hemorrhage. After an acute episode of hemorrhage, a lateral radiograph of the dorsal caudal lung region may reveal an increased bronchointerstitial pattern or localized radioopacity. Radiographic exam is not considered a pathognomonic means of diagnosis.

47. What is the cause of EIPH?

The cause of EIPH is not known with certainty. Accumulating evidence suggests that EIPH is caused by mechanical failure of the walls of the pulmonary capillaries when internal pressure rises to a very high level. The pulmonary vascular pressures of galloping horses reach extremely high levels. Thus, to some extent EIPH is an inevitable consequence of the extremely high cardiac output required by athletes.

48. What is the source of the infection for foals with *Rhodococcus equi* pneumonia?

R. equi is a gram-positive, pleomorphic, facultative, intracellular, obligate aerobic bacterium that lives in feces and soils and is resistant to most chemical and environmental conditions. The organism is found in the intestines of many normal mammals, including horses. Horses are most often infected by inhalation of the organism from the soil or feces of animals, but ingestion and umbilical entry are also possible.

49. What typical radiographic changes are seen with *R. equi* infection?

A prominent interstitial pattern may be seen in acutely or less severely affected foals. However, in more severely affected foals (especially with chronic changes), a prominent alveolar pattern with ill-defined regional consolidation is commonly seen. Nodular lung lesions, especially solitary lesions, and lymphadenopathy are almost pathognomonic in foals. Lesions may become cavitary.

50. What is the recommended treatment for *R. equi* pneumonia?

Successful treatment of *R. equi* pneumonia has been difficult because of the intracellular position of the organism. Recommended treatment is the combination of erythromycin and rifampin. Erythromycin is a macrolide antimicrobial that concentrates in phagocytes and is effective against *R. equi*. It is absorbed orally. Erythromycin causes gastrointestinal irritation and has been responsible for mild-to-severe diarrhea and colic in some foals. The recommended dose is at 25–30 mg/kg of estolate paste orally 4 times/day. Erythromycin phosphate or stearate is dosed at 37 mg/kg orally twice daily. Rifampin is synergistic with erythromycin and penetrates macrophages, neutrophils, and caseous material readily. The dose for rifampin is 5 mg/kg orally twice daily. Rifampin should not be used alone, because resistance may develop rapidly.

51. What is the most common cause of fungal pneumonia in a horse?

Mycotic pneumonia in horses occurs rarely, but when present is due to opportunistic fungi such as *Aspergillus* species. Most cases of fungal pneumonia occur secondarily in a horse with a severe primary disease, particularly enterocolitis. Clinicians must be careful in attributing significance to the presence of fungal elements in a tracheal aspirate or isolation of a fungus from these samples. Fungal hyphae often present either free or in large mononuclear cells in tracheal aspirates from healthy horses or in horses with other respiratory disease (e.g., COPD) due to decreased clearance mechanisms. To be significant, cytologically the fungal elements should be in large numbers and be involved in the inflammatory process within the lung.

52. What is the cause of bronchointerstitial pneumonia and acute respiratory distress in foals several months old?

The cause is unknown. It appears to be a reaction of the lung to a number of insults that result in autodestructive inflammation.

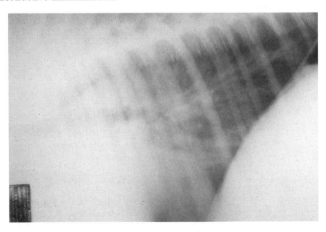

Foal with radiographic evidence of bronchointerstitial pneumonia.

53. What pathologic changes are seen with bronchointerstitial pneumonia and acute respiratory distress in foals several months old?

Histologic changes include severe, diffuse necrotizing bronchiolitis; alveolar septal necrosis; filling of alveolar spaces with mononuclear cells, neutrophils, and other cells; and epitheloid-like cells enmeshed in eosinophilic proteinaceous or fibrinoid material suggestive of hyaline membrane formation; congestion; and edema of interstitium. If the condition is more chronic, interstitial fibrosis may be present.

54. What is the recommended treatment for bronchointerstitial pneumonia and acute respiratory distress in foals several months old?

The cause of bronchointerstitial pneumonia is multifactorial and not known. Thus, treatment needs to address many areas. Oxygen therapy and attention to external thermoregulation are important. Corticosteroids, both parenteral and inhaled, should be considered. Dimethyl sulfoxide and other nonsteroidal antiinflammatory agents are commonly used. Antimicrobial agents should have a broad spectrum. Other possible treatments are antiulcer medication and bronchodilators.

BIBLIOGRAPHY

 1. Ainsworth D, Biller D: Respiratory system. In Reed S, Bayly W (eds): Equine Internal Medicine. Philadelphia, W.B. Saunders, 1998, pp 251–289.
 2. Beech J (ed): Equine Respiratory Disorders. Philadelphia, Lea & Febiger, 1991.
 3. Derksen FJ: Chronic obstructive pulmonary disease. In Beech J (ed): Equine Respiratory Disorders. Philadelphia, Lea & Febiger, 1991, pp 223–235.
 4. Lane JG: Larynx. Traub-Dargatz JL, Brown CM (eds): Equine Endoscopy, 2nd ed. St. Louis, Mosby, 1997, pp 74–96.
 5. Lavoie JP: The respiratory system. In Robinson NE (ed): Current Therapy in Equine Medicine, vol. 4. Philadelphia, W.B. Saunders, 1997, pp 401–465.
 6. Mair TS, Sweeney CR: The investigation of pleural effusion in the horse. Equine Vet Educ 4(2):70–74, 1992.
 7. Rakestraw PC, Hackett RP, Ducharme NG, et al: Arytenoid cartilage movement in resting and exercising horses. Vet Surg 20:122, 1991.
 8. Sweeney CR: Causes of pleural effusion in the horse. Equine Vet Educ 4(2):75–77, 1992.
 9. Sweeney CR: Diseases of the respiratory system. In Smith B (ed): Large Animal Internal Medicine. St. Louis, Mosby, 1996, pp 550–619.
10. Sweeney CR, Benson CE, Whitlock RH, et al: *Streptococcus equi* infection in horses. Part II. Compend Contin Educ 9:689–693, 1987.
11. Sweeney CR, Benson CE, Whitlock RH, et al: *Streptococcus equi* infection in horses. Part II. Compend Contin Educ 9:845–851, 1987.
12. Sweeney CR, Maxson AD: Equine pleuropneumonia: The value of thoracic ultrasongraphy in diagnosis and management. Equine Vet Educ 7(6):330–333, 1995.
13. Wilson WD, Lakritz J: Bronchointerstitial pneumonia and acute respiratory disease. In Robinson NE (ed): Current Therapy in Equine Medicine, vol. 4. Philadelphia, W.B. Saunders, 1997, pp 612–619.

10. GASTROENTEROLOGY

Scott M. Austin, M.S., D.V.M., Dip. ACVIM

MOUTH AND ORAL CAVITY

1. Describe the clinical signs associated with dental disease in the horse.

Clinical Signs of Dental Disease

DENTAL PAIN	ALTERED BEHAVIOR	CHANGE IN GENERAL HEALTH
Quidding	Abnormal head carriage	Unthriftiness
Slow eating or reluctance to eat	Playing with bit	Weight loss
Increased salivation	Resisting the bit	Chronic unilateral nasal discharge
Chewing on one side of mouth only	Head tossing at work	Recurrent colic
Pocketing of feed	Head shyness	Recurrent esophageal obstruction
Halitosis	Change in attitude	(choke)

2. List the eruption times for the permanent teeth of the horse. Why is this information important?

Eruption Times for Permanent Teeth of the Horse

TOOTH	ERUPTION
First incisor	2.5 yr
Second incisor	3.5 yr
Third incisor	4.5 yr
Canine	4–6 yr
First premolar (Wolf tooth)	5–6 mo
Second premolar	2.5 yr
Third premolar	3 yr
Fourth premolar	4 yr
First molar	9-12 mo
Second molar	2 yr
Third molar	3.5–4 yr

The eruption times and wear patterns of permanent incisors are useful to approximate the age of the horse. Veterinarians are frequently asked to render an opinion about the compatibility of the estimated age with the reported age of a horse. Estimated age is also valuable in examining a horse with dental problems; there is some correlation between the age of the horse and the type of problems that may be encountered. The third and fourth premolars have the greatest chance of becoming impacted because of the eruption sequence.

3. Describe how to differentiate between "eruption bumps" and periapical abscessation of the teeth.

While the permanent teeth are erupting, many young horses develop symmetric, nonpainful swellings on the ventral margin of the mandible that are called eruption bumps. These bumps are normal and disappear after the tooth has completely erupted.

Differentiating Features of Eruption Bumps vs. Periapical Abscessation

SIGN	ERUPTION BUMPS	APICAL ABSCESS
Age	1.5–4 yr	Varies
Symmetry	Occur in pairs	Asymmetric, singular
Pain	No	Yes
Draining tracts	Not usually	Common
Radiography	Eruption cyst	Loss of lamina dura dentes
Nasal discharge	No	Yes

4. Where do enamel points develop on the teeth of a horse?

The equid tooth has a long crown and a short root. The majority of the crown is held in reserve and erupts as the tooth is worn. The top jaw is 30% wider than the bottom jaw; therefore, as tooth wear occurs, sharp enamel points form on the outside of the upper arcade and inside of the lower arcade.

5. List the differential diagnoses for increased salivation (ptyalism).

In evaluating a horse with increased salivation, it is essential to differentiate increased production of saliva from failure to swallow saliva (dysphagia). A common cause of ptyalism is ingestion of legumes infected with the mold *Rhizoctonia leguminicola*, which produces the mycotoxin, slaframine. Slaframine causes a syndrome, referred to as "slobbers," that resolves once the offending feed is removed from the diet. Other causes of increased salivation include vesicular stomatitis, mechanical irritation from grass awns or bristle grass, nonsteroidal antiinflammatory drug (NSAID) toxicosis, uremia, blister beetle toxicosis (*Cantharidin* toxin), and migration of *Gasterophilus* or *Habronema* species through tissues of the mouth. Increased salivation also has been observed in some older horses that mouth the bit.

6. What causes cleft palate in a foal? How is it diagnosed and treated?

Cleft palate is caused by failure of the transverse palatal folds to fuse in the roof of the oral cavity and may be an inherited defect. Affected foals demonstrate nasal regurgitation of milk soon after birth, dysphagia, coughing, failure to grow normally, and aspiration pneumonia. The diagnosis is confirmed by visualization of the defect following oral examination or after endoscopy. Surgical repair of the defect is the only method of treatment. Owners should be apprised of the possible hereditary nature of cleft palate and made aware of the complications encountered after repair—aspiration pneumonia and dehiscence of the repair. Minor clefts may occur in the soft palate. They may go unrecognized for substantial periods and be diagnosed coincidentally.

DISEASES OF THE ESOPHAGUS

7. List the risk factors for esophageal obstruction (choke).

Inadequate mastication of food due to poor dentition is one of the most common risk factors for esophageal obstruction. Horses that gulp their food may choke because of insufficient saliva lubrication during swallowing. Occasionally, horses may ingest foreign bodies, such as corn cobs, persimmons, apples, carrots, or bedding, that result in esophageal obstruction. Other risk factors for choke include feeding too soon after sedation or general anesthesia, exhaustion, dehydration, and preexisting esophageal disease. Esophageal abnormalities that increase the risk for choke include strictures, external compression, and esophageal diverticula.

8. What is the typical presentation of a horse with esophageal obstruction?

Clinical signs have an acute onset and may be first recognized while the horse is eating. Owners may describe frequent, ineffectual attempts at swallowing characterized by nasal regurgitation of feed and saliva followed by complete refusal to eat. Other signs include coughing during attempts to swallow, increased salivation, anxiety, periodic stretching of the neck, and retching motions. In some horses, external enlargement of the esophagus may be visible.

9. Describe the management of a horse with choke.

Esophageal obstruction should be regarded as an emergency. Treatment begins upon the veterinarian's first contact with the owner. The owner should be instructed to remove feed and water until the veterinarian arrives; if the horse is trying to eat bedding material, bedding should be removed or the horse should be muzzled. After physical examination, a stomach tube should be passed to confirm the site of the obstruction. Administration of xylazine hydrochloride (1.1 mg/kg/IV) is recommended because it improves patient compliance, relaxes esophageal spasms, and lowers the head, thus decreasing the likelihood of aspiration pneumonia. Often gentle pressure on the stomach tube relieves the obstruction. Forceful attempts to relieve the choke should be avoided because of the potential for esophageal damage, perforation, or movement of the obstruction to a thoracic location, where it is more difficult to treat. If the obstruction is not relieved with gentle pressure, it may be lavaged through the nasogastric tube with warm water or saline. Do *not* use mineral oil. Oxytocin (0.11–0.22 U/kg IV) has been shown to decrease intraluminal esophageal pressure and may be useful in conjunction with other described methods for treating choke. The beneficial effect of oxytocin appears to be restricted to the cranial two-thirds of the esophagus, which has a muscular wall composed of striated muscle.

Hance SR, Noble J, Holcomb S, et al: Treating choke with oxytocin. In Proc Am Assoc Equine Pract 43:338–339, 1997. *Editor's note:* The dose in this article is incorrect; the correct dose is given above.

10. How do you manage refractory cases of choke?

If lavage is not successful or an esophageal foreign body is suspected, an endoscopic examination should be performed to determine the nature of the obstruction. If the obstruction appears to be impacted feed material, more vigorous esophageal lavage may be performed on the sedated horse with a cuffed nasoesophageal tube. If more vigorous lavage is to be undertaken, sometimes it is useful to place a cuffed nasotracheal tube to maintain a patent airway and to avoid worsening of aspiration. If the impaction is not relieved, the horse should be placed in an unbedded stall between lavage attempts. Lubricating agents such as mineral oil or docusate sodium are contraindicated because they may be aspirated. An alternative to the above procedure is vigorous lavage under general anesthesia. A cuffed endotracheal tube is used to prevent aspiration of lavage fluid. If the obstruction is in the proximal esophagus, a nasotracheal tube may be placed to maintain anesthesia, and a manual oral-esophageal examination may be made to remove part of the obstruction. If an esophageal foreign body is identified, treatment options are limited to manual retrieval with an endoscopic snare or surgical removal. Most clinicians consider surgery to be the treatment of last resort because of the poor healing of the esophagus and the high incidence of strictures at the surgical site.

11. What complications are seen after acute esophageal obstruction?

The most common complication after esophageal obstruction is aspiration pneumonia. Broad-spectrum antibiotics should be instituted immediately if (1) tracheal fluid can be auscultated, (2) abnormal lung sounds can be auscultated, or (3) a fever develops after resolution of an esophageal obstruction. Other complications include esophageal stricture, esophageal rupture, and formation of diverticula. Strictures occur secondary to pressure necrosis from prolonged obstruction or trauma. Overzealous attempts to relieve obstruction or sharp, irregular foreign bodies may cause esophageal rupture. Damage to the muscular layers of the esophagus may result in the outpouching of the mucosa through the rent and the formation of a diverticulum. Small diverticula usually are not problematic, but larger ones may fill with feed material and cause intermittent luminal compression of the esophagus.

12. Describe the appropriate care after resolution of esophageal obstruction.

Aftercare includes an endoscopic examination of (1) the trachea to evaluate the potential for aspiration pneumonia and (2) the esophageal mucosa to evaluate damage. If no damage is apparent in the esophagus, the horse may be fed a few handfuls of soaked hay or allowed to graze within a few hours. In horses with mild damage, grass or hay that has been soaked in water or a slurry of moistened pellets may be offered in 24 hours, but other feeds are withheld for 24–72 hours. In instances of severe ulceration or persistent dysphagia, all feed should be withheld and parenteral nutrition should be considered. Endoscopy is essential to evaluate healing. Other aftercare includes correction of dehydration and electrolyte disturbances, monitoring for and treating aspiration pneumonia, and decreasing esophageal inflammation through administration of NSAIDs, such as flunixin meglumine or phenylbutazone.

GASTRIC DISEASES

13. Describe the clinical syndromes in foals with gastric ulceration.

1. **Asymptomatic foals.** Up to 50% of foals less than 50 days of age have endoscopic evidence of gastric ulceration, but most of them remain asymptomatic. Ulcers are generally confined to the squamous portion of the stomach adjacent to the margo plicatus along the greater or lesser curvature of the stomach.

2. **Bruxism and dorsal recumbency.** A minority of all foals with gastric ulcers develop ulcers in the gastric glandular mucosa or the duodenum and display the classic signs of gastric ulceration: bruxism (grinding of the teeth), ptyalism (increased salivation), dorsal recumbency and colic, interrupted nursing, and poor appetite. The presence of clinical signs suggests that the ulceration is severe.

3. **Poor growth and diarrhea.** A third slightly different syndrome is recognized in foals with severe ulceration of the squamous portion of the stomach. Diminished appetite, diarrhea, poor growth, rough hair coat with a "potbelly" appearance, and, in rare cases, bruxism and colic may be seen.

14. What clinical signs suggest a diagnosis of gastric ulceration in yearlings and adult horses?

Yearlings with gastric ulcers may show recurrent bouts of colic, poor body condition with variable appetite, and intermittent diarrhea. Adult horses with clinically significant gastric ulceration experience acute or recurrent colic, loss of body condition, poor appetite, decreases in performance, and attitude changes. Endoscopic examination of affected horses usually demonstrates multifocal ulcers in the squamous mucosa adjacent to the margo plicatus. If lesions are identified in the glandular portion of the stomach, NSAID toxicosis should be suspected as the cause.

15. List the risk factors for the development of gastric ulceration.

Gastric ulceration is a multifactorial disease, and few specific causes have been identified in horses. Although *Helicobacter pylori* has been identified as a primary pathogenic agent in humans, an infectious cause of ulceration has not been identified in horses. Risk factors for horses include stress from illness or hospitalization, NSAID administration, strenuous exercise, and altered eating behavior. Horses that are not eating or are held off feed have greater gastric acidity than horses that are fed. In addition, horses that are fed concentrate have a lower gastric pH than horses consuming roughage. Conditions that delay gastric emptying, such as duodenal strictures, may cause severe ulceration of the stomach. Excessive administration of NSAIDs may cause ulceration of the glandular mucosa of the stomach.

16. How is gastric ulceration treated?

Treatment of gastric ulceration includes decreasing gastric acidity, enhancing mucosal protection, and improving gastric emptying. Histamine type-2 receptor antagonists, proton pump inhibitors, and antacids have been used to decrease gastric acidity. Sucralfate is the primary mucosal protectant used in foals. Sucralfate binds to damaged glandular mucosa, stimulates mucus production, and enhances prostaglandin formation. If gastric emptying is delayed, prokinetic drugs such as metoclopramide or bethanechol may be beneficial. Metoclopramide at the recommended dosages has been associated with nervous excitement, whereas bethanechol has been reported to be beneficial with minimal side effects (although colic and excessive lacrimation may occur).

Drugs Used to Treat Gastric Ulceration

DRUG TYPE	DRUG	DOSAGE
H2 antagonist	Cimetidine	15–20 mg/kg PO every 6–8 hr
	Ranitidine	6.6 mg/kg PO every 8 hr
Proton pump inhibitor	Omeprazole	0.7–1.0 mg/kg* PO daily
Antacid	Aluminum/magnesium hydroxide	40–50 ml/100 kg PO every 2–6 hr
Mucosal protectant	Sucralfate	10–20 mg/kg PO every 6–8 hr
Prokinetic drugs	Metoclopramide	0.1–0.25 mg/kg PO every 6–8 hr
	Bethanechol	0.025–0.30 mg/kg SC every 4–6 hr (titrate dose)
	Bethanechol, maintenance	0.35–0.45 mg/kg PO every 6–8 hr

PO = orally, SC = subcutaneously.
* Prilosec (enteric-coated granules administered by nasogastric tube).

ENTERITIS, COLITIS, AND WEIGHT LOSS

17. How is protein-losing enteropathy diagnosed?
Diagnosis of protein-losing enteropathy is presumptive and requires the exclusion of other causes of decreased serum protein: (1) loss into the urine, (2) loss into a body cavity (pleuritis, peritonitis), (3) decreased protein production due to chronic hepatic disease, or (4) severe starvation. Lesions may be seen in the small intestine, large intestine, or both. Weight loss is the most common concurrent clinical sign. Manure is often soft. Ventral edema may be evident when total protein is less than 4 gm/dl or albumin is less than 1.5 gm/dl.

18. List the differential diagnoses for protein-losing enteropathy.
1. Increased mucosal permeability: enterocolitis, ulceration.
2. Ulceration: NSAID toxicosis
3. Noninfectious infiltrative small bowel disease: granulomatous, plasmacytic/lymphocytic, or eosinophilic enterocolitis.
4. Neoplastic infiltration: lymphoma, adenocarcinoma, squamous cell carcinoma, leiomyoma, leiomyosarcoma.
5. Infectious granulomatous enterocolitis: *Mycobacterium tuberculosis, Mycobacterium paratuberculosis, Aspergillus fumigatus, Histoplasma capsulatum.*
6. Parasitism: cyathostomiasis, strongylosis.

19. What tests are used to evaluate small intestinal absorption?
Either d-glucose or d-xylose absorption tests can be used to evaluate small intestinal absorptive capacity. Both d-glucose and d-xylose (0.5–1 gm/kg, as a 10% solution) are administered by nasogastric tube after an overnight fast, and blood samples are collected at time zero (i.e., before administration) and every 30 minutes for 4 hours. D-glucose is readily available, inexpensive, and easy to analyze. However, glucose is subject to metabolism by the test subject, resulting in some variability in the interpretation of results. D-xylose more accurately estimates small intestinal absorption because it is not metabolized. Disadvantages of d-xylose include increased expense, decreased availability, and lack of laboratories that perform the analysis. Peak absorption should occur within 60–90 minutes after administration. Peak plasma levels in a normal horse should be at least 15 mg/dl greater than baseline values.

20. Describe the five major mechanisms that produce diarrhea.
1. **Maldigestion/malabsorption.** Villous blunting and microvillous damage occur to some degree with most enteric diseases, resulting in loss of brush border enzymes (maldigestion) and loss of surface are (malabsorption).

2. **Osmotic overload.** Malabsorption results in an increase in osmotically active particles, and the absorptive capacity of the intestinal tract is overwhelmed.

3. **Secretory disorders.** Some bacteria, such as *Salmonella* species and *Clostridium perfringens*, may produce enterotoxins that directly stimulate intestinal secretion. Invasive organisms also may trigger a prostaglandin-mediated increase in intestinal secretion.

4. **Abnormal motility.** Primary motility disorders have not been identified in large animals, but inflammation and bowel irritation may cause decreased intestinal transit time.

5. **Increased blood-to-lumen hydraulic pressure.** Hypoalbuminuria (decreased plasma oncotic pressure), heart failure (increased capillary hydraulic pressure), and lymphatic obstruction due to inflammation may cause diarrhea by this mechanism.

21. List the differential diagnoses for foals with diarrhea.

Differential Diagnosis of Diarrhea in Foals

BACTERIA	VIRUS	PARASITES	MISCELLANEOUS
Clostridium perfringens	Rotavirus	*Strongyloides westeri*	Foal heat diarrhea
Clostridium difficile	Adenovirus*	*Strongylus vulgaris*	Overeating
Salmonella species	Coronavirus*	*Giardia* species	Lactase deficiency
Rhodococcus equi	Parvovirus*	*Cryptosporidium* species*	Septicemia
*Escherichia coli**		*E. luekartti*	Antimicrobials
			Ulceration (gastric, duodenal, colonic)

* The significance of these organisms is not known.

22. Describe the risk factors for diarrhea in foals.

Management factors that increase the risk of diarrhea include failure to disinfect foaling stalls between uses, use of shavings as a stall bedding, and failure to wash the mare's udder before nursing occurs. These factors are associated with the build-up of potential pathogens in the environment. Foals receiving prophylactic antibiotics or vitamin injections also are more likely to develop diarrhea than foals that do not receive injections, and this practice should be discouraged. One exception is that foals born to farms with endemic *C. perfringens* problems may be treated prophylactically with procaine penicillin G or metronidazole. If possible, mares should be moved to the farm where they will foal 30–60 days before expected parturition. Sufficient time to acclimate to a new environment and develop antibodies to resident bacteria is important, because foals born to visiting mares are more likely to develop diarrhea than foals born to resident mares.

East LM, Savage CJ, Traub-Dargatz JL, et al: Enterocolitis associated with *Clostridium perfringens* infection in neonate foals: 54 cases (1988–1997). J Am Vet Med Assoc 212:1751–1756, 1998.

Traub-Dargatz JL, Gay CC, Evermann JF, et al: Epidemiologic survey of diarrhea in foals. J Am Vet Med Assoc 192:1533–1556, 1988.

23. Describe the characteristics of foal heat diarrhea.

Foal heat diarrhea has a temporal association with the mare's first heat after foaling and is the most common cause of diarrhea in foals between 7 and 14 days of age. The cause is unknown, but the diarrhea probably results from a physiologic change in intestinal cell populations or from establishment of the normal intestinal population through coprophagia. Previous theories that have been disproved include changes in milk composition, *S. westeri* infection, and estrus secretions on the mare's udder. Affected foals are afebrile, continue to nurse, and have relatively mild diarrhea. No treatment is necessary as long as the foal is bright and alert and continues to nurse. If the diarrhea persists, fever is evident, or the foal becomes depressed, a thorough work-up for other causes of diarrhea should be made.

24. List the causes of necrotizing enterocolitis (i.e., hemorrhagic diarrhea) in neonatal foals.

1. *C. perfringens* types A and C. Exotoxins produced by these bacteria (especially the β-toxin produced by type C) may cause colic, bloody diarrhea, hemorrhagic necrosis of the gut wall, and

rapid progression to death in foals less than 48 hours old. Clinical signs are variable and range from obtunded mentation, mild colic, and mild nonhemorrhagic diarrhea to severe hemorrhagic diarrhea, severe colic, and death.

2. *C. difficile*. These bacteria may cause watery diarrhea in foals from 2–5 days of age. Clinical signs are variable and range from mild diarrhea to severe hemorrhagic enteritis with abdominal cramping and death.

3. *Clostridium septicum*. Endotoxins produced by these bacteria cause symptoms similar to those produced by endotoxins of *C. perfringens*, but in older foals.

4. Necrotizing enterocolitis of premature foals. This syndrome is associated with ischemic hypoxic bowel injury, presence of intraluminal bacteria, and enteral feeding. Ischemia results in a breakdown of mucosal defenses, and intraluminal bacteria invade and multiply within the bowel wall (i.e., intramural bacteria). Enteral feeding provides substrate for bacterial multiplication. Pneumatosis intestinalis (gas within intestinal wall) may develop, and the bowel may rupture.

25. Describe clinical disease caused by rotavirus infection of foals.

Rotavirus is a common cause of diarrhea in foals less than 3 months of age. Clinically affected foals become depressed, febrile, and anorexic. Watery diarrhea is usually evident within 12–24 hours after initial clinical signs. Rotavirus diarrhea may be sporadic or occur as an outbreak involving most foals on a farm. The source of the virus may be adult carriers, asymptomatic foals, and foals recovering from clinical infections. The virus is stable and may persist in the environment for as long as 9 months. Rotavirus infects epithelial cells of the small intestine, causing villous atrophy that results in malabsorption and secondary osmotic diarrhea. Severely affected foals may experience persistent weight loss, poor growth rate, and unthriftiness for some time after resolution of diarrhea.

26. List the four syndromes associated with salmonellosis.

1. **Inapparent infection.** Approximately 10–20% of horses may be inapparently infected and establish a latent (nonshedding) or active (shedding) carrier state. Active carriers are more likely to shed relatively low numbers of bacteria and generally are not thought to represent a significant risk to healthy horses.

2. **Depression, fever, anorexia, and neutropenia without diarrhea or colic.** Affected horses generally recover in several days with specific treatment. However, some horses require intravenous fluids.

3. **Enterocolitis with diarrhea.** This syndrome is characterized by severe fibrinonecrotic typhlocolitis. The initial signs usually are fever and anorexia. Moderate-to-severe neutropenia with a left shift usually occurs concurrently with onset of fever. In many instances, abdominal pain may precede the onset of diarrhea.

4. **Septicemia.** Young horses and foals may develop septicemia and septic osteoarthritis, although concurrent enterocolitis may be present.

27. What are the risk factors for developing salmonellosis?

The risk of clinical salmonellosis depends on the virulence of the bacterial serotype, infective dose of organism, host susceptibility, and environmental factors. Multiple serotypes of *Salmonella* species have been isolated from the horse, although a host-adapted serotype has not been identified. Virulence varies with serotype and among strains of the same serotype. Clinical infection with *Salmonella* species generally requires exposure to millions of organisms. The first risk factor is exposure to a horse with clinical salmonellosis. Other risk factors include exposure to wildlife (rodents or birds), exposure to pigs or chickens, and *Salmonella*-contaminated feed. Stress or illness may compromise host defenses so that infection is possible after exposure to a few thousand organisms. Some of the stresses that have been identified include hospitalization (especially for gastrointestinal disorders), transportation, general anesthesia, antimicrobial therapy, and high environmental temperatures. After stress latent carriers may begin to shed organisms or in some instances may develop enterocolitis.

Tillotson K, Savage CJ, Salmon MD, et al: Outbreak of *Salmonella infantis* infection in a large animal veterinary teaching hospital. J Am Vet Med Assoc 211:1554–1557, 1997.

28. How is a diagnosis of salmonellosis confirmed?

The most common method of diagnosis is a serial culture (5–7 samples) of feces using enrichment media. This technique identifies less than 50% of horses infected with *Salmonella* species. Concurrent culture of rectal biopsy specimens and feces increases the sensitivity to 60–75% of infected horses. A polymerase chain reaction (PCR) has been used to identify *Salmonella* species in feces and appears to be at least as sensitive as culture techniques.

Cohen ND: Use of PCR to detect *Salmonellae* in equine feces and environmental samples from an equine clinic: Detection of bacteria in body fluids using PCR. Proc Annu Vet Med Forum 14:541–542, 1996.

29. Describe the method for collecting rectal biopsies.

Rectal mucosa biopsies are easily obtained, and restraint is similar to that required for rectal palpation (e.g., twitch, stocks, tranquilization). A lubricated gloved hand is passed into the rectum to the level of the wrist, and a uterine forceps is passed into the palm of the cupped hand within the rectum. The thumb and finger grasp a fold of rectal mucosa; samples should be obtained from areas slightly lateral to the dorsal midline to avoid the dorsal vasculature. The jaws of the biopsy instrument are opened, and the instrument is advanced until the mucosal fold is within the jaws. The jaws are closed to obtain a sample of rectal mucosa, which may be placed in formalin for histopathology or enrichment media for bacterial culture.

30. Describe the epidemiology of Potomac horse fever.

Potomac horse fever is caused by the rickettsial organism, *Ehrlichia risticii*. This disease does not appear to be contagious from horse to horse, infections are limited usually to the spring-summer months (March to September), and most cases are found in close proximity to major rivers or waterways. These factors suggest involvement of a vector and intermediate host in the transmission of Potomac horse fever; however, a vector has not yet been identified. Currently it is thought that a coprophagic insect may be involved. The disease can be transmitted by whole blood, but experimental transmission with ticks or biting insects was unsuccessful. Experimental infection has been achieved through oral inoculation of organisms; therefore, oral transmission has not been ruled out.

31. How is the diagnosis of *E. risticii* infection confirmed?

Potomac horse fever clinically resembles other causes of enterocolitis, and clinical signs cannot be used to make the diagnosis. Presumptive evidence of active infection requires the demonstration of a fourfold rise in antibody titers to *E. risticii* on acute and convalescent samples by the indirect fluorescent antibody test, but interpretation of serology is often confusing. Because of the long incubation period, antibody titers may have peaked by the time clinical signs are evident, and a further increase in titer does not occur. A single high titer cannot be used to confirm the diagnosis because horses in endemic areas may have high antibody titers in the absence of disease or titer may be due to vaccination. A California study identified a high rate of false-positive results with the indirect fluorescent antibody test. Recently, a PCR has been developed for *E. risticii*. This test provides a highly sensitive and specific method for identification of *E. risticii* infection in horses with enterocolitis.

Madigan JE, Rikihisa Y, Palmer JE, et al: Evidence for a high rate of false-positive results with the indirect fluorescent antibody test for *Ehrlichia risticii* antibody in horses. J Am Vet Med Assoc 207:1448–1453, 1995.

32. List other causes of acute colitis in adult horses.

Although salmonellosis and Potomac horse fever are the most common causes of acute colitis in adult horses, other causes are occasionally encountered. *C. perfringens* type A has been implicated as a cause of peracute, hemorrhagic, fatal enterocolitis in adult horses. According to one theory, parasitized horses that undergo deworming may have sufficient damage in their intestine to allow anaerobic conditions that provoke *C. perfringens* infection. Antimicrobial therapy may cause colitis secondary to alterations in normal colonic flora. Disruption of the normal flora may result in abnormal volatile fatty acid production and initiate abnormal secretory/absorptive patterns in the colon. Loss of normal bacterial flora also may allow the proliferation of enteropathogens. Parasitism caused by cyathostomes and *Strongylus vulgaris*, ingestion of sand, overuse of NSAIDs, and stress also have been associated with colitis in the adult horse.

33. What are the clinical signs of peritonitis?

Clinical signs of peritonitis are highly variable and depend on the cause of the peritonitis, duration of the process, and extent of peritoneal involvement. Bowel rupture or a rectal tear results in peracute peritonitis that is characterized by severe toxemia and circulatory failure. Typical clinical findings include weakness with muscle fasciculations, depression or severe colic, sweating, weak peripheral pulses, tachycardia, tachypnea, red-to-purple mucous membranes, and prolonged capillary refill time. Reluctance to move, guarding of the abdomen, reluctance to urinate or defecate, and sensitivity to external abdominal pressure may be seen in some cases. The serosal and parietal peritoneum may feel gritty on rectal palpation. Chronic peritonitis is characterized typically by a history of chronic or intermittent colic, depression, loss of appetite, weight loss, intermittent fever, ventral edema, decreased or absent intestinal sounds, and occasionally diarrhea. Diagnosis of peritonitis is usually confirmed with abdominal paracentesis.

34. Formulate a diagnostic plan for a horse with chronic weight loss.

1. Collect a complete history (e.g., affected horse[s], diet, farm management). The clinician must determine the extent and duration of weight loss. A dietary history may reveal that the affected horse does not have access to sufficient amounts of quality feed and water to meet metabolic demands, and the weight loss can be corrected by changing dietary management. Inadequate anthelmintic treatments or lack of routine dental care may suggest parasitism or dental abnormalities as a cause of weight loss.

2. Physical examination. Signs of concurrent disease may suggest a primary disease as the cause of weight loss. Eating behavior should be observed to determine whether the horse is able to prehend, chew, and swallow food normally.

3. Diagnostic evaluation. If a cause of weight loss is not evident after a complete history and thorough physical examination, a diagnostic work-up is warranted:
   - Complete blood count and fibrinogen: evidence of inflammation, eosinophilia, or anemia.
   - Serum chemistry and urinalysis: evidence of organ failure or metabolic derangement.
   - Rectal examination: intraabdominal masses or thickened rectal mucosa. Collect renal mucosal biopsy for histopathology.
   - Fecal examination: fecal flotation, occult blood, or sand.
   - Abdominal paracentesis: peritonitis or neoplasia.
   - Coggin's test

4. Evaluation of small intestinal absorption.

5. Exploratory laparotomy and intestinal biopsy.

35. What are the differential diagnoses for chronic diarrhea in horses?

1. Chronic salmonellosis

2. Gut-associated rhodococci (younger horses [< 2 yr] often have a previous history or concurrent respiratory disease)

3. Chronic parasitism: *S. vulgaris, Strongylus edentatus,* or small strongyles (cyathostomes)

4. Abdominal abscessation or chronic peritonitis

5. Sand enteropathy

6. Cellular infiltrate disorders: granulomatous, eosinophilic, or lymphocytic-plasmacytic enterocolitis

7. Neoplasia: lymphosarcoma

8. Abnormal fermentation

9. Ulceration of bowel

36. Formulate a diagnostic plan for a horse with chronic diarrhea.

The client should be aware that a cause cannot be identified in many cases of chronic diarrhea and that a diagnostic work-up to determine the cause can be expensive.

1. Complete physical examination
2. Collect minimal database: complete blood count, fibrinogen, serum biochemistry profile,
and urinalysis
3. Abdominocentesis
4. Fecal examination: serial culture of feces and/or rectal mucosal biopsies for salmonellosis, PCR for *Salmonella* species, fecal occult blood, fecal parasite assay, direct examination for
strongyle larvae, fecal sedimentation (sand)
5. Rectal mucosal biopsy for histopathology
6. Absorption tests
7. Exploratory laparotomy with biopsy

37. Describe the empirical treatment for chronic diarrhea in horses.

1. Alteration of diet. Simple grass hay or pelleted feed may favorably alter volatile fatty acid
production and facilitate water absorption.
2. Withdrawal of NSAIDs if toxicity is possible.
3. Transfaunation. Recommended when protozoa are absent in the fecal sample or after prolonged antibiotic therapy.
4. Removal of sand. Psyllium, 0.1–0.2 kg daily in feed for 1 week of every month.
5. Lavicidal anthelmintics: ivermectin at 200 μg/kg/day, fenbendazole at 50 mg/kg/day for 5
days.
6. Classify rectal biopsy.
   • Fibrosis and inflammatory changes: potentiated sulfas and iodochlorhydroxyquin
     (Rheaform, 20 mg/kg/day) for 2 weeks. Most horses on Rheaform improve and then
     relapse.
   • Mononuclear infiltrate: dexamethasone (20–30 mg/day; taper dose to 10 mg over 1
     week). If diarrhea improves, continue treatment with prednisolone (600–800 mg/day
     orally; taper over 2 months)

38. How do cyathostomes (small strongyles) cause diarrhea in horses?

Fourth-stage cyathostome larvae migrate through the mucosa of the large colon and form
cysts within the mucosa. Larvae may undergo arrested development (hypobiosis) and remain encysted during the winter months only to emerge in the spring. Simultaneous emergence of large
numbers of larvae causes considerable colonic inflammation, which may cause severe diarrhea.
The diarrhea is typically profuse and watery and may be accompanied by mild-to-severe weight
loss, ventral edema, intermittent fever, and sporadic mild colic. Intestinal protein loss may be significant. Horses of any age may be affected, and clinical signs are usually seen during the late
winter or early spring. Elimination of adult cyathostomes may signal the emergence of encysted
larvae since affected horses often have a history of recent anthelmintic treatment. Fecal egg
counts are often negative because clinical signs are caused by the emergence of larval stages.
Demonstration of large numbers of larvae in the feces is considered to be presumptive evidence
of cyathostome-induced diarrhea.

39. What clinical signs often accompany enterocolitis in horses?

Shock and dehydration are the most common signs that accompany diarrhea in enterocolitis.
Shock represents a decrease in effective circulatory volume that is manifest as decreased jugular
distensibility, cool extremities, increased capillary refill time, increased heart rate, and decreased
pulse pressure. Dehydration develops secondary to fluid losses and is characterized by decreased
skin turgor, dry mucous membranes, sunken eyes, and decreased urine production. Other signs
are due to the presence of endotoxemia as a result of the absorption of endotoxin through damaged intestinal mucosa. Endotoxin causes elevations in respiratory rate, brick-red or cyanotic

mucous membranes, leukopenia, toxic changes in neutrophils, and fever. Other clinical signs include ventral edema secondary to intestinal protein loss and laminitis.

40. Describe how to differentiate between a horse with a strangulating obstruction and a horse with duodenitis/proximal jejunitis (DPJ).

The clinical signs of DPJ closely resemble those of small intestinal obstruction. Some previous reports suggested that the prognosis for horses with DPJ that undergo surgery is poorer compared with horses treated medically; thus it is important to distinguish clinically between the two syndromes. Some veterinarians believe that removing excessive fluid from the small intestine into the large intestine may decrease ileus. Clinical findings that suggest DPJ include (1) elevated temperature; (2) voluminous, fetid, orange-brown gastric reflux; (3) signs of abdominal pain that are replaced by severe depression after gastric decompression; (4) increased peritoneal fluid protein concentration (> 3.5 gm/dl) with mild increases in the peritoneal white blood cell count (< 10,000 cells/μl), and (5) moderately distended small intestine on rectal palpation (compared with often turgid small intestine in patients with a strangulating obstruction).

COLIC

41. Describe the source of visceral pain in a horse with gastrointestinal disease.

Visceral pain originates from one of four basic mechanisms:
1. Stretching of the bowel wall as a result of distention with ingesta, fluid, or gas
2. Displacement or torsion of the bowel that causes tension on the root of the mesentery
3. Infarction or ischemia of the bowel
4. Deep ulcers in stomach or bowel

42. Describe the structures normally identified on rectal palpation.

The rectal examination of the horse should be accomplished in a systematic manner to ensure that all structures are examined. Adequate restraint or sedation is necessary. Structures that can normally be palpated in the horse include urethra and accessory sex glands (male), female reproductive tract (i.e., cervix, uterus, ovaries), urinary bladder, inguinal rings, pelvic flexure, small colon, spleen, left kidney, nephrosplenic ligament, abdominal aorta, root of the mesentery, and ventral band and base of the cecum. The peritoneal surface of the abdomen and abdominal viscera should feel smooth without crepitus or irregularities.

43. Describe abnormal findings on rectal examination.

1. Delayed fecal transport; small, dry fecal balls covered with pasty mucus in the rectum.
2. Intestinal impaction: enlarged bowel with a pasty or doughy consistency. Digital impressions that can felt with the hand remain for some time.
3. Intravaginal inguinal hernia: enlarged loop of small intestine with abnormal fixed position in inguinal area, taut mesentery, and acute pain.
4. Obstruction of small intestine (physical, functional): distended loops of small intestine that are compressible to some degree. Pain may be observed on palpation of distended intestine.
5. Acute dilation of cecum: gas distention or impaction.
6. Displacement of the large colon: recognized by distention of the colon with gas, taut mesenteric bands, or abnormal location of the bowel.
7. Obstruction of the small colon: foreign bodies and fecal concretions often can be palpated at the ventral abdominal wall near the pelvic inlet.
8. Abnormal peritoneal surface: presence of masses or roughening of the surface.

44. What is the incidence of surgical colic in horses?

Estimates suggest that the majority (80%) of colic cases are mild and resolve with medical therapy. Most of these cases are termed simple colic and probably represent transient ileus, gas accumulation, or spasmodic colic, although a specific diagnosis often is not reached. Impaction is the most common diagnosis among cases with an identifiable cause, and affected horses generally have a good prognosis. Of all horses suffering from colic, only 2–3% require surgery. Over the years mortality among horses with surgical colic has improved, and long-term survival is approximately 70%, although the risk for repeat colic is increased compared with the normal population. The case fatality rate among horses with colic is about 7%, and the mortality rate due to colic for the entire population of horses has been estimated at 0.7%.

45. Discuss the risk factors for equine colic.

History of previous colic and abdominal surgery are important risk factors for colic. Other factors that appear to increase the risk of colic include a sudden decrease in the level of activity, sudden changes in diet, and alterations in stabling conditions. Practitioners associate the ingestion of rapidly growing, lush pasture with an increased frequency of gas colic. Feeding a high concentrate diet also increases the risk of colic compared with a diet free of grain. Impaction colic is seen more often when poor-quality roughage or coastal Bermuda grass in fed. Many practitioners associate changes in weather with an increased onset of colic, but results of studies examining this risk factor have been conflicting. Others have suspected a link between recent transport and colic, but this association is still unproved. In certain instances, the recent deworming of horses may be associated with increased instances of colic—especially in young horses, in whom the rapid killing of ascarids may lead to ascarid impaction.

Cohen ND, Matejka PL, Honnas CM, Hooper RN: Case-control study of the association between various management factors and development of colic in horses. J Am Vet Med Assoc 206:667–673, 1995.

46. How do you determine whether a horse with colic should be treated by medical or surgical means?

Common indications for surgery

1. Moderate-to-severe pain that is poorly responsive to appropriate analgesic therapy
2. Identification of small intestinal distention (DPJ also should be considered), intestinal displacement, or an intestinal foreign body on rectal palpation
3. Weak pulse rising over 70 beats/minute
4. Large amounts (> 4 L over priming fluid volume) of greenish nasogastric reflux
5. Absence of borborygmi
6. Peritoneal fluid with increased protein, erythrocytes, and toxic neutrophils
7. Progressive distention of the abdomen

Indications for medical therapy

1. Elevations in rectal temperature suggesting impending enteritis (e.g., DPJ), colitis, pleuritis, or peritonitis
2. Neutropenia with a left shift or marked neutrophilia (also may occur in horses with devitalized bowel in the abdomen)
3. Severe icterus with marked elevation of hepatic enzymes consistent with liver disease
4. Pain replaced by depression after gastric decompression

47. Describe the therapeutic goals for the medical management of colic.

1. Control of pain
2. Decompression of distended bowel: nasogastric intubation or cecal trocharization
3. Correction of fluid and electrolyte disorders
4. Administration of laxatives for resolution of impaction

48. Describe the medial correction of a left dorsal displacement of the colon (i.e., nephrosplenic entrapment).

Left dorsal displacement is characterized by movement of the left colon dorsally between the left body wall and the spleen until it is positioned in the nephrosplenic space (see figure on facing page). Nonsurgical correction may be attempted if the entrapped portion of the colon is not greatly distended with feed material. The horse is anesthetized in right lateral recumbency and slowly rolled into dorsal recumbency. A hoist should be used to lift the horse by the legs, and after 1 minute the horse is returned to dorsal recumbency and then slowly turned to its left side.

Ultrasonic evaluation and rectal palpation may be used to determine whether the displacement has been corrected. Feed restriction has been reported to result in spontaneous correction when only the pelvic flexure is entrapped in the nephrosplenic space. Improved success for this procedure has been reported after administration of phenylephrine (3 µg/kg/min for 15 minutes) to cause splenic contraction before rolling the horse.

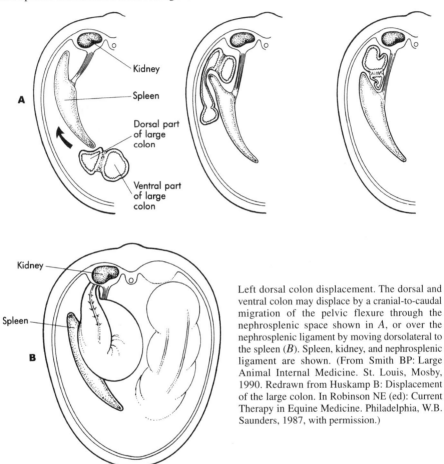

Left dorsal colon displacement. The dorsal and ventral colon may displace by a cranial-to-caudal migration of the pelvic flexure through the nephrosplenic space shown in *A*, or over the nephrosplenic ligament by moving dorsolateral to the spleen (*B*). Spleen, kidney, and nephrosplenic ligament are shown. (From Smith BP: Large Animal Internal Medicine. St. Louis, Mosby, 1990. Redrawn from Huskamp B: Displacement of the large colon. In Robinson NE (ed): Current Therapy in Equine Medicine. Philadelphia, W.B. Saunders, 1987, with permission.)

49. What is right dorsal colitis? How is it managed?

Right dorsal colitis has been described in horses that have received inappropriately high doses of NSAIDs. Clinical signs include intermittent fever, chronic diarrhea, mild intermittent colic, and hypoproteinemia characterized by low serum albumin. Management can be challenging, and in some horses surgical resection of the damaged bowel is necessary for resolution of clinical signs and intestinal protein loss. All NSAIDs (e.g., flunixin meglumine, phenylbutazone, dipyrone, ketoprofen, aspirin) should be discontinued, and serum protein levels are carefully monitored. Medical treatment includes low-bulk, low-roughage diets (i.e., complete or incomplete pelleted feeds) and corn oil. Reduction of fiber decreases the mechanical load on the damaged colon. Corn oil (60–120 ml daily) is high in linoleic acid,which may promote prostaglandin production and enhance mucosal repair.

Cohen ND, Carter GK, Mealey RH, Taylor TS: Medical management of right dorsal colitis in 5 horses: A retrospective study (1987–1993). J Vet Intern Med 9:272–276, 1995.

50. Describe the diagnosis of sand colic.

Several methods to identify sand impaction have been described, including sedimentation of sand in the feces, palpation of a sand-filled viscus on rectal palpation, and identification of radio-dense material of abdominal radiographs. Abdominal auscultation findings characteristic of sand in the large colon also have been described. Auscultation is performed on the ventral abdomen in the area just caudal to the xiphoid process. Sand sounds are gritty in character and of variable duration and intensity. They have been described as resembling the sound generated by partially filling a paper bag with sand and slowly rotating it.

Ragle CA, Meagher DM, Schrader JL, Honnas CM: Abdominal auscultation in the detection of experimentally induced gastrointestinal sand accumulation. J Vet Intern Med 3:12–14, 1989.

51. What are the causes of abdominal distention in a foal?

The causes of abdominal distention usually can be differentiated after abdominal ballottement, simultaneous auscultation and percussion, radiography, and ultrasonography. These procedures can usually determine whether the distention is caused by gas or fluid. However, the greatest difficulty is distinguishing functional obstruction from mechanical obstruction of the intestinal tract.

1. **Mechanical obstructions**
   - Meconium impaction or congenital disorders of the bowel (first few days of life)
   - Fecoliths (miniature horses and pony foals)
   - Ascarid impactions: heavy worm burdens, history of rapidly active anthelmintic usage
2. **Intestinal accidents**
   - Small intestinal volvulus and intussusceptions in foals less than 6 months of age
   - Umbilical, inguinal, scrotal, and diaphragmatic hernias
3. **Functional obstruction (ileus)**
   - Overfeeding
   - Enterotoxemia
   - Enteritis
   - Immaturity
   - Electrolyte imbalances
4. **Distention of the peritoneal cavity with fluid**
   - Peritonitis
   - Uroperitoneum secondary to ruptured bladder

52. What are the clinical features of blister beetle (*Epicauta* species) toxicosis?

1. The toxin cantharidin is absorbed from the digestive tract and causes disruption of cell membranes, resulting in oral, esophageal, gastric, and small and large intestinal ulceration.
2. Colic, diarrhea, dehydration, hypocalcemia, hypomagnesemia, and hypoalbuminemia
3. Cystitis with occasional hematuria
4. Myocarditis and myocardial necrosis
5. Deterioration and death

HEPATIC DISEASES

53. Describe the epidemiology of Theiler's disease (acute hepatic necrosis).

Theiler's disease is an acute necrotic hepatitis that affects only adult horses. It is usually sporadic in nature, but outbreaks have been reported. Most cases occur in the summer and fall. Although the exact cause is not known, a high percentage of cases may occur within 4–10 weeks of receiving an equine-origin biologic agent (e.g., blood, plasma, tetanus, antitoxin), leading to the name *serum-associated hepatitis*. The history, clinical course, and histopathologic findings are similar to hepatitis B in humans, but so far the search for a viral etiology has been unrewarding.

54. What clinical signs suggest a diagnosis of choledocolithiasis?

Choledocolithiasis is recognized most commonly in middle-aged horses (6–15 years). Affected horses frequently present for recurrent colic, intermittent fever, depression, and weight loss. Icterus is almost always present. Signs of hepatic failure may develop during the course of the disease, including photosensitization, petechial hemorrhages, and hepatic encephalopathy. Diagnosis can be confirmed by demonstrating a marked increase in gamma-glutamyl transferase (GGT) and a direct-acting bilirubin fraction that exceeds 25% of the total bilirubin. Ultrasonography of the liver usually reveals dilated bile ducts and occasionally may identify a stone (usually echogenic and shadow-inducing) within the bile duct.

55. Describe how to perform a liver biopsy.

Ultrasonography is the most useful tool for determining the site for liver biopsy; however, a biopsy can be performed in some horses even if ultrasound is not available. Unfortunately, it may not be possible to obtain the biopsy in horses with right-sided hepatic atrophy. The site for blind hepatic biopsy is the 12th–14th intercostal space on the right side of the abdomen at the intersection of a line drawn from the tuber coxae to a point midway between the elbow and the point of the shoulder. The site should be clipped and surgically scrubbed. After infiltration of the area with local anesthetic, a stab incision through the skin is made with a number 15 blade. The biopsy instrument is inserted and directed cranially and ventrally through the diaphragm into the liver. Advancement of the needle through the pleural cavity should coincide with maximal expiration to minimize the opportunity for pulmonary damage. The biopsy samples are placed into 10% buffered formalin for histopathologic examination or into transport media for bacterial culture.

56. What risk factors are associated with hyperlipemia in horses?

Hyperlipemia is recognized most often in ponies, donkeys, and miniature horses that are overweight and undergo a period of negative energy balance. Factors that may cause negative energy balance include late pregnancy, lactation, transport, parasitism, and anorexia due to primary disease. Hyperlipemia is characterized by rapid mobilization of peripheral fat stores, lipemic serum, and fatty liver. Adult horses that are azotemic are also at increased risk of hyperlipemia.

57. How do you distinguish between hyperlipemia and hyperlipidemia?

Hyperlipemic horses are clinically ill and demonstrate complete or partial anorexia, depression, and variable diarrhea, ventral edema, or ataxia. Serum from affected horses is grossly lipemic, and plasma triglycerides exceed 500 mg/ml. In contrast, hyperlipidemia describes a condition of mild-to-moderate serum triglyceride elevation, but levels do not exceed 500 mg/dl. The serum is clear, clinical signs are absent, and there is no evidence of liver pathology.

58. Discuss possible causes of toxic hepatopathy.

Plants associated with toxic hepatopathy include kleingrass, fall panicum, alsike clover, and plants that produce pyrrolizidine alkaloids (*Senecio, Amsinckia,* and *Crotalaria* species). Kleingrass, which is seen primarily in the southwestern United States, may cause hepatic damage leading to icterus and photosensitivity from late spring to early fill. In the eastern portion of the U.S., a similar syndrome has been described in horses grazing fall panicum. Alsike clover, which is seen in the northeastern part of the U.S. and Canada, causes hepatic damage, icterus, and photosensitivity. Disease due to alsike clover is most common during wet parts of the year or when clover is the predominant forage. Pyrrolizidine alkaloid toxicosis occurs months after the ingestion of offending plants, and liver damage occurs once a horse ingests 5% of its body weight of dry plant material. Other causes of toxic hepatitis include ingestion of grains contaminated with the mycotoxin from *Fusarium* species molds. In addition to causing leukoencephalomalacia, this mycotoxin is capable of causing significant liver damage. Iron toxicosis has been reported as a cause of hepatic failure.

59. Describe the characteristic findings of liver biopsy in a horse suffering with pyrrolizidine alkaloid toxicosis.

Pyrrolizidine alkaloids interfere with cell division. Characteristic findings in biopsy samples include megalocytosis, biliary hyperplasia, and focal hepatic necrosis with fibrous replacement

of damaged tissue. Most other plants that cause toxic hepatopathy cause biliary fibrosis, peripor-
tal bridging fibrosis, and moderate bile duct proliferation.

60. Describe the clinical signs in a horse with acute pancreatitis.

Clinical signs in horses with acute pancreatitis are nonspecific and often resemble those seen
with small intestinal obstruction. Examples include severe abdominal pain, shock, gastric reflux,
and gastric rupture. Release of pancreatic enzymes from the inflamed pancreas may cause the
loss of body fluids into the gastrointestinal tract and peritoneal cavity, leading to shock and dehydration. Hypovolemia is further compounded by the release of vasoactive substances such as myocardial depressant factors, tissue thromboplastin, and endotoxin. Signs of cardiovascular
collapse include tachycardia, prolonged capillary refill time, congested mucous membranes, decreased temperature of the ears and distal extremities, and sweating.

61. Describe the advantages and disadvantages of heparin in the treatment of horses with gastrointestinal disease.

Heparin is an anticoagulant that suppresses thrombin-dependent amplification of the clotting cascade by combining with and activating antithrombin III. If administered before antithrombin III consumption, heparin may prevent development of some of the common
complications associated with severe gastrointestinal disease, including venous thrombosis,
laminitis, and disseminated intravascular coagulation. Experimental evidence also suggests that
heparin therapy may attenuate the hemodynamic and hemostatic alterations associated with endotoxic shock. Other beneficial effects of heparin may include a reduction in postoperative complications such as intestinal adhesions.

Complications from heparin therapy include anemia, fatal hemorrhage, thrombocytopenia,
and painful swelling at injection sites. Heparin therapy apparently causes agglutination of red
cells in the microvasculature, and the anemia resolves in 96 hours after discontinuation of therapy. Complications related to overdosage can be reduced through the recognition that the dose-
response relationship for heparin is not linear, and elimination time is prolonged with repeated
administration. Therefore, a regimen of decreasing doses of heparin is recommended to prevent
hemorrhagic complications. The initial recommended dosage is 60–150 U/kg subcutaneously
followed by 40–125 U/kg subcutaneously twice daily for 6 doses. The dose then should be further reduced to 20–100 U/kg to compensate for accumulation of heparin in the plasma.

Moore BR, Hinchcliff KW: Heparin: A review of its pharmacology and therapeutic use in horses. J Vet
Intern Med 8:26–35, 1994.

62. When should antimicrobial therapy be used in horses with diarrhea?

Antimicrobial usage in horses with colitis is controversial. Antimicrobial therapy has been
proved beneficial to horses infected with *E. risticii*. However, there is little indication that antimicrobial therapy alters the course of colitis due to other causes. Although antimicrobial therapy
may not alter the course of colitis, broad-spectrum antimicrobial coverage is indicated in horses
that are neutropenic. Neutropenia increases the risk of septicemia, and antimicrobial treatment
may limit the spread of enteric organisms to other body systems. Antimicrobial therapy may actually prolong bacterial shedding in horses with salmonellosis and increase the severity of diarrhea by destroying normal flora of the gut.

BIBLIOGRAPHY

1. Cohen ND: Use of PCR to detect *Salmonellae* in equine feces and environmental samples from an equine
   clinic: Detection of bacteria in body fluids using PCR. Proc Annu Vet Med Forum 14:541–542,
   1996.
2. Cohen ND, Carter GK, Mealey RH, Taylor TS: Medical management of right dorsal colitis in 5 horses:
   A retrospective study (1987–1993). J Vet Intern Med 9:272–276, 1995.
3. Cohen ND, Matejka PL, Honnas CM, Hooper RN: Case-control study of the association between various
   management factors and development of colic in horses. J Am Vet Med Assoc 206:667–673, 1995.

4. East LM, Savage CJ, Traub-Dargatz JL, et al: Enterocolitis associated with *Clostridium perfringens* infection in neonate foals: 54 cases (1988–1997). J Am Vet Med Assoc 212:1751–1756, 1998.
5. Hance SR, Noble J, Holcomb S, et al: Treating choke with oxytocin. In Proc Am Assoc Equine Pract 43:338–339, 1997.
6. Madigan JE, Rikihisa Y, Palmer JE, et al: Evidence for a high rate of false-positive results with the indirect fluorescent antibody test for *Ehrlichia risticii* antibody in horses. J Am Vet Med Assoc 207:1448–1453, 1995.
7. Moore BR, Hinchcliff KW: Heparin: A review of its pharmacology and therapeutic use in horses. J Vet Intern Med 8:26–35, 1994.
8. Ragle CA, Meagher DM, Schrader JL, Honnas CM: Abdominal auscultation in the detection of experimentally induced gastrointestinal sand accumulation. J Vet Intern Med 3:12–14, 1989.
9. Reed SM, Bayly WM (eds): Equine Internal Medicine. Philadelphia, W.B. Saunders, 1998.
10. Robinson NE (ed): Current Therapy in Equine Medicine, 4th ed. Philadelphia, W.B. Saunders, 1997.
11. Smith BP (ed): Large Animal Internal Medicine, 2nd ed. St. Louis, Mosby, 1996.
12. Taylor FGR, Hillyer MH (eds): Diagnostic Techniques in Equine Medicine. London, W.B. Saunders, 1997.
13. Tillotson K, Savage CJ, Salmon MD, et al: Outbreak of *Salmonella infantis* infection in a large animal veterinary teaching hospital. J Am Vet Med Assoc 211:1554–1557, 1997.
14. Traub-Dargatz JL, Gay CC, Evermann JF, et al: Epidemiologic survey of diarrhea in foals. J Am Vet Med Assoc 192:1533–1556, 1988.
15. White NA (ed): The Equine Acute Abdomen. Philadelphia, Lea & Febiger, 1990.

11. URINARY TRACT

Harold C. Schott, II, D.V.M., Ph.D., Dip. ACVIM

1. What is the most common congenital anomaly of the equine urinary tract? How is it treated?

Patent urachus is the most common malformation of the equine urinary tract and appears to occur more commonly in foals than in other domestic species. The urachus is the conduit for urine passage into the allantoic cavity during gestation and normally closes at the time of parturition. Greater-than-average length and partial torsion of the umbilical cord have been suggested to cause tension on the urachus, leading to dilation and subsequent failure to close at birth. In foals with patent urachus, the umbilicus is moist from birth, and urine leaks in drips or as a stream during micturition. It is important to distinguish a nonseptic patent urachus from infection of the umbilicus, which also may result in a patent urachus within a few hours to days after birth. The former has been termed a congenital anomaly and the latter an acquired patent urachus, but both may be observed from the time of birth.

In the absence of apparent infection, no treatment may be indicated, but affected foals are routinely placed on prophylactic antimicrobials. With an acquired patency (accompanied by local infection or septicemia), broad-spectrum systemic antimicrobial therapy is indicated; resolution of the umbilical infection is accompanied by closure of the urachus. Although application of an antiseptic solution several times may decrease the risk of infection, chemical cauterization to enhance closure of a congenital patent urachus is no longer recommended. Furthermore, chemical cauterization is contraindicated with local sepsis because it may lead to urachal rupture and uroperitoneum. If no decrease in urine leakage from the urachus is observed after a few days of prophylactic medical treatment or if ultrasonographic examination reveals abnormalities of multiple structures within the umbilicus, surgical exploration and resection of the affected urachus and umbilical vessels are usually pursued. Patent urachus also may increase the risk for fusion of the bladder to the abdominal wall at the umbilicus, which may lead to other problems of the lower urinary tract later in life.

2. What congenital anomalies/malformations of the equine urinary tract may lead to renal failure? Describe the management of each.

Congenital anomalies/malformations that may result in renal failure in horses include renal agenesis, renal hypoplasia, renal dysplasia, and polycystic kidney disease. **Renal agenesis** may be unilateral or bilateral. The more frequent descriptions of unilateral anomalies may simply reflect the incompatibility of bilateral agenesis with postnatal life. Unilateral defects may be incidental findings in otherwise healthy horses or may be detected during examination of the reproductive tract, since most are associated with anomalies of the reproductive system. Although no information suggests a hereditary basis in horses, renal agenesis can be a familial disorder in other species; thus it may be advisable to discourage repeat matings of dam and sire if the anomaly is detected.

Renal hypoplasia is diagnosed when one kidney is at least 50% smaller than normal or when the total renal mass is decreased by more than one-third. The anomaly may be confused with **renal dysplasia** (the term used to describe disorganized development of renal tissue due to anomalous differentiation, intrauterine ureteral obstruction, fetal viral infection, or exposure to teratogenic agents). Unilateral renal hypoplasia is usually accompanied by contralateral hypertrophy and normal renal function, whereas bilateral hypoplasia or dysplasia generally leads to chronic renal failure before 5 years of age. One or more renal cysts are occasionally discovered as incidental findings on necropsy examination.

In contrast, **polycystic kidney disease** is a disorder in which numerous cysts of variable sizes are found throughout the cortex and medulla. The condition has been reported in stillborn foals as well as in a few adult horses with chronic insufficiency. In humans, two forms of hereditary polycystic kidney disease have been described. Although a genetic cause has been proposed in some domestic animal species, patterns of inheritance have not been established.

3. What urinary tract problems may result in incontinence in young horses? Describe the management of each.

1. **Anomalous fusion of the bladder to the inner umbilical ring** may occur with absence of the urachus. This malformation precludes normal contraction and evacuation of the bladder, and megavesica or a markedly enlarged bladder may develop. The abdomen may become distended (requiring differentiation from uroperitoneum), and urinary incontinence is noted, especially when foals stand up or lie down. Surgical separation of the bladder from the umbilical ring may restore anatomic and functional integrity of the bladder.

2. **Abnormal distention of the bladder** in compromised neonatal foals, in the absence of anomalous fusion, also has been observed to cause incontinence (another example of overflow bladder). The problem typically resolves within a few days after placement of an indwelling bladder catheter and correction of other primary disease processes.

3. **Ectopic ureter** is a developmental anomaly in which a ureter terminates at a site other than the trigone of the bladder. The ectopic ureter may open into the urethra, vagina, or other part of the reproductive tract and results in incontinence from birth. Although the condition has been diagnosed more often in females than in males, it is unclear whether there is a true sex predilection or whether incontinence and perineal urine scalding are more easily recognized in females. Unless secondary problems such as urinary tract infection or hydronephrosis/pyelonephritis complicate the anomaly, there are usually no other clinical abnormalities and growth is unaffected. The aberrant opening(s) of the ureter can be observed in females via vaginal speculum examination if the ectopic ureter enters the genital tract or by endoscopy if it enters the bladder or urethra aberrantly. Alternatively, contrast excretory urography can be used to diagnose ectopic ureter, but this technique may not be as helpful in localizing the site of entry. With unilateral ectopic ureter, treatment options include unilateral nephrectomy or reimplantation of the ureter by ureterovesicular anastomosis. Bilateral ectopic ureters appear to carry a poorer prognosis, and surgical treatment is limited to ureterovesicular anastomosis.

4. What congenital anomalies/malformations of the equine urinary tract may result in uroperitoneum?

Uroperitoneum may result from bladder rupture during parturition in foals (most commonly males) or from urachal leakage/rupture secondary to infection of the umbilical structures (in both sexes). Retroperitoneal accumulation of urine and uroperitoneum also have been described in foals with ureteral and bladder defects that do not appear to be associated with trauma or sepsis. The cause of such defects is not known, but foals delivered from mares that have been supplemented during gestation with folic acid (as an adjunct treatment for equine protozoal myelitis) may be at greater risk. Ureteral defects may be unilateral or bilateral but have been limited to the proximal third of the ureter. Bladder defects are found in the dorsal or ventral bladder wall and are clinically indistinguishable from ruptured bladders. During surgical repair, however, detection of a smooth margin to the defects, in combination with a lack of appreciable inflammation, suggests anomalous development rather than a traumatic etiology.

5. What are the most common laboratory abnormalities in foals with uroperitoneum? Discuss diagnosis and treatment.

Uroperitoneum leads to a number of clinicopathologic abnormalities, including postrenal azotemia, hyponatremia, hypochloremia, hyperkalemia, and variable changes in acid-base status. Since the peritoneum allows fairly free exchange of uncharged or small molecules, azotemia and electrolyte abnormalities develop as urine (poor in sodium and chloride but rich in potassium) accumulates in the abdomen and effectively expands extracellular fluid volume. Equilibration of the expanded extracellular fluid volume with plasma results in loss of sodium and chloride from plasma into the peritoneal cavity. In contrast, plasma potassium concentration increases as potassium moves from the peritoneal cavity into the vascular space.

A diagnosis of uroperitoneum should be suspected on the basis of signalment (neonatal foal) and clinical signs (inappetance [i.e., loss of suckle], depression, tachycardia, tachypnea, and progressive abdominal distention); the diagnosis is confirmed by either ultrasonographic detection of free urine in the abdomen or documentation of a twofold or greater increase in creatinine concentration in abdominal fluid compared with serum. Measurement of the abdominal fluid-to-serum creatinine ratio is more accurate than the same ratio for urea, a small uncharged molecule that is more freely permeable across the peritoneal membrane. It is important to assess the severity of metabolic alterations in cases of uroperitoneum because hyperkalemia may lead to cardiac arrhythmias, especially when combined with the effects of general anesthetics such as halothane. Consequently, fluid therapy to correct the metabolic disturbances is often more important than immediate surgical correction of the bladder defect.

6. What congenital anomalies/malformations of the equine urinary tract may result in hematuria?

Anomalies of the vascular supply to the equine kidneys (arteriovenous and arterioureteral fistulas) are rare but may result in hematuria in young horses. In some cases the defect may fill with a thrombus and become silent, whereas in other cases significant anemia and/or ureteral obstruction and hydronephrosis may develop. With the latter complications unilateral nephrectomy may be a successful treatment option in nonazotemic patients if an abnormality can be detected via ultrasonographic examination or if hematuria is observed from only one of the ureters during cytoscopic examination.

7. What is different about equine urine in comparison with urine of other species?

Normal equine urine is cloudy and viscid rather than clear and thin. These properties can be attributed to large amounts of crystals and mucus, which also impart a deep yellow-to-tan color and an almost stringy consistency to normal horse urine. Crystals are predominantly calcium carbonate, but calcium phosphate and calcium oxalate crystals also can be found in normal equine urine. The abundance of crystals in horse urine reflects the comparatively greater role that the equine kidneys play in calcium excretion compared with other species. Enough crystals are often present in urine to create a sediment in the ventral aspect of the bladder between urinations, especially in horses fed alfalfa (which is high in calcium). Accumulations of crystalline material have been confused with bladder masses on both rectal and ultrasonographic assessment of the bladder and may form into large concretions (sabulous urolithiasis) with bladder paresis. The presence of this normal urine sediment explains why the character of urine often changes from a clearer, dark yellow to a thicker, milky fluid as urination progresses: crystals are passed to a much greater extent toward the end of urination. Similarly, frequent passage of small volumes of urine by mares in estrus may lead to coating of the perineum with whitish, crystalline material that may be confused with a purulent discharge from the reproductive tract. Mucus is secreted into the renal pelvis and proximal ureter from goblet cells and compound tubular mucus glands; horses have greater numbers of both than other species. Mucus protects ureteral and bladder mucosa from crystal deposition, which may occur rapidly on any area of traumatized or inflamed mucosa or on the surface of any device placed into the bladder lumen (e.g, a Foley catheter).

8. What may cause red urine in apparently normal horses?

The urine of some horses contains compounds (probably porphyrin-like molecules from forages) that can be oxidized after excretion into the environment. Oxidation may impart an orange-red-brown color to shavings or, more dramatically, to snow and occasionally prompts a complaint of hematuria in an otherwise healthy horse. To assuage owners' fears, the veterinarian should have them obtain a "free-catch" sample of urine, which will have normal coloration (i.e., deep yellow to tan).

9. What is the pH of equine urine? What factors influence urine pH?

Equine urine, like that of other herbivores but unlike that of small animals and humans, is alkaline with a normal pH of 8.0–8.5. Urine pH decreases to 7.0–8.0 with high-grain diets and when the flow rate is high (dilute urine). Similarly, foals that are normally polyuric because of the large water intake with a milk diet produce urine with a pH of ~ 7.0. Furthermore, urine may be transiently acidic after high-intensity exercise (racing) and with certain metabolic disorders (paradoxical aciduria with hypochloremic metabolic alkalosis).

10. What is the mechanism of paradoxical aciduria in the face of metabolic alkalosis?

Occasionally, aciduria is detected in a dehydrated or anorectic horse. Such patients typically have hypochloremic metabolic alkalosis. The mechanism for paradoxical aciduria appears to be similar to that described for ruminants with abomasal outflow obstruction. After all chloride has been reabsorbed from the glomerular filtrate, further sodium reabsorption occurs by exchange with (excretion of) potassium or hydrogen ions. Thus, paradoxical aciduria is most likely to occur with concomitant hypokalemia or whole-body potassium depletion.

11. What are the most common presenting complaints for horses with urinary tract disease?

Horses with urinary tract disease typically present for evaluation of weight loss or abnormal urination. Other clinical signs, which vary with the etiology and location of the problem, may include fever, anorexia, depression, ventral edema, oral ulceration, excessive dental tartar, colic, or scalding of the perineum or hindlegs. Weight loss and other systemic signs of disease usually indicate a problem of the upper urinary tract (kidneys and/or ureters), whereas abnormal urination more commonly signals lower urinary tract disease. Although lumbar pain and hindlimb lameness have been attributed to urinary tract disease, a musculoskeletal problem is the usual cause. A decrease in performance may be an early presenting complaint for renal disease, but poor performance probably results from changes accompanying uremia, such as mild anemia and lethargy, rather than from renal pain.

12. What methods for evaluation of the urinary tract are easier to perform in horses than in small animals?

In contrast to small animals, rectal palpation is a relatively easy and informative procedure that should be included in the evaluation of all horses with suspected urinary tract disease. The bladder can be palpated to determine size, wall thickness, and presence of cystic calculi, sabulous material, or mural masses. If the bladder is full, palpation may need to be repeated after bladder catheterization or voiding. The caudal pole of the left kidney can be palpated for size and texture. Ureters are generally not palpable unless enlarged or obstructed by disease, but the dorsal abdomen (retroperitoneal course of ureters) and trigone should be palpated to determine whether the ureters can be detected. Dilation of a ureter may occur with pyelonephritis or ureteral calculi, and in mares palpation of the distal ureters through the vaginal wall may be more rewarding. Furthermore, the ureters can be manually catheterized via the urethra in mares to collect urine samples from each side of the upper urinary tract (although this procedure is best performed endoscopically). The reproductive tract also can be palpated to assess whether a reproductive problem may be the cause of clinical signs. Although radiography of the urinary tract is more informative in small animals than horses, ultrasonography can be equally rewarding in both. Furthermore, endoscopic examination of the lower urinary tract is well tolerated by standing, sedated horses of both sexes, whereas general anesthesia is required to perform the procedure in small animals As well as allowing detailed examination of the urethra and bladder, endoscopy provides qualitative assessment of renal function by observation of flow and character of urine from each ureter. When indicated, ureteral catheterization is also accomplished fairly easily by passing sterile polyethylene tubing via the biopsy channel of the endoscope.

13. What are the two most commonly recognized waste products excreted in urine?

Urea and creatinine.

14. How is urea produced? What affects its concentration in blood? What is the importance of renal excretion?

Urea is produced in the liver from two ammonia ions that are liberated during catabolism of amino acids; for each urea molecule the carbon atom is derived from bicarbonate. Urea synthesized in the liver is released into the blood, and the kidneys are the major pathway of excretion. Urea production by the liver is proportional to dietary protein content; similarly, urinary urea excretion increases in parallel with urea production. Blood urea nitrogen (BUN) concentration depends on age, diet, rate of urea production, and renal function. A low BUN is typically found in neonatal foals because of an anabolic demand for amino acids. In contrast, when levels of dietary protein are higher or when urea is supplemented to the diet, BUN may increase twofold or greater. Urea excretion in urine also accounts for the majority of renal nitrogen elimination. Urea excretion is completely passive, and the high concentrations achieved in urine are merely a consequence of medullary tonicity produced by the countercurrent multiplier function of the loop of Henle. Thus, although variations in dietary protein intake lead to parallel changes in urea excretion, the idea that low-protein diets decrease the work load of the kidney is a fallacy. Urine urea concentration may vary from as low as 50 mg/dl in neonatal foals or horses with primary polydipsia to greater than 2500 mg/dl in normal horse on high-protein diets. Total daily urea excretion usually ranges between 100–300 gm/day in horses with normal renal function.

15. How is creatinine produced? What affects its concentration in blood? What is the importance of renal excretion?

Creatinine is produced by the nonenzymatic, irreversible cyclization and dehydration of creatine, which stores energy in the form of creatine phosphate in muscle and brain. Since 1–2% of the creatine pool is converted to creatinine daily, urinary excretion of creatinine is fairly constant. Creatinine is excreted primarily in urine, but the gastrointestinal (GI) tract provides a secondary route of excretion. In contrast to urea, enterohepatic recycling of creatinine does not occur, and the GI tract may represent a major route of excretion when renal function becomes compromised. Creatinine excreted by the GI tract is rapidly degraded by bacteria; little creatinine is found in feces. As with BUN, serum creatinine concentration may vary with age, level of activity, and renal function. In contrast, dietary protein intake has little influence on creatinine in horses. Newborn foals routinely have creatinine values that are 30–50% higher than values measured in the mare, and values as high as 20–30 mg/dl have been measured in some premature or asphyxiated foals. Such high values may result from immature renal function coupled with limited diffusion of creatinine across the placenta. If the foal appears healthy and all other laboratory values are within reference ranges, an initial creatinine in the range of 5–15 mg/dl should not cause alarm; values should decrease below 3.0 mg/dl with the first 3–5 days of life. After the first week of life, creatinine is actually lower in foals than adults because of the combined effect of rapid growth and the fact that skeletal muscles comprises a lesser percentage of body weight in foals than in adult horses. Other nonrenal factors that may influence creatinine include anorexia, rhabdomyolysis or muscle wasting consequent to disease, and exercise. Although anorexia may increase the measured value for creatinine, a substantial portion of this increase is actually due to other compounds that increase during periods of inappetance and are measured as noncreatinine chromagens in the commonly used Jaffé colorimetric assay for creatinine. In contrast, the increase in creatinine (50–100%) accompanying exercise probably results from the combination of increased release of creatine from muscle and decreased urinary creatinine excretion during the exercise bout. Creatinine is freely filtered at the glomerulus and is concentrated to values of 100–300 mg/dl in equine urine. The result is a total daily urinary excretion of 15–25 gm of creatinine. Only one-tenth as much nitrogen is excreted with creatinine as with urea.

16. Distinguish among azotemia, uremia, and renal failure.

Azotemia is the clinicopathologic abnormality of increased concentrations of urea nitrogen, creatinine, and/or other nonprotein nitrogenous substances in blood. Thus, azotemia is a laboratory finding.

Uremia and **uremic syndrome** describe the multisystemic disorder that results from the effects of uremic toxins on cell metabolism and function. Thus, uremia is the combination of azotemia and clinical signs associated with accumulation of nitrogenous wastes in the blood. Although uremic syndrome was originally attributed to the effects of increased BUN concentration, a number of nitrogenous compounds that accumulate with renal disease contribute to alterations in cell metabolism and function. In fact, the correlation between the severity of uremic syndrome and the magnitude of routine measures of azotemia (BUN and creatinine) is poor.

Renal failure is the term used when the kidneys no longer function adequately to maintain homeostasis. Classically, renal concentrating ability declines after two-thirds to three-fourths of nephrons have become impaired, and azotemia develops after three-fourth of functional renal capacity has been lost. Thus, a polyuric horse may have renal failure in the absence of azotemia or uremia. In such cases, the terms renal insufficiency or compromised renal function are often used interchangeably with renal failure. As the disease progresses, renal failure may be further manifested by development of mild azotemia even if clinical signs (uremia) remain absent. Finally, renal function also may be decreased in the absence of azotemia or any manifestation of renal disease. For example, a 50% decrease in glomerular filtration rate represents a significant decline in renal function; however, function remains adequate for maintenance of homeostasis. Although such cases are rarely detected clinically, they, too, would be described as compromised or impaired renal function.

17. Differentiate among prerenal, renal, and postrenal azotemia.

Azotemia may be prerenal (due to decreased renal perfusion), renal (associated with renal damage), or postrenal (accompanying obstructive diseases or uroperitoneum). Serum chemistry and urinalysis results should always be interpreted in light of hydration status and other presenting signs. For example, dehydration must be detected for azotemia to be deemed prerenal in origin, whereas signs of obstruction or abdominal distention (with uroperitoneum) are consistent with postrenal azotemia. Although no specific threshold values for BUN and creatinine concentrations differentiate renal disease from prerenal azotemia, the magnitude of azotemia is often greater with renal or postrenal azotemia.

Measures of urine concentration and urine-to-serum creatinine ratio provide useful information in the evaluation of azotemic patients. A high urine specific gravity (> 1.035) supports prerenal azotemia, whereas failure to concentrate urine in the face of dehydration supports a diagnosis of renal disease. Measurement of specific gravity is most valid in the urine sample voided before or immediately after fluid therapy is initiated, because successful fluid therapy leads to production of dilute urine. Urine-to-serum creatinine ratios in excess of 50:1 (reflecting concentrated urine) are expected in horses with prerenal azotemia, whereas ratios less than 37:1 were reported in horses with primary renal disease.

In addition to a low specific gravity, detection of proteinuria, glucosuria (in the absence of hyperglycemia), or pigmenturia on reagent strip analysis of urine provides further support that azotemia is renal in origin (in acute but not chronic renal failure). Further biochemical analysis of urine in horses with renal azotemia may reveal increased fractional clearances of sodium, chloride, and phosphorus and increased urinary enzyme activity (enzymuria). Casts and increased numbers of red blood cells may be detected on sediment examination. Finally, evidence to support a postrenal origin of azotemia is usually established by the presenting complaint or further diagnostic evaluation that reveals obstruction or disruption of the lower urinary tract.

18. What is the significance of the BUN-to-creatinine ratio?

Since creatinine is a charged molecule that is less permeable to membranes than urea, acute changes in renal function are more accurately reflected by increases in creatinine than in BUN (the increase in creatinine is proportionately greater than the increase in BUN). Thus the BUN-to-creatinine ratio has been used to differentiate acute from chronic renal insufficiency. With acute renal compromise (prerenal azotemia or acute renal failure), BUN-to-creatinine ratios less than 10:1 are expected, whereas the ratio often exceeds 15:1 with chronic renal failure. Although it may be useful to assess the BUN-to-creatinine ratio, it is not always reliable because BUN may vary considerably with dietary protein intake in horses with chronic renal disease. In such cases, the BUN-to-creatinine ratio also may be used to assess adequacy of dietary protein intake: a value < 10:1 suggests inadequate dietary protein, whereas values > 15:1 suggest that dietary protein intake may be excessive and possibly aggravating the degree of uremia.

19. What is the best measure of renal function?

Glomerular filtration rate (GFR) is considered the best measure of renal function in all species. Classically, GFR must decrease by 75% to result in an increase in serum concentrations of urea or creatinine; thus, the latter are relatively insensitive measures of renal function. Unfortunately, measurement of GFR is often impractical because it requires either a timed urine collection or collection of several blood samples over time to determine the clearance of exogenous (inulin) or endogenous (creatinine) substances by their rate of appearance in urine or rate of disappearance from blood (only exogenous substances).

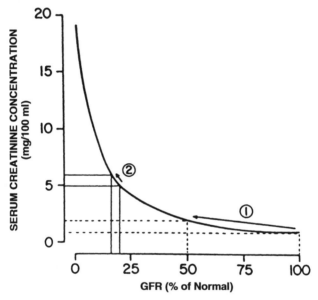

Relationship between GFR and serum creatinine concentration. When renal function is normal, a large decrease in GFR (as with acute renal failure) results in a relatively minor increase in serum creatinine concentration *(arrow 1)*. In contrast, when renal function is decreased (as with chronic renal failure), a much smaller decrease in GFR results in a similar increase in serum creatinine concentration *(arrow 2)*. (From Brezis M, Rosen S, Epstein FH: Acute renal failure. In Brenner BM, Rector FC (eds): The Kidney, vol. 1, 4th ed. Philadelphia, W.B. Saunders, 1991, p 994, with permission.)

20. How is GFR measured in horses?

By definition, GFR is the volume of plasma filtered per unit time and is commonly described in units of ml/min/kg body weight. The GFR of horses and ponies ranges from 1.6–2.0 ml/min/kg; some authors report slightly higher values in ponies. The range is similar in other animals and humans. For a 500-kg horse, a GFR of 1.6–2.0 ml/min/kg equals 800–1000 ml/min or ~ 1200–1400 L/day and represents filtration of the total plasma volume 60–70 times per day. Since urine production is about 10 L/day, more than 99% of the glomerular filtrate is reabsorbed.

Various methods are available to quantitate GFR in horses. Basically, they can separated into plasma disappearance curves or clearance studies involving use of timed urine collections. Generation of plasma disappearance curves requires collection of an initial blood sample, intravenous administration of one of a number of compounds (inulin, creatinine, sodium sulfanilate, phenolsulfonphthalein [phenol red]), or radionuclides), and collection of a series of further blood samples over the subsequent 60–90 minutes. Results can be expressed in terms of an elimination half-life in minutes or as clearance values in ml/min/kg. More traditionally, GFR has been determined by use of timed urine collection periods (to measure urine flow rate) and measurement of plasma and urine concentrations of a test compound. Ideally, the urine collection period should span 24 hours, although for practicality shorter collection periods may be used. All urine produced during the study period is collected, the total volume is recorded, and an aliquot is assayed for the test substance. Similarly, the concentration of the test substance is measured in a blood sample collected near the midpoint of the urine collection period.

For urine collections of 12–24 hours, endogenous creatinine is measured because it is the only substance that does not require administration of a continuous intravenous infusion during the collection period. Although convenient, use of endogenous creatinine typically underestimates GFR because noncreatinine chromagens in plasma artifactually increase plasma creatinine concentration. On the other hand, significant tubular secretion of creatinine may develop as one of the compensatory responses to renal failure and may lead to overestimation of GFR. To avoid these limitations, a number of other filtration markers (inulin, exogenous creatinine, or radionuclides) can be administered as an intravenous infusion throughout the urine collection period. The infusion is started as a bolus to increase the plasma concentration of the test substance to the desired level and subsequently continued as a steady infusion throughout the remainder of the collection period. This type of study is usually performed for a shorter period with the horse restrained in stocks. The bladder should be emptied at the start of the study, and two to three 30-minute urine collection period are subsequently performed. A catheter should be passed, and the bladder should be completely emptied at the end of each 30-minute period. After urine volumes are measured, an aliquot of each urine sample and a blood sample collected at the midpoint of each urine collection period are assayed for the test substance. GFR is calculated as the mean value for the two or three collection periods.

21. What are the most commonly used and most practical clinical measures for assessment of renal function?

Since this test is widely available, **measurement of serum concentrations of BUN and creatinine** is the most common method for clinical assessment of renal function. Furthermore, serial determination of BUN and creatinine during the initial 24–48 hours of therapy provides much greater information about the nature and prognosis of the renal disorder than a single measurement of GFR.

Another readily available measure of renal function is **urine concentration**, usually determined as specific gravity or, more accurately, as osmolality. In a dehydrated horse, assessment of urine concentration is a simple and fairly reliable way to discriminate between prerenal azotemia (concentrated urine with specific gravity of 1.035–1.050 or an osmolality of 900–1500 mOsm/kg) and renal azotemia (dilute urine with specific gravity of 1.005–1.020 or an osmolality of 300–600 mOsm/kg). Unfortunately, most dehydrated equine do not void a urine sample until they have received 10–30 L of fluids during the first few hours of treatment, and fluid therapy typically leads to production of dilute urine. Thus, in most instances adequacy of renal function is assessed by the degree to which azotemia resolves after the initial 12–24 hours of fluid therapy.

Finally, probably the most practical means of assessing renal function in an azotemic, dehydrated horse is **watching for urination in response to fluid therapy**. One of the earliest indicators of acute renal failure, besides dilute urine if an admission sample is obtained, is failure to produce urine within 6 hours after initiation of fluid therapy.

22. What is the normal daily urine production for a horse? What is the normal urine concentration?

Most normal horses produce 5–15 L of urine daily; however, considerable variation may be observed both within an individual horse and between horses under different management regimens. Since the bladder can easily accommodate up to 4 L, horses typically urinate 2–4 times daily. Since over 99% of filtered water is usually reabsorbed in the renal tubules, a small decrease (from 99% to 98% water reabsorption) can result in a dramatic increase in urine production (from 10 to 20 L/day).

Normal urine is typically about 3–4 times more concentrated than plasma (urine specific gravity of 1.030–1.040 or osmolality of 900–1200 mOsm/kg); as with volume, however, wide variation may be observed. Since the kidneys are responsible for fine tuning of water balance, dilute urine or hyposthenuria (specific gravity < 1.010 or osmolality < 300 mOsm/kg) may be detected in horses at pasture (high water content of feed), whereas concentrated urine (specific gravity > 1.035 or osmolality > 1200 mOsm/kg) is expected for hay-fed horses under hot and humid environmental conditions. Similarly, urine is typically quite dilute (specific gravity ~1.005 or osmolality ~200 mOsm/kg) in nursing foals because of the large volumes of milk ingested (250 ml/kg/day). Diets high in protein (alfalfa hay) also increase daily nitrogen intake and urea production and lead to increases in urine volume without a concomitant decrease in urine concentration (because a large daily solute load must be excreted by the kidneys).

With renal disease the ability to produce either concentrated or dilute urine is lost. Thus, horses with chronic renal failure typically manifest isosthenuria: production of urine with an osmolality similar to that of serum (specific gravity of 1.008–1.014). Other disorders that may result in a decreased ability to concentrate urine include pituitary or hypothalamic diseases leading to central diabetes insipidus, diabetes mellitus, septicemia or endotoxemia, washout of the medullary interstitium (with primary polydipsia), or nephrogenic diabetes insipidus.

23. What role do the equine kidneys play in daily water balance?

The kidneys are responsible for fine tuning of body water content to maintain plasma osmolality within a relatively narrow range (270–290 mOsm/kg). Precise balance of body water content is achieved by matching daily water intake with water loss. Water is provided from three sources: (1) drinking, (2) water in feed, and (3) metabolic water. Drinking is the major source of daily water (about 85%), but feed and metabolic water provide about 5% and 10%, respectively. Water is lost by three routes: (1) in urine, (2) in feces, and (3) as insensible losses (evaporation) across the skin and respiratory tract. Horses have a maintenance water requirement of 60–65 ml/kg/day (27–30 L/day for a 500-kg horse). Drinking provides about 50 ml/kg/day. Under mild ambient conditions, urinary and fecal water losses range from 20–55% and 30–55%, respectively, of the total daily water loss. The remaining insensible loss accounts for up to 15–40% of daily water loss. Drinking and renal water excretion are the mechanisms by which water balance is finely tuned. However, they vary widely among individual horses and are also influenced by age, environmental conditions, level of exercise, and diet.

24. What regulates water intake (thirst) and urine concentration?

The two main stimuli for thirst are (1) an increase in plasma osmolality (normal value: ~270–300 mOsm/kg) and (2) hypovolemia and/or hypotension. The former is mediated through osmoreceptors in the hypothalamus, which have a rather high threshold for activation (about 295 mOsm/kg). Hemodynamic stimuli are mediated by both low- and high-pressure baroreceptors. Both osmotic and hemodynamic stimuli may produce a dipsogenic effect, in part by activation of a local renin-angiotensin-aldosterone system in the central nervous system.

Urine concentration is controlled primarily by the action of antidiuretic hormone (ADH; also called arginine vasopressin) on the collecting ducts. ADH is produced in the neurosecretory neurons of the supraoptic nuclei, packaged in granules, and transported down axons for storage in the neurohypophysis (pars nervosa or posterior pituitary). An increase in plasma osmolality and hypovolemia and/or hypotension are the stimuli for ADH release. Osmoreceptors for ADH release are also located in the hypothalamus, adjacent to the osmoreceptors mediating thirst. Activation of these receptors is the signal for ADH release from the neurohypophysis. These osmoreceptors are not equally sensitive to all plasma solutes. For example, increases in plasma sodium concentration and infusion of mannitol are potent stimuli, whereas increases in plasma glucose and urea concentrations are weak stimuli. These differences have led to the suggestion that osmoreceptor activation is caused by an osmotic water shift producing cell shrinkage (which is greater for sodium and mannitol than for glucose or urea). The threshold for ADH release is lower (270–285 mOsm/kg) than that for thirst. Once released, ADH acts on V_2-receptors on the basolateral membrane of collecting duct epithelial cells, leading to insertion of water channels (transmembrane proteins) in the apical membrane. These channels increase the water permeability of the apical membranes and thereby lead to increased water reabsorption. Action of V_2-receptors is mediated via activation of adenyl cyclase and a stimulatory transmembrane G protein. Of interest, V_2-receptor activation can be antagonized by activation of adjacent α_2-adrenoreceptors and by a prostaglandin E_2-mediated effect on an inhibitory G protein. Although effects of these antagonists vary with species and have not been well studied in horses, it is likely that the diuresis associated with administration of α_2-agonists (e.g., xylazine, detomidine) to horses may be attributed to ADH antagonism of the collecting duct.

To summarize, ADH release leading to increased renal water absorption may be viewed as the initial line of defense against a mild increase in plasma osmolality, whereas thirst and drinking are a secondary response to even greater increases in plasma osmolality.

25. How is urinary concentrating ability assessed in horses?

Urinary concentrating ability can be assessed by water deprivation and/or ADH challenge tests. **Water deprivation** is a simple test to determine whether polyuria is due to primary (psychogenic) polydipsia or central or nephrogenic diabetes insipidus (DI). A water deprivation test should not be performed in an animal that is clinically dehydrated or azotemic. A baseline urinalysis and measurement of BUN and creatinine concentrations and body weight should be performed before removal of water (food does not necessarily need to be removed). Urine specific gravity and weight loss are measured after 12 (usually overnight) and 24 hours. Horses with normal renal function typically produce urine with a specific gravity > 1.045 and an osmolality > 1500 mOsm/kg in response to water deprivation of 24–72 hours. Practically the test can be be stopped when specific gravity reaches 1.025 or greater and should be stopped if more than 5% of body weight is lost or dehydration becomes apparent. Horses with long-standing primary polydipsia may not be able to concentrate urine fully (to a specific gravity > 1.025). It is of little benefit to extend the test period beyond 24 hours in such patients. However, affected horses should respond to water deprivation more favorably, producing urine with a higher specific gravity after a period of partial water deprivation (termed a modified water deprivation test) during which daily water intake is restricted to 40 ml/kg for several days. Horses with central or nephrogenic DI cannot concentrate urine in response to a water deprivation test. When DI is suspected, patients should be monitored every few hours because significant dehydration may develop within 6 hours of water deprivation.

In the absence of azotemia or clinical signs of renal failure, an inability to concentrate urine in response to water deprivation supports a diagnosis of DI. However, the test does not distinguish between central and nephrogenic forms. The two can be differentiated by **exogenous administration of ADH**. Typically, intramuscular administration of 0.2 IU/kg of exogenous ADH should produce an increase in specific gravity to > 1.025 for 12 or more hours in horses with central DI, whereas little-to-no response is observed with nephrogenic DI.

26. What is a Hickey-Hare test?

A Hickey-Hare test is an intravenous hypertonic saline challenge that can be used to evaluate horses with polyuria. The goal is to produce an increase in plasma osmolality that triggers release of endogenous ADH and leads to an increase in urine concentration. One protocol is to measure plasma osmolality and endogenous ADH concentrations before and within 30 minutes after administration of 1–2 ml/kg of a 7.5% sodium chloride solution. Horses with primary polydipsia or nephrogenic DI respond with an increased plasma ADH concentration, whereas horses with central DI do not. Urine specific gravity is not expected to increase in response to hypertonic saline administration with either form of DI, but it should increase with primary polydipsia. However, because assays for plasma ADH concentration are not commercially available and because water deprivation is simple to perform, the Hickey-Hare test is rarely used as a diagnostic tool.

27. What role do the equine kidneys play in daily solute balance?

Renal function is traditionally viewed in terms of glomerular filtration, tubular modification of the filtered fluid, and excretion of final urine. This concept accommodates excretion of nitrogenous and organic wastes and the major aspects of regulation of body water content and ionic balance. However, the final urine concentration and volume are also affected by solute excretion. Another way to think about renal function, therefore, is in terms of total solute and water excretion. For example, a horse may produce 6 L of urine daily with an osmolality of 900 mOsm/kg to excrete 5400 mosmoles of solute. If the solute load is doubled to 10,800 mosmoles (e.g., by adding ~ 150 gm of sodium chloride to the diet of a 500-kg horse), 6 L of urine with an osmolality of 1800 mOsm/kg or 12 L of urine with an osmolality of 900 mOsm/kg must be produced to eliminate the additional solute. Thus, urine osmolality reflects the kidney's ability to dilute or concentrate the final urine but does not necessarily provide an accurate estimate of the quantitative ability to excrete solute or retain water. These functions are assessed by calculation of the osmolal (C_{osm}) and free water clearances (C_{H_2O}) and require measurement of urine flow (via timed urine collection) and measurement of both plasma and urine osmolality.

Measures of renal solute and water handling can be conceptualized by considering urine to have two components: one component contains all of the urinary solute in a solution that is isosmotic to plasma (C_{osm}, usually in ml/min or L/day), and the other contains free water with no solute (C_{H_2O} in ml/min or L/day). The sum of these two components is the actual urine flow rate in ml/min or L/day. Since urine is typically more concentrated than plasma, C_{H_2O} typically has a negative value indicative of water conservation. In fact, the inverse of free water clearance is termed renal water reabsorption.

In the above example, excretion of 5400 osmoles requires production of 18 L of urine that is isosmotic with plasma (using a value of 300 mOsm/kg for plasma). However, since 6 L of concentrated urine was actually produced during the time period measured, the kidneys have quantitatively reabsorbed 12 L/day of free water. In contrast, excretion of 10,800 mosmoles requires production of 36 L of urine isosmotic with plasma. Free water clearance is –30 L/day, or 30 L/day of free water is reabsorbed by the kidneys. Thus, although concentrated urine always has a negative value for C_{H_2O}, indicative of renal water reabsorption, and dilute urine always has a positive value for C_{H_2O}, indicative of renal water excretion, quantitative assessment of renal solute and water handling requires measurement of both C_{osm} and C_{H_2O}.

Consideration of the role of the kidneys in excreting a solute load is helpful in understanding water balance in patients with compromised renal function or DI. The ability to excrete an increased solute load may be difficult for horses with a decreased GFR (chronic renal failure), and water retention accompanying the additional solute may lead to edema. Similarly, in patients with DI that cannot concentrate urine, a doubling of the solute load doubles urine output, whereas urine osmolality remains unchanged.

28. What role do the equine kidneys play in daily electrolyte balance?

Intake and loss of electrolytes (like water) must be appropriately matched to maintain body content of electrolytes within relatively narrow ranges. This balance is most important for the exchangeable ions (sodium, potassium, and chloride) because they have minimal tissue (skeletal) reserves for times of need. Electrolytes are provided from three sources: (1) feed, (2) water (usually minimal amounts), and (3) dietary supplements. Electrolytes are also lost by three routes: (1) urine, (2) feces, and (3) sweat (insensible losses).

Horses on a predominantly hay or pasture diet ingest excessive potassium and chloride. In contrast, sodium intake is variable and often marginal. Urinary excretion is the major route for loss of potassium and chloride. Similarly, when excessive sodium is fed, urinary excretion is also the major route of elimination. Thus, on a marginal sodium diet urinary electrolyte concentrations tend to be high for potassium (200–400 mEq/L, intermediate for chloride (25–100 mEq/L), and low for sodium. (undetectable to 10 mEq/L). Although the maintenance sodium requirement for horses is 0.4–0.8 mEq/kg/day (or 200–400 mEq/day [6–12 gm/day] for a 500-kg horse), horses in training have greater dietary sodium and chloride requirements because they lose considerable amounts of sodium in sweat and also may be treated with furosemide. Daily supplementation with 50–75 gm of common salt (sodium chloride [NaCl]) provides 850–1275 mEq (since 1 gm of NaCl provides ~ 17 mEq of both Na^+ and Cl^-); it is a safe and economic method of providing additional sodium and chloride to athletic horses.

Although dietary intake of potassium is usually excessive, equine kidneys do not appear to have a great capacity to conserve potassium during periods of food deprivation or anorexia. Thus, urinary potassium concentration and total excretion can remain substantial in the face of decreased intake. Consequently, horses with decreased feed intake may develop significant total body potassium depletion and, in addition to supplementation with NaCl, often benefit from supplemental oral or nasogastric potassium administration (25–50 gm/day of potassium chloride [KCl] provides 350–700 mEq/L since 1 gm KCL provides ~ 14 mEq of both K^+ and Cl^-).

Finally, in comparison with water intake, salt appetite of horses does not appear to be as closely regulated to balance intake and losses. In fact, when free-choice salt is available, horses often consume more than the maintenance requirement. The excess is eliminated by increasing urinary electrolyte excretion. Although this apparently excessive salt appetite may not seem appropriate, it also may be considered an advantageous response in an exercising horse, which has a greater daily salt requirement.

29. How is electrolyte balance clinically assessed in horses?

As for water and solute, accurate assessment of electrolyte balance requires determination of daily electrolyte intake and output. This determination, in turn, requires knowledge of the electrolyte content of feed, water, and supplements as well as collection of all urine and feces over a 24-hour period. Electrolyte excretion can subsequently be expressed in absolute terms as mEq/day or in terms of the amount of plasma completely cleared of the electrolyte per unit of time (electrolyte clearance). However, a more practical method of assessing electrolyte balance is calculation of fractional electrolyte clearances, which can be determined from urine and plasma samples collected at the same time (timed urine collection can be avoided). Fractional electrolyte clearances are calculated by expressing electrolyte clearance as a percentage of endogenous creatinine clearance, an estimate of GFR that remains stable since delivery of creatinine to the kidneys is relatively constant. The clearance of A (electrolyte or creatinine) is measured as follows:

$$\text{Clearance A} = \frac{[A] \text{ urine}}{[A] \text{ plasma}} \times \text{urine flow}$$

Fractional electrolyte clearance is determined by dividing electrolyte clearance by creatinine clearance and multiplying by 100%:

$$\text{Fractional clearance}_{elec} = \frac{\dfrac{[electrolyte] \text{ urine}}{[electrolyte] \text{ plasma}} \times \text{urine flow}}{\dfrac{[creatinine] \text{ urine}}{[creatinine] \text{ plasma}} \times \text{urine flow}} \times 100\%$$

By rearrangement and cancellation of urine flow from the numerator and denominator, this equation becomes:

$$\text{Fractional clearance}_{elec} = \frac{[electrolyte] \text{ urine}}{[electrolyte] \text{ plasma}} \times \frac{[creatinine] \text{ plasma}}{[creatinine] \text{ urine}} \times 100\%$$

The equine kidneys reabsorb more more than 99% of filtered sodium and chloride, whereas little potassium is conserved. Thus, normal fractional clearance values are less than 1% for sodium and chloride and range from 15–65% for potassium. Values exceeding 1% for sodium and chloride indicate excessive dietary supplementation, whereas a fractional potassium clearance value toward the lower end of the normal range is expected for an anorectic horse. A note of caution is warranted when ion-specific electrodes (instead of a flame photometer) are used to measure urinary potassium concentration because components of equine urine may interfere with the ion-specific electrode and lead to falsely low values. This problem can usually be avoided by performing the analysis on urine diluted with water. Finally, intravenous fluids, certain medications (e.g., furosemide), and low-intensity exercise can result in increases in urine flow and lead to false elevations in fractional sodium and chloride clearances.

30. How is assessment of fractional clearance values useful in horses with renal failure?

Electrolyte reabsorption and secretion are functions of renal tubules; thus, fractional electrolyte clearances can be used to assess renal tubular dysfunction in renal failure. Fractional clearances of sodium, chloride, and phosphorus (FCl_{Na}, FCl_{Cl}, and FCL_P) typically increase to values $> 1\%$ in horses with acute renal failure, and FCl_{Na} may approach 10% in severe cases. However, urine samples used for electrolyte measurement must be collected before fluid therapy is initiated because administration of polyionic fluids increases electrolyte clearances in normal horses. In cases of chronic renal failure that are relatively stable, FCl_{Na}, FCl_{Cl}, and FCl_P are usually within normal ranges because of compensation by remaining nephrons.

31. How can fractional clearance values be used to assess the calcium/phosphorus balance in the diet of young horses?

The equine kidneys play an important role in calcium/phosphorus homeostasis, and renal loss of these ions varies with dietary intake. Fractional clearances of calcium and phosphorus (FCl_{Ca} and FCl_P), therefore, can be used to assess adequacy of dietary intake. Although diet is evaluated more appropriately on a herd basis by feed analyses of hay and concentrates, fractional clearances may be useful in the individual horse or when feed analysis is impractical (e.g., forage consists of pasture). For example, excessive dietary phosphorus intake (which may lead to nutritional secondary hyperparathyroidism) leads to an increase in FCl_P. Evaluation of FCl_{Ca} is hampered by the fact that the majority of calcium in equine urine is in the form of calcium carbonate crystals. To determine a reliable measure of urinary calcium concentration, the entire contents of the bladder must be collected during voiding or via catheterization to ensure that both initial crystal-poor and final crystal-rich fractions are collected. Subsequently, a well-mixed aliquot of urine is treated with acetic or nitric acid to solubilize the crystals. FCl_{Ca} values $> 2.5\%$ and FCl_P values $< 4\%$ are considered to be consistent with adequate dietary intake (adequate calcium intake with phosphorus intake that is not excessive). However, because rather wide ranges for FCl_{Ca} and FCl_P have been reported for normal horses, use of fractional clearances may not be sensitive enough to detect minor dietary imbalances.

32. How is assessment of fractional clearance values useful in horses with recurrent rhabdomyolysis?

Determination of fractional electrolyte clearance values has been advocated in the evaluation of horses with recurrent rhabdomyolysis because low sodium and potassium clearances have been reported in some affected horses. Whether these low fractional clearance values reflect total body electrolyte depletion (as a consequence of repeated bouts of exercise in hot weather) or a true predisposition to rhabdomyolysis has not been determined. Nevertheless, low fractional clearance values document the need for electrolyte supplementation in equine athletes. Another population of horses with recurrent rhabdomyolysis may have an increase in fractional phosphorus clearance, which has been reported to respond to dietary supplementation with ground limestone. Thus, although determination of fractional electrolyte clearances may be a useful adjunct in the evaluation of horses with recurrent rhabdomyolysis, only a small portion of affected horses are likely to show significant clinical improvement in response to dietary electrolyte supplementation alone.

33. What are the most common causes of acute renal failure (ARF) in horses?

ARF is a clinical syndrome characterized by a sustained decrease in GFR that results in azotemia and disturbances in fluid, electrolyte, and acid-base homeostasis. In horses, ARF is most commonly due to hemodynamic or nephrotoxic insults. A reduction in renal blood flow (RBF) usually accompanies acute enterocolitis, severe colic, endotoxemia/septicemia, acute blood loss, or prolonged exercise and leads to decreases in GFR and urine output. If the decrements in RBF and GFR are severe and/or prolonged, ischemic injury to renal tubules and interstitium may occur, resulting in hemodynamically mediated ARF. Important nephrotoxins include antimicrobials (primarily aminoglycosides and, to a lesser degree, tetracyclines, sulfonamides, cephalosporins, and polymixin B), nonsteroidal antiinflammatory drugs (NSAIDs), endogenous pigments (myoglobin or hemoglobin), heavy metals (mercury in counterirritants or blisters, lead, arsenic, cadmium, and gold), vitamin D or K (menadione), blister beetles (cantharidin), and acorns. Acute glomerulonephritis (a component of immune-mediated vasculitis syndromes, including purpura hemorrhagica), interstitial nephritis associated with septicemia or ascending renal infections, leptospirosis, and renal microvascular injury (hemolytic uremic-like syndrome) are less common causes of ARF.

34. What is the mechanism of aminoglycoside nephrotoxicity?

Nephrotoxicity results from accumulation of aminoglycosides within the renal cortex. After filtration at the glomerulus, aminoglycoside antimicrobials bind to phospholipids on the brush border of proximal tubular cells and are subsequently reabsorbed. Accumulation of aminoglycosides in proximal tubular cells interferes with lysosomal, mitochondrial, and sodium-potassium-adenosine triphosphatase function. Binding to the brush border is saturable; thus, sustained exposure of proximal tubular cells to the drug, as may occur with multiple daily dosing regimens and/or prolonged use, results in greater accumulation and increased nephrotoxicity. Therefore, a once-daily dosing regimen that results in high peak concentrations and low trough concentrations in serum maintains, or even improves, therapeutic efficacy and should attenuate the risk of nephrotoxicosis.

35. What is the mechanism of NSAID nephrotoxicity?

Although NSAIDs are more likely to result in clinical problems of the GI tract than the kidneys, ARF has been reported as a complication of both high doses of phenylbutazone (4–8 gm/day) and routine doses in dehydrated patients. Along with the beneficial effect of blocking prostaglandin production at sites of inflammation, NSAIDs also suppress renal prostaglandin synthesis. Although prostaglandins (PGs) play only a minor role in maintenance of RBF in the normal state, PGE_2 and PGI_2 are important vasodilatory mediators of autoregulation of RBF under conditions of renal hypoperfusion. Thus, administration of NSAIDs to dehydrated or toxemic patients may further contribute to ischemic renal injury by exacerbating a decrease in RBF. Furthermore, the renal medulla receives less than 20% of total RBF. As a consequence, the inner medullary tissue normally functions in a relatively hypoxic environment, and the lesion associated with NSAID toxicity is renal medullary crest or papillary necrosis.

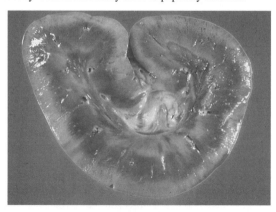

Equine kidney following acute renal failure after NSAID administration and "tying up."

36. How is measurement of urinary enzyme activity useful in assessing nephrotoxicity of certain medications?

Renal tubules are metabolically active; they are responsible for absorption or excretion of a wide range of substances. Transport of these compounds is facilitated by a number of enzymes, which are found in large amounts in lysosomes within or in the luminal brush borders of tubular epithelial cells. Regular turnover of these cells and release of endocytotic vesicles and lysosomes into the tubular lumen result in enzyme activity in urine (enzymuria). In horses, normal values have been established for activities of gammaglutamyl transferase (GGT), alkaline phosphatase (AP), N-acetyl-b-D-glucosaminidase (NAG), lactate dehydrogenase (LDH), and kallikrein. Inflammation or necrosis of tubular epithelial cells results in elevated urinary activity of lysosomal and brush border enzymes.

GGT is a membrane-associated enzyme found primarily in the brush border of the proximal tubular epithelium. Its activity in distal tubular epithelium is negligible. Although elevations in serum GGT activity are typically associated with hepatic disease, GGT is not filtered at the glomerulus; thus, elevated activity in urine is presumed to originate from the kidneys. To correct for urine concentration, values for urine GGT activity are expressed as a ratio of urine GGT activity per gram of urine creatinine (Cr) concentration using the following formula;

$$GGT/Cr = \frac{GGT \text{ activity in urine (IU/L)}}{\text{Urine Cr (mg/dl)}} \times 0.01$$

A value < 25 is considered normal. Determination of GGT-to-Cr ratio in equine urine has been advocated as an early indicator of proximal tubular damage as well as a tool for monitoring horses on nephrotoxic drug therapy. Unfortunately, elevated urine GGT-to-Cr ratios can be found with dehydration and after the initial dose or two of nephrotoxic medications. Thus, although results may reflect renal tubular damage, in practical situations the ratio has sometimes been considered too sensitive and is not currently used as much as when the test was originally described. However, in studies of gentamicin nephrotoxicity, GGT-to-Cr ratios exceeding 100 IU/gm were consistently found to precede increases in serum creatinine concentration. Thus, such values warrant reassessment of aminoglycoside usage (including measurement of peak and trough concentrations via therapeutic drug monitoring) and hydration status of the patient. LDH is a more ubiquitous tubular epithelial enzyme than GGT; it is as active in distal tubules and medullary papillae as in proximal tubular epithelium. Consequently, urine LDH activity has been studied in conjunction with NSAID nephrotoxicity but is not currently in clinical use.

37. Is it safe to give gentamicin to a dehydrated patient?

This is a common concern among equine clinicians, but the answer is clearly yes. Since gentamicin nephrotoxicosis is a cumulative toxicity, minimal damage is associated with gentamicin administration, even in an azotemic patient. Especially in a septicemic neonatal foal, delay in administration of the aminoglycoside during the initial hours of hospitalization (while fluid therapy is pursued) may increase the severity and potentiate complications of sepsis. If azotemia persists, antimicrobial usage may be changed or the gentamicin dosage interval prolonged (without decreasing the dose) in conjunction with measurement of trough serum gentamicin concentrations using therapeutic drug monitoring techniques.

38. What are positive and negative prognostic factors in horses with ARF?

The prognosis for ARF in horses depends on the underlying cause, duration of renal failure, response to initial treatment, and development of secondary complications such as laminitis, thrombophlebitis, and diarrhea. Regardless of the cause, duration of renal failure before initiation of therapy is one of the most important determinants of prognosis. In addition to prompt recognition and treatment, other positive prognostic factors are young age, suspected nephrotoxic cause, lack of oliguria, and rapid (within first 12 hours) induction of polyuria in response to intravenous fluid therapy. Negative prognostic factors include older age, suspected hemodynamic/ischemic cause, persistent oliguria/anuria, concurrent sepsis, and history of preexisting renal disease.

39. What is the expected response to fluid therapy in an azotemic horse?

The expected response to fluid therapy in patients with prerenal azotemia (serum creatinine typically < 5 mg/dl) is rapid resolution of azotemia over the initial day or two of treatment. Patients with a favorable prognosis for recovery from intrinsic ARF (serum creatinine may range from 5–15 mg/dl) have a more gradual decline in serum creatinine over 3–7 days. When oliguric ARF persists past the initial 48–72 hours of treatment, the prognosis is poor even with dialysis. Azotemia in such cases is usually severe (creatinine may exceed 15 mg/dl), and the incidence of serious complications, including thrombophlebitis and laminitis, is high.

40. What is the approach to treatment of oliguric ARF?

In most horses with prerenal and renal azotemia, initial treatment consists of large volumes of intravenous fluids for the primary disease (e.g., duodenitis-proximal jejunitis, enterocolitis, colic), and oliguria typically progresses to polyuria. However, when significant renal damage has been sustained, persistence of oliguric ARF is usually recognized as failure to produce a significant volume of urine in response to fluid therapy, along with minimal change in the degree of azotemia over the initial day of treatment. If patients are not carefully monitored (ideally by serial measurement of body weight or central venous pressure), fluid retention may lead to development of subcutaneous and pulmonary edema. Other clinical signs may include tachycardia, hyperemic mucous membranes, pyrexia, mild colic, laminitis, and occasionally neurologic deficits.

When oliguria persists after rehydration, treatment with diuretics and/or vasodilators may be attempted. **Mannitol** (0.25–1.0 gm/kg as a 20% solution administered IV over 15–20 minutes), furosemide (0.5–2.0 mg/kg IV every 3–6 hours), or dopamine (3–5 μg/kg/min IV in 5% dextrose solution) have been advocated for treatment of oliguric ARF. As an osmotic diuretic, mannitol decreases cell swelling, increases tubular flow, and helps to prevent tubular obstruction or collapse. Mannitol also may improve RBF and GFR by vasodilatory effects that are mediated via prostaglandin synthesis or by inducing release of atrial natriuretic peptide.

The use of an osmotic diuretic agent is contraindicated in an overhydrated patient because the associated increase in intravascular volume may precipitate pulmonary edema. **Furosemide** is a potent diuretic agent that acts by blocking the sodium-potassium-chloride cotransporter in the ascending limb of the loop of Henle. However, furosemide must be filtered at the glomerulus to exert its action in the tubule; consequently, patients with intrinsic ARF and marked decreases in GFR may respond poorly. Patients who respond to furosemide require close observation for exacerbations of volume depletion, which potentiate an ischemic or toxic insult. For example, furosemide administration has been demonstrated to exacerbate gentamicin toxicity and probably should be avoided in patients with ARF caused by aminoglycoside usage.

Dopamine is a potent renal vasodilating agent that acts via specific dopamine receptors on renal arterioles. It is best administered with an infusion pump through a separate intravenous line. Addition of 120 mg of dopamine to 1 L of 0.9% NaCl or 5% dextrose results in a dopamine concentration of 120 μg/ml. A 500-kg horse requires 12.5 ml of this solution per minute (i.e., 750 ml/hour) for a desired infusion rate of 3 μg/kg/min. Although this recommended infusion rate has minimal effects on systemic hemodynamics, dopamine may induce arrhythmias. Therefore, heart rate and rhythm should be monitored regularly during infusion.

Administration of **furosemide in combination with dopamine** appears to be more effective in increasing RBF and inducing diuresis than the use of either agent alone.

If use of fluid therapy and one or more of the above agents fails to reestablish urine flow, **peritoneal dialysis** may be used as a means of short-term support to allow time for nephron repair and hypertrophy. Peritoneal dialysis also may be warranted in horses with aminoglycoside-induced ARF if plasma concentrations of the drug remain elevated after discontinuation of therapy. Hemodialysis is not available for adult horses but has been used in the treatment of ARF in neonatal foals.

41. What are the most common causes of chronic renal failure (CRF) in horses?

Although most horses (85%) with CRF have acquired disease, congenital anomalies (renal aplasia, hypoplasia, dysplasia, or polycystic kidney disease) should not be overlooked because they are the most important cause of CRF in horses less than 5 years of age. With acquired disease, glomerulonephritis, chronic interstitial nephritis, and end-stage kidney disease are responsible for 50%, 40%, and 10% of cases, respectively. Other less common causes of CRF include amyloidosis and neoplasia. Amyloidosis is most commonly recognized in horses hyperimmunized for antiserum production, and hepatic and splenic involvement appears to be more common than renal involvement.

42. What clinical and laboratory features differentiate ARF from CRF in horses?

ARF is usually a consequence of nephrotoxin exposure or a complication of a number of primary disease processes that result in hypovolemia and ischemic renal damage. In contrast, the most common presenting complaint for horses with CRF is weight loss. Partial anorexia, rough hair coat, and lethargy or poor athletic performance are other concerns voiced by owners. Ventral edema and polyuria/polydipsia can be detected in about 50% of cases, and horses with advanced CRF may develop excessive dental tartar along with a characteristic odor that likely results from the combined effects of uremic halitosis and increased urea secretion in sweat. The kidneys of horses with ARF are usually normal to increased in size, whereas the kidneys of horses with CRF are typically small with irregular surfaces. In addition to laboratory findings common to both ARF and CRF (azotemia, hyponatremia, hypochloremia, and variable hyperkalemia), anemia (packed cell volume = 20–30% because of decreases in erythropoietin production) is a frequent laboratory finding in horses with CRF. Hypercalcemia and hypophosphatemia, which are somewhat unique findings in horses with CRF, occur in about two-thirds of equine patients. Finally, because the ability to produce concentrated and dilute urine is lost with CRF, isosthenuria (specific gravity = 1.008–1.014) is a consistent feature of the syndrome unless accompanied by heavy proteinuria (which may increase urine specific gravity to 1.020).

43. What is normal urinary protein excretion? How is proteinuria assessed in horses with CRF?

With glomerular injury alterations in the integrity of the highly anionic glomerular filtration barrier leads to loss of protein, predominantly albumin, in the urine. Few quantitative data about urinary protein loss are available for horses with CRF because proteinuria has been assessed most commonly with urine reagent strips or the semiquantitative sulfosalicylic acid precipitation test. Reagent strip results of +++ or ++++ correlate to protein concentrations of 100–300 to 1000–2000 mg/dl, depending on the reagent strip used. In a horse with CRF that produces 20 L of urine daily, these values yield a wide range of 20–400 gm of urinary protein loss daily. A loss of 400 gm would approach 25% of the total protein content of plasma and is not realistic. In humans with CRF, urinary protein loss exceeding 50 mg/kg/day is classified as nephrotic-range proteinuria, and some people with heavy proteinuria may lose in excess of 200 mg/kg/day.

When measured quantitatively (with colorimetric assays such as the Coomassie brilliant blue dye method or other assays routinely used with cerebrospinal fluid), the upper limit of normal urinary protein excretion in several species, including horses, is about 20 mg/kg/day. Using these values, estimates for the upper acceptable limit for urinary protein loss and nephrotic-range proteinuria in a 500-kg horse are 10 and > 25 gm/day, respectively.

Another way to document proteinuria is by determining the ratio of urinary protein (in mg/dl with a colorimetric assay) to urinary creatinine (mg/dl). This technique is more practical because it avoids the need for a timed urine collection period. Although a normal range has not yet been reported for horses, values in excess of 1.0 and 3.5 are considered above normal and indicative of nephrotic-range proteinuria in dogs and humans. Thus, a urine protein-to-creatinine ratio greater than 2.0 probably supports significant proteinuria in a horse with CRF.

Finally, a horse with CRF and heavy proteinuria (> 200 mg/kg/day) may excrete as much as 100 gm of protein daily (5–7% of total plasma protein). Proteinuria of this magnitude may increase urine specific gravity to 1.020 or greater. Furthermore, it would certainly be great enough to lead to a decline in serum albumin and total protein concentration despite increased hepatic albumin production.

44. What are the mechanisms of hypercalcemia and hypophosphatemia in CRF?

Hypercalcemia and hypophosphatemia (Williams-Smith syndrome) are fairly common findings in horses with CRF, and the magnitude of hypercalcemia appears to vary with the amount of calcium in the diet. Since the equine kidney is an important route of calcium excretion (via calcium carbonate crystals), impaired tubular function in the face of continued intestinal absorption is the most common explanation for calcium accumulation in blood. This observation is supported by the rapid development of hypercalcemia after experimental bilateral nephrectomy in ponies fed alfalfa hay. In contrast, nephrectomized ponies fed grass hay did not become hypercalcemic. The influence of dietary calcium can be further demonstrated by changing the type of hay fed to horses with CRF. In horses with serum calcium concentrations > 20 mg/dl on a predominantly alfalfa diet, serum calcium concentrations may return to the normal range within a few days of changing the diet to grass hay.

In the few cases in which parathormone has been measured, serum concentration was low in horses with CRF and hypercalcemia; thus, hyperparathyroidism does *not* appear to play a role. However, parathormone clearance by the kidney is reduced with CRF and may be associated with a change in the regulatory set point for calcium in uremic humans.

Although an important complication of CRF in other species, renal osteodystrophy has not been described in horses. Furthermore, it is not known whether hypercalcemia is associated with exacerbation of renal disease or tissue mineralization in horses with CRF. The cause of hypophosphatemia in horses with CRF also remains undocumented, although it has been explained by the law of mass action, which leads to a decrease in serum phosphate concentration in association with hypercalcemia. However, a similar response is not observed in horses eating *Cestrum diurnum* (leading to a syndrome of hypervitaminosis D), which develop hypercalcemia without hypophosphatemia. Another possibility is that hypophosphatemia may be a consequence of long-standing anorexia accompanying CRF. Regardless of the cause, clinical problems associated with hypophosphatemia have not yet been recognized in horses with CRF.

45. What are the expected alterations in acid-base status in horses with CRF?

A degree of metabolic acidosis accompanies CRF in humans and small animals and is attributed to a decreased ability of failing kidneys to excrete hydrogen ions and regenerate bicarbonate. Normally, acid-base balance is maintained by reabsorption of filtered bicarbonate and excretion of hydrogen ions in combination with ammonia and phosphate. As renal function declines in the early stages of renal failure, hydrogen ion excretion via renal ammoniagenesis and ammonium excretion may actually increase. However, as renal failure progresses, both compromised renal ammoniagenesis and decreased medullary recycling of ammonia probably contribute to impaired ammonium excretion and development of metabolic acidosis. Metabolic acidosis further contributes to a number of the clinical signs of uremic syndrome and may exacerbate some of the electrolyte imbalances (e.g., hyperkalemia) accompanying CRF. Although metabolic acidosis has been reported in a limited number of horses with CRF, most horses are able to maintain relatively normal acid-base status until the terminal stages of CRF.

46. Why is the plasma of horses with advanced CRF lipemic?

Horses with CRF may develop hypercholesterolemia and hyperlipidemia (hypertriglyceridemia), and an occasional horse with advanced CRF may have grossly lipemic plasma (hyperlipemia). With azotemia, hyperlipidemia may develop as a result of increased synthesis, increased mobilization of triglycerides from fat stores, and/or decreased tissue utilization. Decreased lipoprotein lipase activity (decreasing tissue utilization) has received the greatest attention in horses, probably because heparin treatment (40 IU/kg subcutaneously every 8 hours) has been advocated for stimulation of lipoprotein lipase in an attempt to clear the serum. Hypercholesterolemia and hyperlipidemia also stimulate mesangial cell proliferation and matrix production in diseased glomeruli and thereby accelerate progression to glomerulosclerosis. As a consequence, there has been considerable interest in modification in dietary lipids as a means of slowing the progression of CRF.

47. What causes glomerulonephritis (GN)? What disease processes have been implicated in equine GN?

GN is initiated by deposition of circulating immune complexes or autoantibodies along the glomerular basement membrane (GBM) and in the mesangium, leading to complement activation and leukocyte infiltration. The inflammatory response is characterized by endothelial and epithelial cell swelling (with fusion of foot processes), formation of microthrombi in glomerular capillaries, and mesangial cell proliferation. Furthermore, the GBM proliferates to surround the immune deposits, leading to thickening of the filtration barrier. With immune complex disease, immunofluorescent staining with antiimmunoglobulin G (anti-IgG) and anticomplement (anti-C3) antibodies reveals an irregular (granular or "lumpy bumpy") staining pattern. In the much rarer true autoimmune GN, immunofluorescent staining shows a more regular or smooth, linear pattern. Despite widening of the filtration barrier and a decline in GFR in both instances, size-selective and charge-selective filtration properties are compromised, leading to proteinuria.

A number of systemic inflammatory and infectious disease processes may produce GN in horses, but progression to CRF appears to be a rare sequela. For example, experimental *Leptospira pomona* infection produced subacute GN characterized by hypercellularity and edema of capillary tufts, but leptospirosis is a rare cause of clinical renal disease in horses. Similarly, experimental infection with equine infectious anemia (EIA) virus produced histologic and immunofluorescent evidence of GN in 75% and 78% of infected horses, respectively. Immunoglobulins with anti-EIA activity were eluted from glomeruli collected from experimentally infected horses, but none of the horses showed clinical signs of renal disease. Poststreptococcal GN is a well-recognized cause of GN in humans, and group-C streptococcal antigens also have been eluted from immune complex deposits in glomeruli collected from horses with CRF.

Autoimmune GN also has been described as one of the manifestations of systemic lupus erythematosus in horses. Another immune mechanism of GN in horses is production of mixed or monoclonal cryoglobulins and deposition of antibody-antibody immune complexes along the GBM. Cryoglobulinemia may be a more important initiator of GN than previously recognized, since electron microscopic examination is required to demonstrate characteristic fibrillar or crystalline intracapillary and subendothelial deposits.

48. What is the difference between proliferative and membranous GN?

Although a number of terms are used to describe the specific morphologic changes accompanying glomerular injury, GN is most broadly categorized histologically as proliferative or membranous. **Proliferative (or mesangioproliferative) GN** describes glomerular injury associated with influx of inflammatory cells and proliferation of mesangial cells. The predominant histologic finding is increased cellularity in glomeruli. This lesion tends to be associated with the more acute stages of GN, during which immune complexes are deposited in a predominantly subendothelial location.

Membranous GN describes glomerular injury accompanied by marked thickening of the capillary wall and GBM. The predominant histologic finding is an increase in periodic acid-Schiff (PAS) staining material in the mesangial area and on the GBM. Thickening of the GBM can be seen further with a methenamine silver stain. Membranous GN tends to be associated more soluble immune complexes or autoantibodies that can pass through the GBM and localize in a predominantly subepithelial location, resulting in less infiltration of the inflammatory cells.

As expected, a wide spectrum of lesions can be seen in naturally occurring GN and leads to varying histologic descriptions of the disease, including **membranoproliferative GN**. As glomerular injury progresses, proliferation of the parietal epithelium also occurs, probably in response to filtration of macromolecules and cellular debris. Lesions associated with parietal cell proliferation may include layering of epithelial cells, termed "crescents," on the inner aspect of Bowman's capsule, adhesion formation between the glomerular tuft and Bowman's capsule, and tuft collapse. **Glomerulosclerosis** describes the end stage of progressive, irreversible glomerular injury in which replacement of glomerular components with hyaline material is observed histologically.

49. What causes chronic interstitial nephritis (CIN)? What disease processes have been implicated in equine CIN?

CIN is defined most strictly by clinical signs of renal disease associated with histologic changes of tubular damage and an interstitial inflammatory cell infiltrate. Inflammatory cells include lymphocytes, monocytes, and occasional plasma cells. Neutrophils are uncommon; however, eosinophilic infiltrates suggest adverse drug reactions in humans. Major glomerular and vascular lesions are not apparent. The hallmark distinguishing CIN from acute tubular and interstitial disease is the presence of interstitial fibrosis. Although CIN has a fairly strict histologic definition, a number of disease processes can lead to tubulointerstitial damage; for all practical purposes, CIN is used as as catch-all term for nonglomerular causes of CRF.

In horses, CIN usually results from acute tubular necrosis subsequent to ischemia, sepsis, and/or exposure to nephrotoxic compounds. CIN also may develop secondary to ascending urinary tract infection, resulting in pyelonephritis or bilateral obstructive disease due to ureteroliths and/or nephroliths. When the history is not well documented, an initiating cause of the tubular disease may be difficult to identify. Since a number of disease processes may result in CIN, gross findings in affected horses vary dramatically. For example, NSAID toxicity may produce papillary necrosis manifested by hematuria in the early stages of disease. Chronic cases may develop nephrolithiasis and hydronephrosis, which develop because the area of papillary necrosis acts as a nidus for nephrolith formation and subsequent obstructive disease leads to hydronephrosis. Similarly, upper urinary tract infection may lead to major changes in the architecture of the kidneys, including abscess and nephrolith formation. Although CIN may be expected to be accompanied by evidence of tubular dysfunction (enzymuria, glucosuria, increased fractional electrolyte clearance values), these abnormalities are rarely detected because of chronicity and compensation by remaining functional nephrons. Finally, proteinuria, the hallmark of glomerular disease, is not an expected feature of CIN.

50. What is end-stage kidney disease (ESKD)?

ESKD describes the severe gross and histologic changes in kidneys collected from animals in the final stages of CRF. Grossly, the kidneys are typically pale, shrunken, and firm and may have an irregular surface with an adherent capsule. Histologically, severe glomerulosclerosis and hyalinization are accompanied by extensive interstitial fibrosis. The presence of end-stage lesions makes it essentially impossible to determine the initiating cause of renal disease.

51. Is oxalate nephropathy a cause of CRF in horses?

Several early cases of CRF in horses have been attributed to oxalate poisoning because oxalate crystals were observed in renal tubules. However, horses appear to be more resistant to oxalate-induced renal damage than other domestic species. Experimental administration of various forms of oxalate (in high doses) produces hypocalcemia and GI signs rather than renal failure. In fact, the early reports of "oxalate nephropathy" failed to demonstrate exposure of the affected horses to oxalates. Furthermore, chronic ingestion of oxalate-containing plants produces fibrous osteodystrophy (oxalates bind calcium in the intestinal tract, thus decreasing intestinal calcium absorption), but renal damage in affected horses has been minimal. It is now recognized that formation of oxalate crystals in diseased equine kidneys is a secondary change probably related to stasis of urine flow in damaged renal tubules; thus oxalate nephropathy is a consequence rather than a cause of CRF.

52. What are the indications for renal biopsy in horses? What risks are involved?

In theory, renal biopsy is a useful diagnostic technique for determining the affected region of the nephron, the type of lesion, and the chronicity and severity of the disease. Although the procedure is relatively safe when performed with ultrasonographic guidance, its inherent risks include perirenal hemorrhage and/or hematuria and, less commonly, penetration of the bowel. In humans, perinephric hematomas are common and have been detected in 57–85% of patients on the day after biopsy. Microscopic hematuria occurs in virtually all patients for the first few days after biopsy, and gross hematuria is observed in 5–10% of patients. Most of these complications are inconsequential but have resulted in the need for postbiopsy transfusions in 1–3% of patients. Similar complications, including fatal hemorrhage, have been anecdotally reported in horses. Thus, renal biopsies should be approached with caution and are indicated only when results will alter the therapeutic plan and/or prognosis. Information about the impact of renal biopsy results on therapy and outcome of renal disease in humans is limited; however, in one prospective study biopsy results were found to influence physicians' decisions in about one-half of the patients on which the technique was performed. In general, renal biopsy is pursued more aggressively in humans with ARF than in humans with CRF, especially when it is difficult to determine the type of renal disease based on results of urinalysis and sediment examination. Unlike in humans, in horses glomerular disease (which often requires electron microscopic examination in addition to routine histopathology) is infrequently recognized as the cause of ARF; consequently, renal biopsy in horses with ARF is probably best used in cases in which a hemodynamic or nephrotoxic insult is not apparent.

Although in theory renal biopsy results should provide more useful diagnostic and prognostic information about the type of renal disease in horses with ARF (glomerulonephritis, tubular necrosis, or interstitial nephritis), they more often have been used to confirm the presence of chronic disease in horses with CRF. In most cases of CRF, the inciting cause cannot be detected unless it can be associated with a historical event or immunofluorescent testing is pursued. This limitation can be attributed to the fact that pathologic lesions are widespread at this point, and involvement of all nephron segments as well as the interstitium often leads to an interpretation of ESKD. In occasional horses, biopsy results may aid in separating infectious (pyelonephritis) or congenital (renal dysplasia) from nonspecific causes of renal failure. Although such results may assist in the therapeutic approach, the limitations and risk of renal biopsy should be considered before it is performed in horses with CRF.

53. How is a renal biopsy performed in horses?

A renal biopsy should be performed with the horse sedated and restrained in stocks. A Tru-cut biopsy needle or, preferably, an automated biopsy device (e.g., Monopty, Bard Radiology Division, Covington, GA 30014) should be used. Penetration of the needle into the renal parenchyma is imaged ultrasonographically by triangulating the ultrasound beam with the biopsy instrument and kidney. The tissue collected should be placed in formalin for histopathologic and possible electron microscopic evaluation. If desired, additional samples may be collected for bacterial culture and immunofluorescent testing. Check with the testing laboratory for preferred media.

54. What is the prognosis for equine CRF?

Because of the progressive and irreversible nature of CRF, the long-term prognosis is poor. Specific corrective treatment (renal transplantation) is not available for horses, and maintenance by peritoneal dialysis or hemodialysis is not practical except for short-term support during treatment of ARF. Pyelonephritis may be considered an exception because antimicrobial treatment, in theory, may lead to resolution of infection and improvement in renal function. Unfortunately, significant renal damage has already occurred by the time most cases of bilateral pyelonephritis are diagnosed; thus, the prognosis for a return to normal renal function is guarded to poor. In contrast, the short-term prognosis may be more favorable. Some horses with CRF may maintain serum creatinine concentration below 5 mg/dl for months with minimal deterioration. Prediction of which cases will deteriorate more rapidly is difficult, but recent history, ability to counteract weight loss with improved management, and change in creatinine over the first few months are useful indicators. In general, horses that eat well and maintain reasonable body condition carry the best short-term prognosis and may still be able to perform a limited amount of work. The goal in each case is to provide appropriate supportive care and to monitor the horse closely to provide humane euthanasia before the horse reaches a state of uremic decompensation.

55. Describe the treatment of equine CRF.

Management of horses with CRF involves palliative efforts to minimize further loss of renal function. The goals are to prevent complicating conditions such as lack of water availability, to discontinue administration of nephrotoxic agents, and to provide a palatable diet (with lower calcium and possibly lower protein levels) to encourage appetite and minimize further weight loss. Supportive care also may include supplementation of sodium bicarbonate (50–150 gm/day) when serum bicarbonate concentration is consistently below 20 mEq/L. Eliminating high calcium and protein feed sources such as alfalfa hay and substituting good-quality grass hay and carbohydrates (corn and oats) may help to control hypercalcemia and azotemia. Ideally, the hay and grain should have an adequate, but not excessive, amount of protein (less than 10% crude protein), which should maintain the BUN-to-creatinine ratio within a target range of 10:1–15:1. It is important to provide unlimited access to fresh water and to encourage adequate energy intake by offering a variety of palatable feeds. In fact, if appetite for grass hay deteriorates, it is preferable to offer less ideal feeds such as alfalfa hay or increased amounts of concentrate to meet energy requirements and lessen the rate of weight loss. Often horses continue to graze at pasture when their hay appetite is diminished. Administration of B vitamins and/or anabolic steroids for their putative appetite-stimulating effects may be of benefit in some animals. Although dietary fat supplementation may provide a dense source of calories, it must be approached judiciously in patients with hyperlipidemia and hypercholesterolemia.

The progressive renal injury that occurs in CRF is associated with continued damage to glomerular and tubular membranes that is mediated by ongoing activation of the inflammatory cascade. Although not supported by experimental data in horses, treatment with antioxidant medications and free radical scavengers may be of theoretical benefit. Similarly, there has been considerable interest in the role of dietary fatty acids as precursors of eicosanoids. Specifically, dietary supplementation with sources rich in omega-3 fatty acids (linolenic acid) as opposed to omega-6 fatty acids (linoleic acid) appears to decrease generation of more damaging fatty acid metabolites during activation of the inflammatory cascade. In horses, dietary supplementation with omega-3 fatty acids in the form of linseed oil has been effective in ameliorating the effects of endotoxin in in vitro studies, and supplementation with fish oil (another rich source of omega-3 fatty acids) slowed the progression of renal failure in laboratory animals. Finally, there is considerable interest in developing therapeutic strategies that may modulate or limit renal fibrosis. Current studies of the effects of cytokines, lymphokines, and proteoglycans on matrix synthesis and degradation by mesangial cells and on fibroblast activation in damaged glomeruli may lead to novel treatment options in the future.

56. What clinical measures are used to assess severity and monitor progression of CRF?

The magnitude of azotemia is the most readily available and practical measure to assess the severity of CRF in horses. Serum creatinine concentrations in the range of 5–10 mg/dl indicate a marked decline in renal function, and values exceeding 15 mg/dl are consistent with a grave prognosis. In contrast, horses with creatinine < 5 mg/dl may exhibit few clinical signs and can be managed for months or years. Plotting the inverse of serum creatinine concentration (1/Cr) over time also has been used to monitor progression of CRF in an attempt to predict the endpoint of the disease process. Unfortunately, these plots are subject to considerable variation and have not proved to be of any more value than monitoring creatinine over time. Measurement of GFR provides the most accurate quantitative assessment of renal function, but it is infrequently pursued because it is more time-consuming and technically demanding than measurement of creatinine. Since tubular creatinine secretion may develop in horses in the earlier stages of CRF, GFR may be overestimated when measured by endogenous creatine clearance (Cl_{Cr}). Despite this limitation, repeated measurement of Cl_{Cr} in the same animal can be a useful method to monitor progression of CRF over time.

57. What types of urinary tract infections (UTIs) occur in horses?

Bacterial UTI is recognized much less commonly in horses than in small animals and humans. Nevertheless, cystitis and pyelonephritis occur in horses but are almost always associated with a predisposing anatomic defect (persistent urachal attachment of the bladder to the ventral abdomen), functional deficit (bladder paresis), or obstruction. A quantitative urine culture should be included in the minimal database for equine patients with signs consistent with lower (stranguria, pollakuria, hematuria) and upper (inappetance, fever, depression) UTI. Furthermore, a quantitative culture may be rewarding in detection of silent UTI with other disorders, such as ARF, CRF, urolithiasis, bladder paresis and incontinence, neoplasia, and hyperadrenocorticism (pituitary adenoma). Parasitic UTIs with the nematode *Halicephalobus deletrix* and the coccidia *Klossiella equi* also may be detected in horses. The former is a rare disease, usually detected at postmortem examination, that presents with verminous meningoencephalomyelitis. Renal lesions, although extensive, are often silent. Similarly, infection with *K. equi* has not been recognized to cause clinical signs of UTI, but it has been found worldwide in horses, ponies, donkeys, burros, and zebras.

58. What types of uroliths are found in horses?

Cystoliths or bladder stones are the most common urolith in horses. Two general types, both predominantly calcium carbonate in composition, are found: (1) larger, spherical-to-ovoid stones that are usually yellow to green with rough or spiculated surfaces and (2) smaller, often irregular stones that are usually gray to white with smooth surfaces. The former constitute more than 90% of cystoliths; fortunately, most are rather porous and can be crushed to facilitate removal. However, their rough surfaces often adhere to bladder mucosa, and significant mucosal damage can be complicated by UTI. In contrast, the less common stones contain a greater amount of phosphorus (although still predominantly calcium carbonate in composition) and are often quite dense and refractory to crushing. Recurrence after removal of cystoliths may approach 40%. This relatively high rate is probably due to the combined effects of predisposing anatomic or physiologic problems (typically not documented), damage to bladder mucosa, and poor ability to acidify equine urine.

Nephroliths and ureteroliths, which also are composed primarily of calcium carbonate, occur less commonly in horses and are rarely detected until signs of CRF develop secondary to bilateral obstruction. In contrast to primary nephrolithiasis in humans, nephroliths and ureteroliths in horses are more likely a consequence of previous renal damage (NSAID nephropathy, sequelae of neonatal septicemia) or concurrent renal disease (renal dysplasia, polycystic kidney disease, or pyelonephritis). They may be incidental findings at necropsy in horses with unilateral disease or may cause signs of recurrent abdominal pain. Nephrectomy is the treatment of choice for unilateral disease (in the absence of azotemia) because obstruction typically leads to complete loss of function of the kidney on the affected side.

Urethral calculi are an occasional cause of stranguria in male horses and may cause signs of moderate-to-severe colic when obstruction is complete. They are commonly found at the level of the ischial arch where the urethra narrows and turns cranioventrally. They are most commonly secondary to a urethral lesion (e.g., neoplasia or stricture from a previous perineal urethrotomy) or disorders higher in the urinary tract (e.g., cystolith or unilateral pyelonephritis). When they are detected, a full evaluation of the upper and lower urinary tract is warranted after relief of the obstruction.

59. What are the differential diagnoses for polyuria/polydipsia (PU/PD) in horses?

The major causes of PU/PD in horses include CRF, pituitary adenoma, and primary (psychogenic) polydipsia. Less common causes include excessive salt consumption, central and nephrogenic DI, diabetes mellitus due to pancreatic insufficiency, sepsis and/or endotoxemia, ARF, and iatrogenic causes (sedation with α-2 agonists, corticosteroid therapy, or diuretic usage). PU/PD is reported in some, but not all, horses with CRF, because the magnitude of polyuria is typically much less than with primary polydipsia or DI. With CRF azotemia is present, and urinalysis consistently reveals isosthenuria (urine specific gravity of 1.008–1.014). Pituitary adenomas are common in older horses and may lead to a moderate degree of polyuria. Although PU/PD has been reported in some horses with sepsis or endotoxemia, other clinical signs such as fever, abdominal pain, and weight loss predominate. The mechanism is unclear but may be a consequence of endotoxin-induced prostaglandin production, since prostaglandin E_2 can antagonize the effects of ADH on collecting ducts.

60. What is the most common cause of PU/PD in adult horses? How is it diagnosed and managed?

Primary polydipsia is probably the most common cause of PU/PD in adult horses and appears to be a stable vice in most affected horses. Typically, primary polydipsia results in more dramatic polyuria than either renal failure or pituitary adenoma. Horses exhibiting this behavior are usually in good body condition, are not azotemic, and have hyposthenuria (urine specific gravity < 1.008). The diagnosis of primary polydipsia is made by exclusion and response to water deprivation (urine specific gravity should exceed 1.025 after 24 hours). Management typically involves restricting water intake to meet maintenance, work, and environmental requirements along with increasing the amount of exercise or turn-out time. PU/PD also may be associated with excessive salt consumption, which is suspected to be another psychogenic or behavioral problem. Affected horses usually have an increased fractional sodium clearance. The problem can be controlled by reducing salt availability.

61. How does DI lead to PU/PD?

DI may be central or nephrogenic in origin. Central DI results from failure in production, transport, or release of ADH and leads to limited ability to concentrate urine in response to water deprivation. Azotemia is not apparent, and the remaining urinalysis results are normal. The condition has been reported in association with viral encephalomyelitis and as an idiopathic disorder. Since the kidneys are normal with central DI, affected horses respond to parenteral administration of ADH. Horses that fail to concentrate urine in response to exogenous ADH may have nephrogenic DI, in which ADH production is normal but the collecting ducts are insensitive to its effects. Nephrogenic DI may be a hereditary disorder in people, and a similar hereditary disease has been described in sibling Thoroughbred colts.

62. What is the mechanism of PU/PD in horses with pituitary adenomas?

Pituitary adenomas are common in older horses and may lead to PU/PD by several mechanisms:

1. Polyuria may be a consequence of actions of hormones derived from proopiomelanocortin (POMC), most specifically adrenocorticotropin (ACTH). Hyperadrenocorticism resulting from excessive ACTH activity leads to hyperglycemia, which may exceed the renal tubular threshold for reabsorption. The resultant glucosuria leads to osmotic diuresis. Although commonly implicated as the cause of polyuria in horses with pituitary adenomas, glucosuria was found in only 1 of 5 affected horses in a recent clinical report.

2. People and dogs appear to experience a potent thirst response to exogenous corticoids; thus, polydipsia may be an important cause of polyuria. In horses on chronic dexamethasone treatment for immune-mediated disorders, profound glucosuria (2–3 gm/dl) may be observed, contributing to osmotic diuresis, but increased thirst has not been described.

3. Polyuria may result from antagonism of the action of ADH on the collecting ducts by cortisol. Although commonly cited as the mechanism of polyuria in canine hyperadrenocorticism, experimental evidence to support this mechanism is limited in both dogs and horses.

4. Growth of the adenoma may lead to impingement on the posterior pituitary and hypothalamic nuclei (located immediately dorsal to the pituitary gland), the sites of ADH storage and production, respectively. Decreased ADH production and release would result in a partial central DI as the fourth mechanism for polyuria. Central DI, however, is not likely to be the primary cause of polyuria in all cases because some affected horses can concentrate urine when deprived of water. Consequently, the PU/PD seen in many, but not all, horses with pituitary adenomas is probably a combined effect of several mechanisms.

63. What are the differential diagnoses for glucosuria in horses?

Although the renal threshold for glucose has not been critically evaluated in horses, an early study suggested that it may be lower (about 150–175 mg/dl) than in small animals and humans (200 mg/dl). Thus, glucosuria may accompany a number of stressful conditions (e.g., colic, endotoxemia, laminitis) in which catecholamine release may lead to hyperglycemia. Similarly, glucosuria is transiently observed in 5–10% of horses after racing. Glucosuria also may be observed with administration of dextrose-containing fluids or parenteral nutrition products, sedation with α-2 agonists (e.g., xylazine, detomidine), or exogenous corticosteroid administration. When glucosuria is detected in the absence of hyperglycemia, primary tubular dysfunction should be suspected. Glucosuria has been detected more commonly in horses with ARF (mostly in experimental models of nephrotoxicity) than in horses with chronic renal disease. Other problems resulting in hyperglycemia and glucosuria include pituitary adenoma and diabetes mellitus (DM). Both insulin-dependent DM (type I) and non–insulin-dependent DM (type II) that were not caused by a pituitary adenoma and that resulted in PU/PD (consequent to glucosuria) as one of the presenting complaints have been reported in a few horses.

64. What is renal tubular acidosis (RTA)? What are the causes and clinical signs?

RTA is an uncommon disorder of renal tubular function that results in decreased urinary acid excretion and metabolic acidosis. Two types of RTA occur in horses. Type 1 is defined as failure of distal tubular epithelial cells to secrete hydrogen ions against a pH gradient and type 2 as wasting of bicarbonate by proximal tubular cells. Inciting causes of the tubular defect(s) may include renal insufficiency, autoimmune diseases, drug reactions, pyelonephritis, or obstructive disorders. Although a hereditary form has been suggested, a foal produced from a mare and stallion affected with type 1 RTA did not have the disease. Clinical signs are related to the degree of metabolic acidosis and range from mild weakness and anorexia to profound depression and ataxia. Other complaints may include weight loss or mild abdominal pain. Laboratory evaluation characteristically reveals hyperchloremia (up to 120 mEq/L) and metabolic acidosis (blood pH as low as 7.0 with a bicarbonate concentration of 7–10 mEq/L). Hypokalemia also may be present. Urine usually remains alkaline despite acidemia, indicative of an inability to retain bicarbonate. Replacement of lost bicarbonate, in part by chloride ions, leads to hyperchloremia. An important diagnostic criterion for RTA is recurrence of the metabolic derangements after withdrawal of therapy.

65. How is RTA treated?

Both types of RTA affecting horses appear to resolve with supportive therapy, including intravenous fluids supplemented with sodium bicarbonate to correct the base deficit. Potassium chloride also may be added to fluids or administered via nasogastric intubation to replace potassium deficits. Once the metabolic acidosis has been corrected, the horse can be managed successfully with oral supplementation of sodium bicarbonate (baking soda, 100–150 gm 2 or 3 times/day). Bicarbonate therapy may need to be continued for an extended period (12–24 months) or for the life of the horse, depending on persistence of the tubular defect. With type 2 RTA, massive bicarbonate wasting is less responsive to supplementation.

66. What are the differential diagnoses for pigmenturia in horses?

Grossly red-to-brown discoloration of urine may result from hematuria, hemoglobinuria, methemoglobinuria, or myoglobinuria; until the source is established, it is best termed pigmenturia. Similarly, a positive result for blood on a urine reagent strip may result from the presence of hemoglobin, methemoglobin, myoglobin, or intact red blood cells in the urine sample. Evaluation of serum for hemolysis and creatine kinase activity and examination of urine sediment for red blood cells may help to differentiate these pigments. Although rarely necessary because of presenting clinical signs, an ammonium sulfate precipitation test (Blondheim test) also may be used to differentiate hemoglobinuria from myoglobinuria. Gross pigmenturia throughout urination is consistent with rhabdomyolysis, hemolysis, or hemorrhage from the kidneys, ureters, or bladder, whereas pigmenturia (usually hematuria) at the beginning or end of urination may be associated with lesions in the distal or proximal urethra, respectively. Rhabdomyolysis and hemolysis are generally accompanied by other clinical signs, whereas hematuria throughout urination may be the presenting complaint for UTI (cystitis or pyelonephritis), urolithiasis, urinary tract neoplasia, idiopathic renal hematuria, or drug toxicity (NSAIDs, particularly phenylbutazone). A peculiar cause of hematuria in geldings (predominantly Quarter Horses) is a tear or defect of the urethra at the level of the ischial arch, which results in hemorrhage from the corpus spongiosum penis. Hematuria is observed as bright red squirts of blood at the end of urination in association with contractions of the urethralis muscle. Glomerular and tubular damage accompanying ARF also typically results in microscopic pigmenturia/hematuria and occasionally grossly discolored urine, whereas pigmenturia is rarely detected with CRF unless accompanied by infection or lithiasis. Finally, microscopic hematuria almost always accompanies high-intensity exercise, but exercise-associated hematuria is a rare complaint unless gross hematuria, usually due to trauma to bladder mucosa, is observed.

67. What are the causes of urinary incontinence in horses? What is the treatment?

Incontinence has been described with a number of disorders in horses, including bladder paralysis, ectopic ureter, vaginal injuries or polyps, and hypoestrogenism. Horses with incontinence may have intermittent or continuous dribbling of urine unrelated to micturition. Mares tend to be at increased risk because of the combination of a short urethra with an increased likelihood of acquiring lower urinary tract abnormalities during breeding or parturition. In mares, urine scalding and dermatitis of the medial aspects of both hindlegs may accompany incontinence, whereas soiling of the dorsal aspect of the hindlegs and ventral abdomen may be observed in males. In both sexes a strong urine odor may be present. Incontinence is typically exacerbated by factors that increase intraabdominal pressure; in fact, it is often first observed during exercise or in association with coughing. Bladder paralysis leads to bladder distention and overflow of urine. Horses with incontinence due to bladder paralysis may have other neurologic signs, including hindlimb ataxia and atrophy or loss of tail or anal tone. Rectal palpation reveals a moderately enlarged bladder (lower motor neuron bladder) that can be expressed via rectal manipulation. However, incomplete emptying or complete paralysis may lead to accumulation of urine sediment in the ventral aspect of the bladder, termed sabulous urolithiasis, that may be confused with a bladder mass. Vaginal malformations, such as postfoaling strictures or polyps, have been associated with incontinence, possibly by impairing function of the external urethral sphincter or by causing urine pooling in the vagina. Lastly, although hypoestrogenism is a common cause of incontinence in companion animals, few cases of estrogen-responsive incontinence in horses have been well documented.

68. How is urinary incontinence treated?

Treatment of incontinence includes correction of primary problems (surgery for ectopic ureter or vaginal problems) and supportive care. The latter usually includes antimicrobial prophylaxis against UTIs and repeated manual expression or bladder catheterization in an attempt to allow recovery of detrusor function (most helpful in acute cases). Surgical removal of sabulous material via perineal urethrotomy, combined with irrigation or lavage with large volumes of fluid, may result in temporary improvement but is rarely curative. In horses with bladder distention in which some detrusor activity is apparent, medical treatment with phenoxybenzamine (0.7 mg/kg orally every 6 hours to decrease urethral tone) and bethanechol (0.25–0.75 mg/kg subcutaneously or orally every 6–8 hours to stimulate detrusor muscle activity) may be tried but are rarely rewarding because of long-standing paresis or paralysis at the time of presentation. The prognosis for recovery of bladder function in horses with incontinence is generally poor, unless the problem can be attributed to a specific neurologic disease such as equine herpes virus 1 or equine protozoal myeloencephalitis. (See also question 3.)

69. What are the most common neoplasms of the equine urinary tract?

Neoplasia is a rare disorder of the equine urinary tract. However, because it may affect all levels of the urinary tract, presenting complaints vary from anorexia and weight loss to hematuria with or without stranguria. Lesions of the distal penis may result in a swollen or malodorous sheath as well as produce dysuria. The most common neoplasm affecting the equine kidney is renal cell carcinoma. This tumor is most effectively treated by unilateral nephrectomy, providing that function of the contralateral kidney is normal. Other neoplastic disorders of the upper urinary tract include renal adenocarcinoma, nephroblastoma, or metastatic lymphoma or melanoma. They may be suspected when an enlarged kidney is palpated on rectal examination. The most common neoplasm affecting the bladder and urethra is squamous cell carcinoma. Transitional cell carcinoma, leiomyoma, and leiomyosarcoma also have been described as causes of hematuria and/or stranguria. Although surgical resection of the affected portion of the bladder or penis may be curative, its results only in temporary improvement if the neoplastic tissue cannot be completely excised. Topical 5-fluorouracil also may be of benefit in horses with urogenital squamous cell carcinoma or sarcoids when surgical excision is impractical or incomplete. The penis and prepuce or vulvar areas also may be affected by sarcoids or melanomas.

BIBLIOGRAPHY

1. Bayly WM: A practitioner's approach to the diagnosis and treatment of renal failure in horses. Vet Med 86:632–639, 1991.
2. Divers TJ: Chronic renal failure in horses. Compend Cont Educ Pract Vet 5:S310–S317, 1983.
3. Divers TJ: Disease of the renal system. In Smith BP (ed): Large Animal Internal Medicine, 2nd ed. St. Louis, Mosby, 1996, pp 953–974.
4. Divers TJ, Whitlock RH, Byars TD, et al: Acute renal failure in six horses resulting from hemodynamic causes. Equine Vet J 19:178–184, 1987.
5. Grossman BS, Brobst DF, Kramer JW, et al: Urinary indices for differentiation of prerenal azotemia and renal azotemia in horses. J Am Vet Med Assoc 180:284, 1982.
6. Hoffman KL, Wood AKW, McCarthy PH: Sonographic-anatomic correlation and imaging protocol for the kidneys of horses. Am J Vet Res 56:1403–1412, 1995.
7. Kiper ML, Traub-Dargatz JL, Wrigley RH: Renal ultrasonography in horses. Compend Cont Educ Pract Vet 12:993–1000, 1990.
8. Kohn CW, Chew DJ: Laboratory diagnosis and characterization of renal disease in horses. Vet Clin North Am Equine Pract 3:585–615, 1987.
9. Koterba AM, Coffman JR: Acute and chronic renal disease in the horse. Compend Cont Educ Pract Vet 3:S461–S469, 1981.
10. Laverty S, Pascoe JR, Ling GV, et al: Urolithiasis in 68 horses. Vet Surg 21:56–62, 1992.
11. Matthews HK, Andrews FM, Daniel GB, Jacobs WR: Measuring renal function in horses. Vet Med 88:349–356, 1993.
12. Schmitz DG: Toxic nephropathy in horses. Compend Cont Educ Pract Vet 10:104–111, 1988.
13. Schott HC, Varner DD: Urinary tract. In Brown CM, Traub-Dargatz J (eds): Equine Endoscopy, 2nd ed. St. Louis, Mosby, 1996, pp 238–259.
14. Schott HC: The urinary system. In Robinson NE (ed): Current Therapy in Equine Medicine, 4th ed. Philadelphia, W.B. Saunders, 1997, pp 467–497.
15. Schott HC, Bayly WM: Urinary tract diseases. In Reed SM, Bayly WM (eds): Equine Internal Medicine. Philadelphia, W.B. Saunders, 1997, pp 807–911.

12. THE MUSCULAR SYSTEM

Stephanie J. Valberg, D.V.M., Ph.D., Dip. ACVIM, and
Jennifer M. MacLeay, D.V.M., Dip. ACVIM

1. What is embryologic origin of skeletal muscle and the connective tissue surrounding the muscle fibers?

Muscle fibers derive from paired embryonic somites; connective tissue arises from the somatopleure. The somatic mesoderm migrates and splits sequentially to form the arrangement of individual muscles. Myoblasts sequentially develop into myotubes and mature muscle fibers. Motor neurons establish neuromuscular junctions with myotubes and facilitate normal development of the muscle fiber. Tendons are established independently, and elongating muscle becomes continuous with the tendons.

Snow DH, Valberg SJ: Muscle anatomy, physiology and adaptations to exercise and training. In Hodgson DR, Rose RJ (eds): The Athletic Horse: Principles and Practice of Equine Sports Medicine. Philadelphia, W.B. Saunders, 1994, pp 129–144.

2. Detail the organization of skeletal muscle contractile proteins from the gross anatomic level to the molecular level.

A muscle consists of fascicles that contain groups of individual muscle cells or muscle fibers. Muscle fibers contain parallel arrays of myofibrils that are composed of sarcomeres stacked end to end. Sarcomeres are composed primarily of the myofilaments actin and myosin and form the basic contractile unit.

Snow DH, Valberg SJ: Muscle anatomy, physiology and adaptations to exercise and training. In Hodgson DR, Rose RJ (eds): The Athletic Horse: Principles and Practice of Equine Sports Medicine. Philadelphia, W.B. Saunders, 1994, pp 129–144.

3. What are the events in excitation-contraction coupling?

Electrical impulses travel down a motor neuron to the neuromuscular junction at the motor endplate. Acetylcholine is released and traverses the synaptic cleft and binds to nicotinic receptors on the sarcolemma. Increased sodium and potassium conductance in the endplate membrane leads to generation of an endplate action potential. The action potential is conducted along the sarcolemma and t-tubule system. Depolarization leads to activation of the voltage-sensitive dihydropyridine receptor, which in turn triggers the ryanodine receptor in the terminal cisternae of sarcoplasmic reticulum to release calcium into the sarcoplasm. Calcium binds to troponin C, changing its configuration and exposing the myosin binding site on the actin filament. The globular myosin heads bind to actin, thereby forming a cross-bridge. Myosin adenosine triphosphatase (ATPase) cleaves a phosphate from adenosine triphosphate (ATP) to form adenosine diphosphate (ADP), and subsequently myosin draws the actin filaments toward the center of the sarcomere. Each sarcomere shortens in unison.

Snow DH, Valberg SJ: Muscle anatomy, physiology and adaptations to exercise and training. In Hodgson DR, Rose RJ (eds): The Athletic Horse: Principles and Practice of Equine Sports Medicine. Philadelphia, W.B. Saunders, 1994, pp 129–144.

4. Why are muscles contracted in rigor mortis?

ATP is necessary to fuel the calcium-ATPase pump, which pumps calcium back into the sarcoplasmic reticulum from the sarcoplasm. This is the major step in relaxation. After death ATP and phosphorylcreatine are depleted, whereas sarcoplasmic calcium concentrations remain elevated. In the presence of calcium, actin and myosin maintain the cross-bridge; hence rigor mortis.

Ganong WF: Excitable tissue. In Ganong WF (ed): Review of Medical Physiology. Norwalk, CT, Appleton & Lange, 1989, pp 50–66.

5. What are the major types of fiber in locomotor skeletal muscle and their oxidative and glycolytic capacities?

Type I (i.e., slow-twitch fibers) and types IIA and IIB (i.e., fast-twitch fibers) are the major types of contractile fibers. In an untrained muscle, type I fibers have the slowest contractile speed, tend to have a small cross-sectional area, and have lower glycolytic capacity and higher oxidative capacity than fast-twitch fibers. Type IIA fibers have a faster speed of contraction, an intermediate cross-sectional area, high glycolytic capacity, and moderate oxidative capacity. Type IIB fibers have the fastest speed of contraction, largest cross-sectional area, highest glycolytic capacity, and lowest oxidative capacity.

Ganong WF: Excitable tissue. In Ganong WF (ed): Review of Medical Physiology. Norwalk, CT, Appleton & Lange, 1989, pp 50–66.

6. What muscle fiber adaptations are seen in response to training?

With regular training, muscle fibers become more oxidative because of increased numbers of mitochondria. The specific fiber type adaptation varies with the intensity of exercise. Training of type IIB fibers requires exercise at high speed. Fiber cross-sectional areas become more uniform among all fiber types, and capillarization is increased.

Ganong WF: Excitable tissue. In Ganong WF (ed): Review of Medical Physiology. Norwalk, Connecticut, Appleton & Lange, 1989, pp 50–66.

7. What is responsible for muscle fatigue?

In high-intensity exercise, increased muscle temperature slows metabolic functions, especially calcium reuptake by the sarcoplasmic reticulum. When energy demands are high, energy is supplied primarily by glycolysis with formation of lactate from pyruvate instead of oxidation of pyruvate by the tricarboxylic acid (TCA) cycle. Lactate accumulation contributes to fatigue through intracellular acidosis. This acidosis impairs glycolysis, generation of force by contractile proteins, and calcium release and reuptake by the sarcoplasmic reticulum. Acidosis also activates adenosine monophosphate (AMP) deaminase. When ATP is depleted by contractile activity, the accumulated ADP molecules are combined to form ATP and AMP. Deamination of AMP drives this reaction forward and thus leads to accumulation of inosine 5'-monophosphate (IMP). IMP cannot be reaminated quickly to AMP, and depletion of the total nucleotide pool available for contraction and relaxation contributes to fatigue. Decreased availability of glycogen does not normally limit short-term high-intensity exercise.

With prolonged low-intensity or submaximal exercise, aerobic metabolism of free fatty acids and glycogen provide energy. Over time, depletion of glycogen is involved in the onset of fatigue. In addition, hyperthermia, electrolyte depletion, and myalgia contribute to fatigue at moderate-to-low intensity. Lactic acidosis does not occur at these speeds.

Ganong WF: Excitable tissue. In Ganong WF (ed): Review of Medical Physiology. Norwalk, Connecticut, Appleton & Lange, 1989, pp 50–66.

Snow DH, Valberg SJ: Muscle anatomy, physiology and adaptations to exercise and training. In Hodgson DR, Rose RJ (eds): The Athletic Horse: Principles and Practice of Equine Sports Medicine. Philadelphia, W.B. Saunders, 1994, pp 129–144.

8. Define the term *tied-up*. What other terms are used for the same syndrome?

Tied-up and *tying-up* are lay terms to describe horses with painful muscle cramping to the point that the muscles are hard and firm when palpated. The term usually describes a syndrome of exertional rhabdomyolysis. Exertional rhabdomyolysis is literally the dissolution of striated muscle fibers in response to exercise. Other terms frequently used for exertional rhabdomyolysis include set fast, azoturia, Monday morning disease, chronic intermittent rhabdomyolysis, and equine rhabdomyolytic syndrome.

Snow DH, Valberg SJ: Muscle anatomy, physiology and adaptations to exercise and training. In Hodgson DR, Rose RJ (eds): The Athletic Horse: Principles and Practice of Equine Sports Medicine. Philadelphia, W.B. Saunders, 1994, pp 129–144.

9. What causes the syndrome of exertional rhabdomyolysis?

It is appropriate to consider exertional rhabdomyolysis as a syndrome characterized by clinical signs of muscle dysfunction or damage. There are numerous causes, although a definitive etiologic agent remains unknown. Horses with exertional rhabdomyolysis may have a sporadic form or a recurrent form. Sporadic exertional rhabdomyolysis is most commonly associated with electrolyte aberrations, muscle strain, and exercise beyond the fitness level of the horse. With appropriate diet and training, horses may not have further episodes. Recurrent exertional rhabdomyolysis may be caused by at least two specific diseases: (1) polysaccharide storage myopathy (PSSM) in Quarter Horse-related breeds, Drafts, and Warmbloods or an abnormality in muscle contractility (putative) in Thoroughbreds, Arabians, and Standardbreds.

Nonexertional rhabdomyolysis may result from recumbency, prolonged anesthesia, malignant hyperthermia, immune-mediated myositis triggered by *Streptococcus equi* var. *equi*, vitamin E and selenium deficiencies, toxins (white snake root, rayless golden rod, cassia), ear ticks (*Otobius megnini*), and trauma (capture myopathy).

Beech J, Lindborg S, Fletcher JE, et al: Caffeine contractures, twitch characteristics and the threshold for Ca^{2+} induced Ca^{2+} release in skeletal muscle from horses with chronic intermittent rhabdomyolysis. Res Vet Sci 54:110, 1993.

Harris P: Equine rhabdomyolysis syndrome. In Robinson EN (ed): Current Therapy in Equine Medicine. Philadelphia, W.B. Saunders, 1997, pp 115–120.

Hodgson DR: Exercise-associated myopathy: Is calcium the culprit? Equine Vet J 25:1–3, 1995.

10. What clinical signs are associated with exertional rhabdomyolysis?

Signs range from mild to severe and involve muscle contracture and firm hard muscles that are electrically silent on electromyographic (EMG) examination. The primary muscle groups involved include the epaxial, gluteal, biceps femoris, semitendinosus, and semimembranosus muscles. The gait is characterized by a short, stiff stride and lameness that progresses to complete refusal to move or recumbency. Hindlimbs are usually affected to a greater extent than forelimbs, but some horses have involvement of the triceps muscles. Affected horses sweat profusely, have an anxious attitude, and may paw and appear to have colic. Severe pain and thrashing may occur. In some horses, areas of fluctuant swelling in muscle may be seen, indicating muscle tearing. Endurance horses often show concurrent signs of depression, exhaustion, and electrolyte abnormalities. Such horses may have other signs, including rapid heart and respiratory rates, diaphragmatic flutter, dehydration, hyperthermia, acute renal failure, and collapse. Differential diagnoses include colic, laminitis, snakebite, and hypocalcemic tetany.

Harris P: Equine rhabdomyolysis syndrome. In Robinson EN (ed): Current Therapy in Equine Medicine. Philadelphia, W.B. Saunders, 1997, pp 115–120.

Snow DH, Valberg SJ: Muscle anatomy, physiology and adaptations to exercise and training. In Hodgson DR, Rose RJ (eds): The Athletic Horse: Principles and Practice of Equine Sports Medicine. 1994, pp 129–144.

11. How are episodes of exertional rhabdomyolysis diagnosed?

A history of exercise-associated muscle cramping, clinical signs described in question 10, and laboratory confirmation of elevated muscle enzyme concentrations in serum are required to support a diagnosis of exertional rhabdomyolysis. Serum can be analyzed for elevations in the activity of the muscle enzymes creatine kinase (CK), which peaks at 4–6 hours, and aspartate aminotransferase (AST), which peaks at 24–48 hours. Clinical signs are usually associated with peak levels of CK > 20,000 U/L (normal: < 380 U/L). Muscle damage leads to immediate release of myoglobin into the circulation. Myoglobin is filtered by the kidneys, and when the threshold for resorption is overcome by the renal tubular cells, the urine may be occultly or grossly positive for myoglobinuria using nonspecific dipstick tests for hemoglobin. CK and myoglobin may be cleared from the circulation by 48–72 hours after the episode once damage to the muscle has ceased. If the episode is moderate to severe but not repeated, AST levels return to normal after 2 weeks.

Snow DH, Valberg SJ: Muscle anatomy, physiology and adaptations to exercise and training. In Hodgson DR, Rose RJ (eds): The Athletic Horse: Principles and Practice of Equine Sports Medicine. 1994, pp 129–144.

12. How is an acute episode of exertional rhabdomyolysis treated?

The primary aim is to relieve anxiety, muscle pain, and dehydration (if present). Horses with skin tenting or gross myoglobinuria should receive intravenous fluids. In normal to only mildly dehydrated horses acepromazine can be given immediately to increase blood flow to muscles and to decrease anxiety; it has the best effect on increasing the horse's comfort. Acepromazine should not be used in severely dehydrated animals because of its hypotensive effects until the horse has been provided with cardiovascular support (i.e., intravenous fluids). Nonsteroidal antiinflammatory drugs (NSAIDs) such as flunixin meglumine can be used in hydrated animals. Dehydrated animals are more prone to develop renal failure due to myoglobin accumulation in renal tubules. Therefore, nasogastric and/or intravenous fluid therapy is of great importance and should be taken before use of NSAIDs. The horse should be kept warm and not moved unless necessary. With severe rhabdomyolysis hyponatremia, hypochloremia, hypocalcemia, hyperkalemia, and hyperphosphatemia develop because of loss of the major intracellular fluid compartment. Electrolyte abnormalities should be corrected. The horse should be rested with daily turn-out until the serum CK level normalizes; then exercise may be reintroduced gradually.

Snow DH, Valberg SJ: Muscle anatomy, physiology and adaptations to exercise and training. In Hodgson DR, Rose RJ (eds): The Athletic Horse: Principles and Practice of Equine Sports Medicine. 1994, pp 129–144.

13. What is the most effective treatment to prevent recurrent exertional rhabdomyolysis?

It is a myth that any one drug or nutritional supplement will cure a horse of recurrent exertional rhabdomyolysis. Many different defects in muscle function lead to recurrent bouts of rhabdomyolysis; therefore, a single vitamin, mineral, or feed supplement cannot prevent rhabdomyolysis in all horses. Changes in diet and training regimens are the best methods of management.

14. What are the dietary causes of sporadic exertional rhabdomyolysis?

Excessive carbohydrates (> 6 lb [> 2.7 kg] sweet feed/day), low sodium, low calcium/high phosphorus (i.e., low calcium-to-phosphorus ratio), and low vitamin E/selenium status have been associated with sporadic exertional rhabdomyolysis.

Harris PA, Snow DH: Role of electrolyte imbalances in the pathophysiology of the equine rhabdomyolysis syndrome. In Persson SGB, Jeffcott LB, Lindholm A (eds): Equine Exercise Pathology, vol. 3. Davis, CA, ICEEP Publications, 1991, pp 435–442.

Valberg SJ, Hodgson DR: Diseases of muscle. In Smith BP (ed): Large Animal Internal Medicine, 2nd ed. St. Louis, Mosby, 1996, pp 1489–1518.

15. What is polysaccharide storage myopathy (PSSM)?

Excessive storage of glycogen and visualization of an abnormal polysaccharide on periodic acid-Schiff (PAS) stains of muscle fibers are seen in some horses with recurrent exertional rhabdomyolysis. Diagnosis of the disease is based on (1) the presence of abnormal glycogen on frozen sections of muscle stained with PAS; (2) clinical history consistent with recurrent exertional rhabdomyolysis; and (3) documentation of elevations in CK or AST in association with clinical signs (may remain elevated for weeks). To date, the disease has been documented in American Quarter Horses (QH) or QH-related breeds, Warmbloods, and Drafts. QHs show evidence of a familial pattern of inheritance. The defect appears to involve enhanced glucose uptake into skeletal muscle of affected horses.

Valberg SJ: Muscular causes of exercise intolerance in horses. In Gaughan EM (ed): Veterinary Clinics of North America—Equine Practice. Exercise Intolerance. Philadelphia, W.B. Saunders, 1996, pp 495–515.

Valentine BA, Credille KM, Lavoie JP, et al: Severe polysaccharide storage myopathy in Belgian and Percheron draught horses. Equine Vet J 29:220–225, 1997.

16. How is PSSM managed or cured?

Affected horses can be managed but not cured. Horses with PSSM are mildly to severely exercise-intolerant. Horses should be put into exercise gradually and incrementally, starting with only 5 minutes of work in a round pen or on a longe line. Gradual increases in training allow the horse to become more fit and decrease glycogen storage. Some form of daily exercise is extremely important, whether it be turn-out or riding. Elimination of high-carbohydrate feeds such as corn and molasses-based sweet feeds is necessary. Additional calories can be provided in the form of fat supplements, such as rice bran or corn oil. A high-quality grass hay with a balanced vitamin and mineral supplement is recommended. Extra calories in the form of grains or other fats should be minimal.

Valberg SJ, MacLeay JM, Mickelson JR: Exertional rhabdomyolysis and polysaccharide storage myopathy in horses. Compend Cont Educ 19:1077–1085, 1997.

Valentine BA, Hintz HF, Freels KM, et al: Dietary control of exertional rhabdomyolysis in horses. J Am Vet Med Assoc 212:1588–1593, 1998.

17. What defect is associated with exertional rhabdomyolysis in Thoroughbreds?

Most Thoroughbred horses with recurrent exertional rhabdomyolysis (RER) develop intermittent clinical signs of muscle damage, usually when they are fit, and become stressed or nervous. The high incidence of anesthetic myopathies in Thoroughbred horses and in vitro muscle contracture studies suggest that this form of rhabdomyolysis may be due to abnormalities in muscle contractility. The episodes are seen most commonly in nervous horses, especially females and animals on diets that are high in sweet feed. Standardbred and many Arabian horses appear to have a similar underlying etiology for recurrent tying-up.

Beech J, Lindborg S, Fletcher JE, et al: Caffeine contractures, twitch characteristics and the threshold for Ca^{2+} induced Ca^{2+} release in skeletal muscle from horses with chronic intermittent rhabdomyolysis. Res Vet Sci 54:110, 1993.

18. How are Thoroughbreds with RER managed?

Thoroughbreds with RER are managed to minimize the frequency of episodes of rhabdomyolysis. Management strategies that minimize the amount of calories supplied by sweet feed; balance electrolytes and provide vitamin E and selenium in the diet; and minimize stressful conditions seem to help the most. Replacement of calories with fat-based feeds such as rice bran provides needed calories for performance and has been shown to have a calming effect on some nervous horses. Corn oil also may be used to provide calories (e.g., 60 ml twice daily). Relocation of horses to quiet areas of the barn, training them first and at regular times, and minimization of routine changes to prevent stress are also helpful strategies. Avoiding days off and turn-out are important. When horses are transported to competition, they should get light exercise on the day of transport. Use of tranquilizers such as acepromazine during training also may decrease the frequency of episodes but must be administered cautiously to avoid danger of injury to horse and rider. Phenytoin or dantrolene may affect intracellular calcium concentrations and prevent episodes to some extent.

19. Are any supplements or medications used to prevent RER in Thoroughbreds?

Supplements have not been shown to prevent RER completely in most Thoroughbreds. Dantrolene sodium, a drug that decreases calcium release from the sarcoplasmic reticulum by the ryanodine receptor, may provide some protection against acute episodes in some horses prone to RER if given 1 hour before exercise (2.2 mg/kg orally). All performance horses should receive a diet that provides adequate amounts of electrolytes and minerals, including selenium. Fractional clearance of electrolytes can be performed to determine whether electrolyte imbalances are present.

Valberg SJ, Hodgson DR: Diseases of muscle. In Smith BP (ed): Large Animal Internal Medicine, 2nd ed. St. Louis, Mosby, 1996, pp 1489–1518.

20. What is the diagnostic work-up when an owner complains of a horse's decreased ability to perform and mild muscle cramping after exercise?

1. Complete and thorough physical, lameness, and neurologic examinations
2. Complete blood count and serum chemistry profile, including CK and AST
3. Urine sample obtained within 30 minutes of the serum electrolyte sample to calculate renal fractional clearance of electrolytes, especially sodium, potassium, and calcium
4. Exercise challenge involving 15–30 minutes of trotting to evaluate exercise tolerance, to observe for muscle cramping, and to determine the change in CK activity 4 hours after exercise (to quantitate subclinical muscle damage)
5. Muscle biopsy of the middle gluteal or semimembranosus/semitendinosus muscles (in horses with a history of RER with exercise)
6. Muscle biopsy of any other muscles that appear atrophied

7. Biopsy analysis that includes histochemistry on frozen section by specialized laboratories to provide the most valuable information

8. EMG evaluation, if warranted by neurologic examination, history of fasciculations, myotonic dimpling, or muscle biopsy findings

21. How are muscle biopsies obtained?

Muscle biopsies of the middle gluteal are obtained using a 5-mm punch biopsy needle. Biopsies are taken from a standardized site 18 cm along a line from the dorsum of the tuber coxae to the base of the tail (in an adult horse). After surgical preparation and infiltration of the skin with a local anesthetic such as 2% lidocaine, a stab skin incision is made with a no. 15 scalpel blade. Anesthetic should not be introduced into the muscle so that artifact formation is prevented. The biopsy is taken from a depth of 6 cm, and a 200–400-mg sample is obtained.

An open biopsy technique also may be done over the semimembranosus or semitendinosus muscles. The site is located about 13 cm distal and medial to the tuber ischii over the muscle belly in adult horses. The site is surgically prepared, and the skin and subcutaneous tissues are anesthetized with 2% lidocaine. A 4.5-cm vertical incision is made, and the fascia is undermined for 1.5 cm on either side of the incision. Two vertical incisions, each 1.5 cm deep and 2 cm long, are made into the muscle about 1 cm apart. A horizontal incision is made dorsally to connect the vertical incisions. The muscle is grasped dorsally with forceps, and slight tension is applied as the sample is dissected free from the underlying muscle belly. Then the sample is transected ventrally and removed. The sample should be handled gently and placed on gauze lightly moistened with 0.9% saline until it is submitted on ice packs or dry ice for evaluation. The fascia is closed with absorbable sutures, and the skin is closed with intracuticular sutures to discourage rubbing and contamination by fecal material.

22. What is the preferred method of handling skeletal muscle biopsies in horses?

Muscle biopsies for histologic examination should be chilled and submitted to a specialized neuromuscular laboratory (e.g., Room 225, VTH, Departments of CAPS, College of Veterinary Medicine, 1365 Gortner Avenue, St. Paul, MN 55108) for mounting in cross-section and freezing in isopentane chilled in liquid nitrogen. Samples may be frozen first in liquid nitrogen and then thawed completely before mounting and freezing in isopentane. Samples for biochemistry should be snap-frozen in liquid nitrogen and stored at 80° C. Formalin fixation is *not* useful because it results in inability to type fiber, leaches muscle glycogen, and prevents the use of histochemical stains or biochemical analysis.

Valberg SJ, MacLeay JM, Mickelson JR: Exertional rhabdomyolysis and polysaccharide storage myopathy in horses. Compend Cont Educ 19:1077–1085, 1997.

23. What is the difference between horses with exertional rhabdomyolysis and horses with hyperkalemic periodic paresis or paralysis (HYPP)?

HYPP is a dominant heritable defect resulting from a point mutation in the gene encoding for the skeletal muscle sodium channel alpha subunit. This mutation brings the resting membrane potential closer to firing than in normal horses, and with depolarization the sodium channel may remain open longer, leading to persistent depolarization of the cell and thus weakness. Clinical signs are usually manifest as intermittent episodes of fasciculations, sweating, and anxiety that may progress to dog-sitting and flaccid recumbency. Between episodes horses appear and perform normally. Episodes are more common in horses on high-potassium feeds (e.g., alfalfa) and may be brought on by stress, travel, or fasting. Many episodes occur at night and are unobserved apart from dried sweat in the morning. Clinical signs do not include stiffness and muscle contractures, as in exertional rhabdomyolysis. In addition, serum CK is not elevated above 1500 U/L; increased AST and myoglobinuria are not associated with episodes of HYPP.

Rudoef JA, Spier SJ, Byrns G, et al: Periodic paralysis in Quarter horses: A sodium channel mutation disseminated by selective breeding. Nature Genet 7:141–147, 1992.

Spier SJ, Carlson GP, Holliday TA, et al: Hyperkalemic periodic paralysis in horses. J Am Vet Med Assoc 197:1009–1017, 1990.

24. How is HYPP managed?

HYPP is inherited as an autosomal dominant trait. Heterozygous horses may be asymptomatic or mildly to moderately affected. Homozygous HYPP horses usually show more severe signs, respiratory stridor, and more frequent episodes. Use of the potassium-wasting diuretic, acetazolamide (1–4 mg/kg every 12–24 hours), is helpful in the management of HYPP. Low-potassium diets are also helpful. First cuttings of grass hay and any alfalfa are usually too high in potassium for horses with HYPP, as are molasses and sweet feeds. Grass hay is highly variable in potassium content and should be tested before being fed to horses undergoing frequent episodes. Special diets with a controlled potassium content are available at feed stores for horses with HYPP.

Nayler JM: Equine hyperkalemic periodic paralysis: Review and implications. Can Vet J 35:279–285, 1994.

Spier SJ, Carlson GP, Holliday TA, et al: Hyperkalemic periodic paralysis in horses. J Am Vet Med Assoc 197:1009–1017, 1990.

25. How is HYPP prevented?

Since HYPP is an inherited disease expressed as a dominant trait, the only way to prevent it is not to breed affected animals. A genetic test that uses whole blood can be used to identify normal horses (NN), heterozygotes (HN), and homozygotes (HH). At least 50% of the offspring of horses with HYPP are affected with the disorder, even if they are bred to a normal horse. The American Quarter Horse Association now requires HYPP status on registration papers.

Spier SJ, Carlson GP, Holliday TA, et al: Hyperkalemic periodic paralysis in horses. J Am Vet Med Assoc 197:1009–1017, 1990.

26. What causes inflammatory myositis?

Clostridial infections of the muscle secondary to injections or, more rarely, blunt trauma can be severe and life-threatening. *C. chauvoei, C. septicum, C. sordellii, C. novyi* type B, *C. perfringens* type A, and *C. carnis* or mixed bacterial infections are most common. Equine influenza virus A2 and equine herpesvirus-1 have been associated with muscle soreness and rhabdomyolysis. A few encysted *Sarcocystis fayeri* frequently can be seen in equine muscles. Severe infestations may lead to muscle inflammation and necrosis. Treatment with trimethoprim sulfa and pyrimithamine was successful in one case. Immune-mediated streptococcal infections secondary to *S. equi* have been documented and may cause severe rhabdomyolysis. In addition, some horses develop marked atrophy of the epaxial and gluteal muscles after exposure to strangles.

Traub-Dargatz JL, Schlipf JW, Granstrom DE, et al: Multifocal myositis associated with *Sarcocystis* sp. in a horse. J Am Vet Med Assoc 205:1574–1576, 1994.

Valberg SJ, Hodgson DR: Diseases of muscle. In Smith BP (ed): Large Animal Internal Medicine, 2nd ed. St. Louis, Mosby, 1996, pp 1489–1518.

27. Which two clostridial species affect muscle contraction? What is their mechanism of action?

C. botulinum and *C. tetani*, both of which are gram-positive, are spore-forming obligate anaerobes. *C. botulinum* causes a flaccid paralysis due to decreased acetylcholine release from the presynaptic membrane of the cholinergic neuromuscular junction. *C. tetani* causes a rigid paralysis due to binding of the tentanospasmin toxin to interneurons in the spinal cord, and subsequent lack of inhibition of motor neurons.

Whitlock RH, Buckley C: Botulism. Vet Clin North Am Equine Pract 13:107–128, 1997.

28. *C. botulinum* causes three forms of botulism. What are they?

The three types of botulism are (1) forage poisoning, (2) wound botulism, and (3) toxicoinfectious botulism. Forage poisoning occurs when the horse consumes forage containing preformed toxin. Toxin accumulates in the forage as result of decaying forage or decaying carcasses (e.g., rodents). Wound botulism has been described in horses. Toxicoinfectious botulism is seen almost exclusively in foals as a result of toxin production by bacteria in the intestinal tract. Toxin is then absorbed into the circulation.

Mitten LA, Hinchcliff KW, Holcombe SJ, et al: Mechanical ventilation and management of botulism secondary to an injection abscess in an adult horse. Equine Vet J 26:420–423, 1994.

Whitlock RH, Buckley C: Botulism. Vet Clin North Am Equine Pract 13:107–128, 1997.

29. What is the pathogenesis of botulism?

Once absorbed systemically, the neurotoxin acts presynaptically at peripheral cholinergic neuromuscular junctions and blocks evoked release of acetylcholine. The toxin binds rapidly and irreversibly to the receptors on the presynaptic nerve terminal. The prevention of acetylcholine release produces flaccid paralysis. Since binding is irreversible, neuromuscular function improves only with regeneration of a new endplate, which takes approximately 4–10 days.

Whitlock RH, Buckley C: Botulism. Vet Clin North Am Equine Pract 13:107–128, 1997.

30. What are the types of botulism toxin? Which are most common?

Eight toxin types have been identified: A, B, C_1, C_2, D, E, F, and G. Types B and C cause forage poisoning. Type B more commonly results from vegetative decay, whereas type C is less common and usually produced from decay of animal carcasses. Type B botulism also may occur after *C. botulinum* infects a wound and produces toxin. Toxicoinfectious botulism is usually due to type B toxin. The most common type affecting horses depends on the geographic location. Type B spores predominate in the mid-Atlantic states, type A in the western United States.

Whitlock RH, Buckley C: Botulism. Vet Clin North Am Equine Pract 13:107–128, 1997.

31. How is botulism diagnosed?

Clinical signs in one or more animals associated with feeding of ensiled feeds provides strong circumstantial evidence for botulism. Similarly, finding a dead animal in the grain or hay stack is also strong evidence. Identifying preformed toxin is more difficult when the cause of contamination is not apparent. The mouse bioassay is most commonly used. Five milliliters of plasma or serum are obtained from a horse early in the disease. The problem with this assay is that the level of circulating toxin in an affected horse is often below the threshold for detection, because horses are extremely sensitive to the toxins of *C. botulinum*. Detection of *C. botulinum* spores in feedstuff recently eaten by affected horses or in the feces of affected horses may be an alternative technique to detect spores. This assay may detect spores in up to 35–40% of affected horses, but selective media and special laboratory facilities are required. Antibodies against *C. botulinum* can be detected in the plasma of animals recovering from disease.

Whitlock RH, Buckley C: Botulism. Vet Clin North Am Equine Pract 13:107–128, 1997.

32. What are the clinical signs of botulism?

Foals and adults show the same clinical signs, no matter what the source of the toxin. Severity of clinical signs depends on type and amount of toxin to which the animal is exposed. Signs begin 12 hours to 10 days after exposure. Horses display symmetric, progressive motor paralysis. Paralysis is often first noticed as dysphagia with a decrease in tongue tone, which may progress to systemic weakness, fasciculations, recumbency, and respiratory distress or failure. Mydriasis and ptosis may be observed in conjunction with slow pupillary light responses. Decreased tail tone also may be noted.

Whitlock RH, Buckley C: Botulism. Vet Clin North Am Equine Pract 13:107–128, 1997.

33. How is botulism treated?

Medical treatment depends on the source of the toxin. Antimicrobial therapy is indicated only for wound botulism because it is the only case in which the bacteria are within the body. Systemic antimicrobials do not affect gastrointestinal flora in cases of toxicoinfectious botulism. However, if secondary problems, such as pneumonia, develop, broad-spectrum antimicrobial therapy is indicated. Mineral oil may help to prevent constipation, and H_2 receptor antagonists and sucralfate are indicated in foals to prevent gastric ulceration. Sedation may be necessary in animals that struggle in recumbency. Protection of the eyes is necessary to prevent corneal trauma, and mechanical ventilation is indicated in animals showing respiratory paralysis. Polyvalent plasma rich in antibodies against the toxins can be obtained for administration to affected horses. Because of the irreversible binding of the toxin to the presynaptic membrane of the cholinergic neuromuscular junction, the plasma only helps to remove circulating toxin and limits progression of the disease. Therefore, antitoxin plasma should be administered as early in the course of disease as possible.

Nursing care involves prevention of esophageal obstruction from attempts to eat, nutritional support in the form of enteral feeding by nasogastric intubation or parenteral support, oral or intravenous fluids to maintain hydration, and prevention of bed sores by frequent rolling and maintenance on deep bedding.

Whitlock RH, Buckley C: Botulism. Vet Clin North Am Equine Pract 13:107–128, 1997.

34. How is botulism prevented?

Prevention of botulism involves protection of feedstuffs from rodent contamination and spoilage at the levels of manufacturing, transport, and storage in the barn. Ensiled foods should be avoided. A type B toxoid vaccination is now available and effectively prevents infection with type B botulism. However, it does not prevent other types of botulism.

Whitlock RH, Buckley C: Botulism. Vet Clin North Am Equine Pract 13:107–128, 1997.

35. What is myotonia?

Myotonic muscle disorders consist of a heterogeneous group of clinically similar diseases that share the clinical sign of delayed relaxation of muscle after mechanical stimulation or voluntary contraction.

36. What ion channelopathies occur in horses?

Myotonia congenita, myotonia dystrophica, and HYPP.

37. What clinical signs are associated with myotonia congenita?

Affected horses have well-developed musculature and usually are identified during the first year of life. Pelvic limb stiffness is evident as exercise begins and diminishes as it continues. Percussion of the thigh, rump, and shoulder muscles causes muscle contraction and dimpling. Signs do not progress after 6–12 months of age. Quarter Horses appear to have a form similar to myotonia dystrophica and show progression of clinical signs and failure of other organ systems.

Jamison JM, Baird JD, Smith-Maxie LL, et al: A congenital form of myotonia with dystrophic changes in a Quarter Horse. Equine Vet J 19:353–358, 1987.

Valberg SJ, Hodgson DR: Diseases of muscle. In Smith BP (ed): Large Animal Internal Medicine, 2nd ed. St. Louis, Mosby, 1996, pp 1489–1518.

38. How is myotonia congenita diagnosed?

Definitive diagnosis of myotonia is based on electromyography (EMG). Affected horses manifest pathognomonic, crescendo-decrescendo, high-frequency repetitive bursts with a characteristic "dive bomber" sound. The muscle fibers fire repetitively with insertion of the electrodes.

Valberg SJ, Hodgson DR: Diseases of muscle. In Smith BP (ed): Large Animal Internal Medicine, 2nd ed. St. Louis, Mosby, 1996, pp 1489–1518.

39. What is thumps? How is it treated?

Thumps is synchronous diaphragmatic flutter. The phrenic nerve is irritable because of electrolyte derangements. When the heart contracts, the phrenic nerve is stimulated, causing the diaphragm to contract. The horse has the appearance of hiccuping; flank contractions or twitching occurs in synchrony with the heart rate. Inciting causes include endurance exercise or gastrointestinal disturbances, such as esophageal obstruction, that lead to hypokalemia, hypochloremia, and/or metabolic alkalosis with hypomagnesemia. Low serum ionized calcium due to primary hypocalcemia or secondary to metabolic alkalosis is the likely mechanism. Correction of acid-base and electrolyte status resolves the problem.

Carlson GP: Synchronous diaphragmatic flutter. In Robinson NE (ed): Current Veterinary Therapy in Equine Medicine, vol. 2. Philadelphia, W.B. Saunders, 1987, pp 485–486.

40. Describe the signs and treatment of hypocalcemia.

Clinical signs are variable and include increased muscle tone, stiff gait, rear limb ataxia, muscle fasciculations (especially of the masseter and triceps muscles), profuse sweating, tachycardia, convulsions, coma, and death. Corrected serum calcium levels between 5–8 mg/dl are associated with tetanic spasms and incoordination. Levels below 5 mg/dl are associated with recumbency and stupor. Total serum calcium concentrations must be corrected for the albumin concentration (see chapter 20). Hypocalcemia is associated with prolonged transportation with decreased food intake, lactation, ingestion of blister beetles, pancreatitis, and severe rhabdomyolysis.

Treatment of documented, severe hypocalcemia in horses involves the administration of 500 ml of 23% calcium borogluconate diluted in isotonic fluids. It is wise to dilute the 500 ml of calcium borogluconate in at least 5 liters of isotonic fluid, but the exact formulation depends on the severity of clinical signs and laboratory values for corrected calcium (and/or ionized calcium). It is essential to auscultate the horse's heart during administration of the above solution or 23% calcium borogluconate. After the acute period, 80–125 ml of 23% calcium borogluconate can be added per 5-liter bag of isotonic fluids for intravenous administration. The horse also should be fed a ration with an increased calcium concentration (e.g., calcium supplementation, alfalfa).

Valberg SJ, Hodgson DR: Diseases of muscle. In Smith BP (ed): Large Animal Internal Medicine, 2nd ed. St. Louis, Mosby, 1996, pp 1489–1518.

41. Describe the signs and treatment of ear tick-associated muscle cramping.

Horses with *Otobius megnini* infestations may show intermittent signs of severe, painful muscle cramping of the major muscle groups. Cases may resemble recurrent colic episodes. Percussion of the muscle groups results in a myotonic cramp. Horses have increased serum CK levels (> 10,000 U/L). Numerous ticks are usually located in the ears; if pyrethrins are administered in the ear, signs abate within 24–72 hours.

Madigan JE, Valberg SJ, Ragle C, et al: Intermittent painful muscle spasms in five horses associated with ear tick *(Otobius megnini)* manifestations. J Am Vet Med Assoc 207:74–76, 1995.

42. What is the cause of fibrotic myopathy?

Fibrotic myopathy is an acquired disorder resulting from trauma, inflammation, and subsequent fibrosis. Trauma to the semimembranosus and semitendinosus at the origin of the Achilles' tendon is most common and may result from injections or exercise requiring sliding stops and abrupt turns. Horses that get caught in fences or ropes may struggle violently and tear muscle, resulting in fibrous scarring of the muscle when it heals. Permanent distortion of the gait with a shortened anterior phase (goose-stepping) results. Transection of the fibrotic tissue may provide some relief.

Valberg SJ, Hodgson DR: Diseases of muscle. In Smith BP (ed): Large Animal Internal Medicine, 2nd ed. St. Louis, Mosby, 1996, pp 1489–1518.

43. What is the cause of white muscle disease?

Also known as nutritional myodegeneration, white muscle disease is most commonly associated with deficiency of selenium and/or vitamin E. Dams that consume a deficient diet are highly prone to having affected offspring. It is most commonly seen in young, rapidly growing animals.

44. What presenting clinical signs are associated with white muscle disease?

Muscle stiffness, stilted gait, hunched back, recumbency and difficulty in rising, pneumonia, and rapid heart rate with potential arrhythmias are common presenting signs. An uncommon clinical sign is dysphagia with milk exiting the nares.

45. How is white muscle disease diagnosed?

Serum CK and AST activities are elevated. Whole blood selenium and/or selenium-dependent glutathione peroxidase levels in red blood cells can be measured to evaluate selenium status. Vitamin E is measured as alpha tocopherol in serum samples. Vitamin E is highly labile, and samples should be placed on ice, protected from light, and promptly analyzed. Muscle biopsies from affected neonates are often grossly pale and show scattered necrotic and calcified fibers. Postmortem examination reveals large muscle masses that may have gritty, white streaks representing coagulation necrosis, fibrosis, and/or calcification.

Valberg SJ, Hodgson DR: Diseases of muscle. In Smith BP (ed): Large Animal Internal Medicine, 2nd ed. St. Louis, Mosby, 1996, pp 1489–1518.

46. How is white muscle disease managed?

Inject vitamin E and selenium into the pectoral muscles, and repeat in 4 days if necessary. Correct any changes in electrolyte concentrations. Potassium-wasting diuretics and mineralocorticoids are most effective for hyperkalemia because the intracellular compartment is often largely destroyed, causing refractory responses to insulin and glucose. Oral supplementation with commercial vitamin E and selenium products is also advisable. All other foals on the premises should receive either an injection or oral supplementation of vitamin E and selenium. Ensuring adequate dietary supplementation of pregnant mares prevents the disease.

Valberg SJ, Hodgson DR: Diseases of muscle. In Smith BP (ed): Large Animal Internal Medicine, 2nd ed. St. Louis, Mosby, 1996, pp 1489–1518.

47. What are the most common ionophores associated with toxicosis in horses?

Monensin, rumensin, and lasalocid.

48. What clinical signs are associated with ionophore toxicity?

Acute toxicity is most commonly associated with feed refusal and colic. Diarrhea, myoglobinuria, elevations in serum CK and AST, and signs of acute heart failure also may be seen. In chronic cases, in which exposure occurred weeks to months previously, signs of progressive myogenic heart failure predominate. Heart fractions of CK can be measured using electrophoresis techniques to determine whether acute damage to the heart muscle is present.

Plumlee KH: Toxicology of organic compounds. In Smith BP (ed): Large Animal Internal Medicine, 2nd ed. St. Louis, Mosby, 1996, pp 997–1917.

49. What is atrophy? What are the different types?

Atrophy is the decrease in size of an organ or tissue. Muscular atrophy is associated with a reduction in muscle fiber diameter or cross-sectional area and may be neurogenic or myogenic. Neurogenic atrophy is attributed to damage to the innervation of muscle fibers. Without neural stimulus the muscle fiber mass cannot be maintained. Myogenic atrophy results from disuse, malnutrition, cachexia, endocrine imbalances, and immune-mediated diseases.

Valberg SJ, Hodgson DR: Diseases of muscle. In Smith BP (ed): Large Animal Internal Medicine, 2nd ed. St. Louis, Mosby, 1996, pp 1489–1518.

50. How can you tell the difference between myogenic and neurogenic atrophy?

Histologic evaluation of muscle and/or nerve biopsies is used to to differentiate the two types of atrophy. Denervated muscle shows atrophy of all fiber types, including type I fibers, whereas most cases of myogenic atrophy involve only type II fibers. EMG and nerve conduction studies also may be used to help differentiate neurogenic and myogenic atrophy. Five days after denervation, abnormalities on EMG include increased insertional activity, positive sharp waves, and bizarre high-frequency discharges and fibrillation potentials. Nerve conduction velocities are decreased with neurogenic disorders.

Valberg SJ, Hodgson DR: Diseases of muscle. In Smith BP (ed): Large Animal Internal Medicine, 2nd ed. St. Louis, Mosby, 1996, pp 1489–1518.

51. Give several examples of diseases or incidents that may result in atrophy.

Unexercised horses have smaller-than-average musculature, but the muscle fibers are not particularly atrophied on histologic evaluation. Potential causes of neurogenic atrophy include sweeney (traumatic damage to the suprascapular nerve), lower motor neuron disease, and equine protozoal myelitis. An inflammatory cause of muscular atrophy is *Streptococcus equi*-associated myositis. Disuse atrophy may be associated with prolonged lameness or casting. Cushing's disease, caused by pituitary adenoma/hyperplasia, results in type II fiber atrophy. Prolonged illnesses associated with decreased feed intake, such as pleuritis, are often associated with cachexia due to severe catabolism of fat and muscle in the body.

Valberg SJ, Hodgson DR: Diseases of muscle. In Smith BP (ed): Large Animal Internal Medicine, 2nd ed. St. Louis, Mosby, 1996, pp 1489–1518.

52. What is the difference in speed of onset between myogenic and neurogenic atrophy?

In myogenic atrophy due to malnutrition, 30–50% of muscle mass may be lost in the first 1–2 months. In neurogenic atrophy, 50% of muscle mass may be lost in the first 2–3 weeks. Immune-mediated myositis may result in extremely rapid loss of muscle mass (50% in 1 week).

Valberg SJ, Hodgson DR: Diseases of muscle. In Smith BP (ed): Large Animal Internal Medicine, 2nd ed. St. Louis, Mosby, 1996, pp 1489–1518.

BIBLIOGRAPHY

1. Beech J, Lindborg S, Fletcher JE, et al: Caffeine contractures, twitch characteristics and the threshold for Ca^{2+} induced Ca^{2+} release in skeletal muscle from horses with chronic intermittent rhabdomyolysis. Res Vet Sci 54:110, 1993.
2. Carlson GP: Synchronous diaphragmatic flutter. In Robinson NE (ed): Current Veterinary Therapy in Equine Medicine, vol. 2. Philadelphia, W.B. Saunders, 1987, pp 485–486.
2a. Ganong WF: Excitable tissue. In Ganong WF (ed): Review of Medical Physiology. Norwalk, Connecticut, Appleton & Lange, 1989, pp 50–66.
3. Harris P: Equine rhabdomyolysis syndrome. In Robinson EN (ed): Current Therapy in Equine Medicine. Philadelphia, W.B. Saunders, 1997, pp 115–120.
4. Harris PA, Snow DH: Role of electrolyte imbalances in the pathophysiology of the equine rhabdomyolysis syndrome. In Persson SGB, Jeffcott LB, Lindholm A (eds): Equine Exercise Pathology, vol. 3. Davis, CA, ICEEP Publications, 1991, pp 435–442.
5. Hodgson DR: Exercise-associated myopathy: Is calcium the culprit? Equine Vet J 25:1–3, 1995.
6. Jamison JM, Baird JD, Smith-Maxie LL, et al: A congenital form of myotonia with dystrophic changes in a Quarter Horse. Equine Vet J 19:353–358, 1987.
7. Madigan JE, Valberg SJ, Ragle C, et al: Intermittent painful muscle spasms in five horses associated with ear tick *(Otobius megnini)* manifestations. J Am Vet Med Assoc 207:74–76, 1995.
8. Mitten LA, Hinchcliff KW, Holcombe SJ, et al: Mechanical ventilation and management of botulism secondary to an injection abscess in an adult horse. Equine Vet J 26:420–423, 1994.
9. Nayler JM: Equine hyperkalemic periodic paralysis: Review and implications. Can Vet J 35:279–285, 1994.
10. Plumlee KH: Toxicology of organic compounds. In Smith BP (ed): Large Animal Internal Medicine, 2nd ed. St. Louis, Mosby, 1996, pp 997–1917.
11. Rudoef JA, Spier SJ, Byrns G, et al: Periodic paralysis in Quarter horses: A sodium channel mutation disseminated by selective breeding. Nature Genet 7:141–147, 1992.
12. Snow DH, Valberg SJ: Muscle anatomy, physiology and adaptations to exercise and training. In Hodgson DR, Rose RJ (eds): The Athletic Horse: Principles and Practice of Equine Sports Medicine. 1994, pp 129–144.
13. Spier SJ, Carlson GP, Holliday TA, et al: Hyperkalemic periodic paralysis in horses. J Am Vet Med Assoc 197:1009–1017, 1990.
14. Traub-Dargatz JL, Schlipf JW, Granstrom DE, et al: Multifocal myositis associated with *Sarcocystis* sp. in a horse. J Am Vet Med Assoc 205:1574–1576, 1994.
15. Valberg SJ: Muscular causes of exercise intolerance in horses. In Gaughan EM (ed): Veterinary Clinics of North America—Equine Practice. Exercise Intolerance. Philadelphia, W.B. Saunders, 1996, pp 495–515.
16. Valberg SJ, Hodgson DR: Diseases of muscle. In Smith BP (ed): Large Animal Internal Medicine, 2nd ed. St. Louis, Mosby, 1996, pp 1489–1518.
17. Valberg SJ, MacLeay JM, Mickelson JR: Exertional rhabdomyolysis and polysaccharide storage myopathy in horses. Compend Cont Educ 19:1077–1085, 1997.
18. Valentine BA, Credille KM, Lavoie JP, et al: Severe polysaccharide storage myopathy in Belgian and Percheron draught horses. Equine Vet J 29:220–225, 1997.
19. Valentine BA, Hintz HF, Freels KM, et al: Dietary control of exertional rhabdomyolysis in horses. J Am Vet Med Assoc 212:1588–1593, 1998.
20. Whitlock RH, Buckley C: Botulism. Vet Clin North Am Equine Pract 13:107–128, 1997.

13. ORTHOPEDICS

C. E. *Kawcak*, D.V.M., M.S., Di*p*. ACVS

LAMENESS

1. Visual examination of the equine patient from a distance is essential early in a lameness examination. What aspects should be visually examined in a horse in which the primary complaint is lameness?

The first step is to evaluate the whole body conformation of the horse. The hind end, midsection, and neck should divide equally into three parts. Muscle atrophy also should be assessed, which may give the clinician insight into the site of lameness. Individual limbs also should be visualized and evaluated for straightness and proper joint angulation.

2. A complete examination of the foot area, which is the most common source of lameness in any breed of horse, is required for proper diagnosis. What structures in the foot area should be inspected during examination? Why?

With the hoof on the ground, the palmar digital artery, vein, and nerve should be palpated. The pulse should be just palpable and compared with pulse strength in the opposite foot. Increase in pulse strength is a good indicator of a problem in the affected foot. The heel bulbs, deep digital flexor tendon, and the coronary band should be palpated for heat, swelling, and pain. The hoof wall should be inspected and palpated for defects. It also may be percussed with hooftesters to detect pain. With the hoof off the ground and in hand, the hoof first should be cleaned thoroughly and then evaluated for proper size and alignment. The frog, sole, and heel bulbs should be inspected visually and manually with a probe or fingers. Hooftesters can then be applied to detect pain in the sole or frog areas. Results of this process can be obtained rapidly and will direct the clinician to further parts of the examination.

3. In general, how should a horse's limb be examined? What structures can be identified during a lameness examination?

The limb should be examined in a manner similar to the hoof (see question 2). The examination should be conducted in a methodical fashion and commence with the foot on the ground. All bone structures, joints, tendons, ligaments, and tendon sheaths should be palpated for heat, pain and swelling, starting at the distal aspect of the limb. Knowledge of the location of these structures and their normal appearance is essential to interpret the findings properly. Most clinicians start at the distal aspect of the limb and systematically work proximally, following a routine so as not to miss any areas. The same method should be used for inspection with the limb off the ground. This portion of the examination is essential because some structures, such as tendons and ligaments, are easier to palpate with the limb held off the ground; thus more information can be obtained.

4. Subtle lameness that only slightly impedes performance of high-level performance horses are difficult to identify. How may it be possible to diagnose accurately the cause of subtle lameness in a horse?

Diagnostic tests such as flexion tests, use of hooftesters, lunging, and manipulative tests can aid in detecting subtle lameness. The aim is to manipulate the limb or potential area of pain to make the pain worse. This aim can be achieved in a horse with any severity of lameness but is essential for identifying the cause of lameness in subtle cases. For instance, flexing the respective joint for 30–60 seconds before jogging the horse can worsen mildly painful conditions in that area. Worsening of the lameness is a sign of pain in that joint area. However, caution must be used in interpretation, especially in the hind limbs, because other joints and structures may be flexed or stressed unknowingly and hence provoke pain. For instance, a positive fetlock flexion test can indicate pain in the pastern or coffin joints, and a positive hock flexion may indicate pain in the stifle. The author performs digital, fetlock, and carpal flexion tests for 30 seconds and spavin (stifle and tarsus) tests for 60 seconds.

5. The lameness of a jogging horse mildly worsens for 3 steps after flexion of the carpus. Does the horse feel pain in the flexed carpus?

The horse does not necessarily feel pain in the flexed carpus, because almost all horses show mild lameness for about 3 steps after flexion of any joint—especially young racehorses in which intense exercise has commenced, placing increased forces on the joints. The results of such flexion tests must be compared with the results in other joints, such as the contralateral carpus in the present example. Any asymmetry in results may indicate the presence of a disease process.

6. A 15-year-old performance horse (e.g., Western Pleasure Quarter Horse) is presented with the complaint of shoulder stiffness and lameness. What is your diagnostic plan?

Visual inspection, palpation of the limbs (in the standing and flexed positions), use of hooftesters, visual inspection at a walk and then a jog, and manipulative tests (i.e., flexion tests and lunging) should be performed. Usually the area of pain can be identified from these basic procedures. Diagnostic nerve blocks can then be used to locate the area of pain objectively sometimes by exclusion. Once the area of pain is located, other diagnostic procedures, such as radiography and ultrasonography, can be performed. This diagnostic plan is essential for the novice clinician and is tailored by more veteran clinicians, who can often recognize the source of pain just by visual inspection. However, even senior clinicians often find it necessary to perform nerve blocks to identify the source of pain objectively. In most cases, horses that show shoulder pain are primarily lame elsewhere in the limb; the shoulder pain is compensatory because they usually move differently in the lame limb. If lower limb blocks do not eliminate the lameness, intraarticular anesthesia of upper limb joints should be performed. Other more sophisticated diagnostic tests, such as nuclear scintigraphy and upper limb radiographs, are often necessary and usually must be performed at a referral center.

7. Why are some horses with bone spavin sore in the back?

Horses with bone spavin that continue to perform are usually sore in the back because of compensation for the lameness, especially if the condition is allowed to go untreated. The pain from the hock joints causes the horse to adjust its way of moving and thus to use its back differently; this adjustment often leads to pain. Secondary or compensatory pain in the upper body of the horse may result from a variety of lamenesses in any limb.

8. Describe the significance of the site of a nail puncture into a hoof.

Any nail puncture into the bottom of a hoof is a potentially serious problem, but the consequences are different. Punctures into the sole area rarely penetrate any vital structures (e.g., joint, bursa, or tendon sheath) except for the coffin bone (third phalanx). Puncture and penetration of the coffin bone may result in abscess formation or osteomyelitis. Punctures into the frog and sulci areas may result in penetration of the navicular bursa, coffin joint, and/or digital sheath, all of which are synovial structures that can harbor infection. Prompt treatment of this condition is critical of a successful outcome (see figure on top of facing page).

9. What is the appropriate treatment in a horse whose hoof has been penetrated by a nail? The puncture is in the frog area.

Adequate control of the horse is needed during all phases of the examination, and the use of sedatives is necessary to obtain control. Visual examination of the foot is the first step in evaluation. If the nail is still in the hoof, radiography of the foot should be performed to determine the structures that may be involved with the nail. The radiographs can be developed later after initial

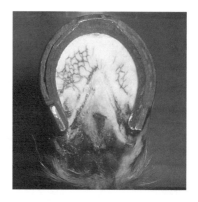

Normal, cleaned cadaver hoof. Cleaning is essential to evaluate sole, frog, and sulci for puncture wounds.

diagnostic and therapeutic procedures are performed. The nail should be removed and its size noted. The hoof should be thoroughly cleaned and disinfected, and the penetration site should be debrided to allow for drainage. Tetanus toxoid status of the horse should be assessed, and vaccination should be given if there is any doubt about the status. The horse should be placed on broad-spectrum antimicrobials. Considerable controversy surrounds the use of nonsteroidal antiinflammatory drugs (NSAIDs) in horses that may have joint penetration and subsequent infection. Some clinicians believe that only very low doses of NSAIDs should be given so that increased lameness can be detected when the joint, bursa, or tendon sheath becomes infected. The author places such horses on NSAIDs for pain and closely monitors the horse for joint or tendon sheath swelling. Intraarticular infusion of sterile saline and observance of the saline at the debrided puncture site also may help in the identification of joint, bursa, or tendon sheath involvement. Referral of such cases is usually best, especially if radiographs detect the involvement of vital structures.

10. Describe the grades of lameness developed by the American Association of Equine Practitioners (AAEP).

Grade 1   Difficult to observe; not consistently apparent regardless of circumstances (e.g., weight-carrying, circling, inclines, hard surfaces).

Grade 2   Difficult to observe at a walk or in trotting a straight line; consistently apparent under certain circumstances (e.g., weight-carrying, circling, inclines, hard surfaces).

Grade 3   Consistently observable at a trot under all circumstances.

Grade 4   Obvious lameness with marked nodding, hitching, or shortened stride.

Grade 5   Minimal weight-bearing in motion and/or at rest; inability to move.

American Association of Equine Practitioners: Definition and classification of lameness. In Guide for Veterinary Service and Judging of Equestrian Events. Lexington, KY, American Association of Equine Practitioners, 1991, p 19.

11. What are the causes of carpal valgus in a foal?

There are four potential causes of carpal valgus in a foal: (1) immaturity and ligament laxity; (2) incomplete ossification and malformation of carpal bones, which may result in carpal collapse, especially of the third and fourth carpal bones; (3) luxation or fracture of carpal bones due to trauma; and (4) asymmetric growth of the distal radial physis, causing malalignment of the epiphysis.

12. What pharmacologic agents are commonly used for perineural and intraarticular anesthesia in horses?

The three most commonly used local anesthetics are (1) lidocaine, (2) mepivicaine, and (3) bupivicaine. Lidocaine has the quickest onset and consequently the shortest duration of action (30–60 minutes). Mepivicaine, which takes slightly longer to work but has a longer duration of action (1.5–2 hours), is the most commonly used local anesthetic for diagnostic nerve blocks in horses. Bupivicaine has the longest duration of effect and is usually reserved for therapeutic purposes or for performing diagnostic anesthetic procedures on horses that require sedation or general anesthesia.

Riebold TW (ed): Veterinary Clinics of North America Equine Practice—Principles and Techniques of Equine Anesthesia. Philadelphia, W.B. Saunders, 1990.

13. What are the complications of perineural anesthesia of the tibial and peroneal nerves?

The tibial and peroneal nerves are responsible for motor function of the lower hind limb. Consequently, proper application of anesthetic agents to these nerves results in occasional loss of the horse's ability to extend the foot properly. This loss results in a "knuckling-over" effect as the horse walks and jogs, which may allow damage to the dorsum of the fetlock; therefore, it is routine to apply a cotton bandage to the fetlock joint of the blocked limb to avoid trauma. Perineural anesthesia of these nerves also is potentially harmful in young racehorses that may have an undiagnosed tibial stress fracture. This condition may worsen after the block is performed. In such cases, the horse may need to be sedated and placed into a box stall until the agent has worn off; the required time depends on the agent.

14. What structures are anesthetized by a palmar digital nerve block?

Structures that are usually desensitized by a palmar digital nerve block are (1) the navicular bone and bursa, (2) the distal aspect of the deep digital flexor tendon, (3) the palmar wings of the third phalanx, (4) the digital cushion, (5) the sensitive frog and sole, (6) the laminar corium, and (7) the coronet. Structures that are occasionally desensitized include (1) the middle and superficial distal sesamoidean ligaments and (2) parts of the coffin joint.

15. How do you test to see if a nerve block is working?

If the skin overlying the area of interest is desensitized, the area is most likely anesthetized. However, especially in more proximal sites in the limb, the deeper structures are often desensitized while the skin is not. Therefore, repetition of manipulative tests, such as use of hooftesters, palpation, and flexion tests, is necessary to determine whether the pain is gone. If pain remains, one of two explanations is possible: (1) the block did not work or (2) the site of pain is elsewhere in the limb. Confidence in the ability of a particular block to work is often subjective and depends on the clinician's experience with the blocking technique.

16. What are the potential complications of intraarticular anesthesia?

Potential complications of intraarticular anesthesia are threefold: (1) sepsis, (2) inability to identify the exact site of disease, and (3) destabilization of incomplete fractures. Intraarticular anesthesia must be approached like any other intraarticular injection. Sepsis is the primary complication from intraarticular injection of any substance. Therefore, correct preparation and injection technique must be followed during this procedure. In addition, the communication pathways that a particular joint makes with other structures must be appreciated. For instance, the tarsometatarsal and distal intertarsal joints communicate in a certain percentage of horses (8–38%); therefore, the clinician must appreciate the fact that injection of the tarsometatarsal joint in a particular horse may communicate with the distal intertarsal joint. Consequently, it may be difficult to identify exactly the site of disease. However, intraarticular anesthesia allows the clinician to gain important information about the general area of pain and the effectiveness of medicating the specific area. Destabilization of hidden, incomplete fractures also may occur with intraarticular anesthesia. For instance, an incomplete, midsagittal fracture of the first phalanx may worsen after intraarticular anesthesia.

McIlwraith CE, Trotter GW (eds): Joint Disease in the Horse. Philadelphia, W.B. Saunders, 1996.

17. How should the skin be prepared before injection of anesthetic agents into a joint?

This subject is controversial. In general an antiseptic scrub (such as betadine or chlorhexidine) should be applied for 7–10 minutes over three applications, alternating with a rinse of alcohol.

Some clinicians prefer to clip the area before injection, other do not. Both sides make good arguments for or against clipping, and the decision depends on the clinician's preference. Some clinicians claim that clippers may introduce more potential pathogens to the injection site than the hair at the site. Other clinicians claim that it is impossible to prepare the site adequately with the hair intact. After injection, some clinicians apply a light bandage, others apply a light ointment, and some apply nothing. Again, the decision is based on the clinician's experience. Some clinicians believe that it is necessary to keep the area sterile under a bandage for at least 24 hours until the injection site closes, others believe that the injection site can be kept adequately clean with ointment, and some believe that pathogens cannot enter the joint through the injection site.

FOOT DISEASE

18. What is the proper technique for removing a horseshoe?

Although the exact means of removing a shoe is controversial, the basic idea is to remove the nail clinches to minimize hoof wall damage with removal of the shoe. The nail clinches are the part of the nail that is folded over to secure the nail and shoe to the hoof wall. Basically, the clinches are removed or bent up with a hammer and clinch cutter. Some people use a rasp to grind down the clinches. The nails can then be removed individually with a nail puller, or the shoe can be removed with a shoe puller. The puller is placed under the shoe at the heels and elevated forward until the shoe comes loose.

19. What is an egg-bar shoe?

An egg-bar shoe is completely round. It is used to give more support to the foot, especially in the heel region where support is usually lacking. It is a common form of treatment for horses with navicular disease and is used prophylactically in some horses.

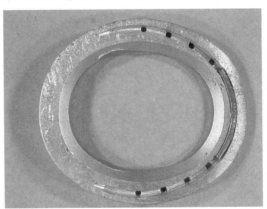

Egg-bar shoe.

20. What are contracted heels?

In contracted heels the heel bulbs are close together. This condition may result from chronic lameness, as the subtle decrease in use of the limb reduces the forces that keep the heel bulbs apart with normal activity. Contracted heels are usually associated with an upright heel, again because of the lack of use. Identification of this abnormality often leads to identification of a potential problem in the affected limb.

21. What are sheared heels?

Sheared heels exhibit unevenness between the heel bulbs (e.g., one heel bulb is higher than the other). An imbalance in the hoof may cause increased pressure on one heel, resulting in shearing forces between the two heel bulbs. This condition may result in heel soreness and cracks on the side of the hoof that is highest (e.g., pushed up).

22. How should a hoof abscess be treated?

Basically, the abscess should be identified and the borders defined. Because an abscess often migrates to another part of the hoof, the extent of the abscess should be determined by radiography, which reveals a gas shadow, or by debridement and visual examination. Adequate drainage should be supplied, and antiseptic packing should be placed into the defect. Some veterinarians make a metronidazole packing to ensure coverage against anaerobic bacteria, and some treat with systemic antimicrobials, whereas others do not. Some clinicians believe that antimicrobial therapy may cause the infection to recede and become latent, only to reappear later when the drugs are discontinued. Soaking the hoof in water with a 1% betadine solution and epsom salts may help to draw out deeper-infected tracts in the hoof. If the abscess is resistive to therapy, other tracts may be present, or the horse may have osteomyelitis of the third phalanx, which requires radiographic examination for diagnosis.

23. How do you prepare a hoof for a radiographic examination of the navicular bone?

The shoe must be removed, and the sole, frog, and sulci must be cleaned. It is best to use a wire brush to clean the hoof wall and sole areas. A packing agent that reduces the air-hoof interface (e.g., Playdo) should be packed into the sulci and any cracks in the sole and frog.

24. What views are needed to evaluate a navicular bone radiographically?

Three views are essential for adequate evaluation of the navicular bone: (1) a 60° dorsoproximal-palmarodistal oblique view, (2) a palmaroproximal-palmarodistal view, and (3) a lateromedial view. A 60° dorsoproximal-palmarodistal oblique view allows the clinician to view the navicular bone in the dorsal-palmar plane (Fig. A). The 45° palmaroproximal-palmarodistal view

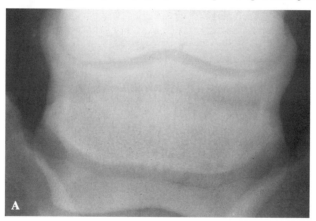

gives the clinician a "skyline" view of the navicular bone (Figs. B and C, top of facing page). The lateromedial view gives the clinician a lateral-to-medial view of the navicular bone. Other views help the clinician to visualize other structures in the foot, but these three are essential for adequate evaluation of the navicular bone.

Figure B (facing page) from Park RD, Lebel JL: Equine radiology. In Stashak TS (ed): Adams' Lameness in Horses, 4th ed. Philadelphia, Lea & Febiger, 1987, with permission.

25. What are the radiographic signs of navicular disease?

This topic is quite controversial. In recent years large studies have shown that radiographic changes that once were thought significant are commonly found in sound horses. However, some radiographic changes are significant, especially if the horse has clinical signs of navicular disease.

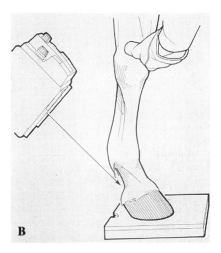

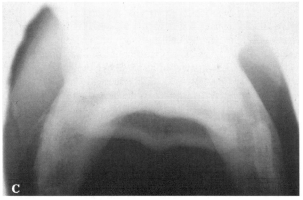

Any fracture of the navicular bone is significant but must be distinguished from separate centers of ossification. Large cysts are also significant. Erosion of the caudal border of the navicular bone or sclerosis of the medullary cavity as seen on the skyline projection (the 45° palmaroproximal-palmarodistal view) are also considered significant. Enlarged vascular foramina may be a radiographic sign of navicular disease, but they also may be seen in horses without clinical signs consistent with navicular disease and hence are a controversial finding.

26. How is navicular disease treated?

Any problem with conformation or shoeing must be addressed first. Shoeing changes are often the best form of therapy for navicular disease; no other therapy usually helps unless the hoof is adequately trimmed and shod. Egg-bar or wide-webbed shoes may be placed on the hooves to provide more support. The toes of these shoes may then be rolled to provide easy breakover of the hoof. Wedge pads may be used if the hoof is too low in the heels. Other forms of therapy include improving blood flow into and out of the navicular area. Isoxsuprine hydrochloride, a peripheral vasodilator, is often used for this purpose. If the soft tissues surrounding the navicular bone are believed to be involved and if the horse improves with a coffin joint block, then intraarticular medication (hyaluronic acid and/or corticosteroids) may be placed within the coffin joint to relieve inflammation. Other newer forms of therapy have also been found to help. Oral glycosaminoglycans (Cosequin) and systemic therapy with glycosaminoglycans (Adequan) and hyaluronic acid (Legend) have been found to be beneficial. If a horse is unresponsive to all forms of medication, a palmar digital neurectomy may be performed to desensitize the navicular region. The disease is rarely curable and can only be contained.

27. What is the prognosis for a horse that required a palmar digital neurectomy for treatment of navicular disease?

The latest study shows that 74% of horses are sound 1 year after a palmar digital neurectomy and 64% are sound after 2 years.

Jackman BR, Baxter GM, Doran RE, et al: Palmar digital neurectomy in horses: 57 cases (1984–1990). Vet Surg 22:285–288, 1993.

28. What are the causes of laminitis?

Laminitis may be caused by a number of local or systemic factors. Local factors include overuse of a limb, as when the contralateral limb was fractured. Systemic derangements, such as endotoxemia, grain/carbohydrate overload (often with endotoxemia), and Cushing's disease (i.e., pituitary hyperplasia/adenoma) also may cause laminitis. Systemic medications, particularly corticosteroids, have been associated with the onset of laminitis. Environmental factors such as black walnut shavings also cause laminitis. Laminitis appears to be more prevalent in older horses.

29. What treatment should be used for the acute phases of laminitis?

The primary goal is to eliminate the causative agent if possible. Horses that have overeaten grain or carbohydrate should be given (1) nasogastric lavage if overload occurred in the last 2–6 hours; (2) mineral oil to reduce the amount of bacterial overgrowth and absorption of endotoxin by the intestines, the effects of lipopolysaccharide released from gram-negative bacteria in the colon, and inflammatory mediators released from the bacteria; (3) systemic NSAIDs or 5–10% dimethyl sulfoxide (DMSO) in intravenous fluids, but not corticosteroids, to further reduce inflammation in the laminae of the hoof; (4) frog support, which is essential and can be achieved by having the horse stand on a sand floor or by application of a commercially available "lily pad"; (5) vasodilators such as acepromazine or isoxuprine hydrochloride to restore normal hemodynamics within the foot; and (6) antithrombotic agents such as aspirin or heparin. Controversy surrounds the efficacy of isoxuprine hydrochloride and heparin regimens.

Bertone JJ (ed): Veterinary Clinics of North America—Emergency Treatment of the Adult Horse. Philadelphia, W.B. Saunders, 1994.

30. What methods can be used to determine the prognosis for a horse with acute laminitis?

The degree of third phalanx rotation on radiographic evaluation, the severity of lameness, and the response to treatment have been used to determine the prognosis of horses with acute laminitis. The degree of rotation of the third phalanx compared with the dorsal hoof wall, as measured on lateromedial radiographic projections, was once believed to be the best method of determining the prognosis for horses with laminitis. Horses with less than 5.5° rotation returned to former athletic function, whereas those with more than 11.5° of rotation did not. This point has since been disputed in a study in which the degree of pain was determined to be the best indicator of laminar damage and hence prognosis. Other clinicians have based prognosis on the speed with which a horse responds to treatment. All three methods have their merits and should be taken into account in determining prognosis. Third phalanx sinking is a sign of poor prognosis.

Stick JA, Jalm HW, Scott EA, Robinson NE: Pedal bone rotation as a prognostic sign in laminitis of horses. J Am Vet Med Assoc 188:251–253, 1982.

Hunt RJ: A retrospective evaluation of laminitis in horses. Equine Vet J 25:61–64, 1993.

31. Describe the grading system to determine the severity of laminitis.

The severity of laminitis is based on the Obel grading scale:

Grade 1   The horse lifts its feet incessantly, often every few seconds

Grade 2   The horse moves willingly at a walk, but the gait is characteristic of laminitis.
           A forefoot may be lifted without difficulty.

Grade 3   The horse vigorously resists attempts to lift a forefoot because of pain in the
            contralateral digit and moves reluctantly.
Grade 4   The horse must be forced to move and may be recumbent.

SOFT TISSUE DISEASES

32. Is a mild pain response on palpation of a proximal suspensory ligament significant?

Some horses with normal suspensory ligaments show a mild pain response on palpation. The key is to be sure that the response is equal on both forelimbs and to ensure that the horse does not jog lamely after palpation. Perineural anesthesia may be needed if the significance of the finding is in question.

33. Which ultrasound probe is used to scan soft tissues of the distal limb?

A 7.5- or 10 MHz probe is most appropriate for evaluating soft tissue structures in the distal limbs of horses. The suspensory ligament can be viewed directly, but the more superficial structures require a standoff pad for visualization.

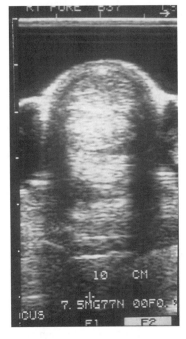

34. What are the signs of acute tendinitis of the superficial digital flexor (SDF) tendon?

The signs depend on the use of the animal, the cause of the injury, and the severity of the lesion. Injuries due to bandaging or direct trauma manifest themselves immediately. The limbs become hot, swollen, and painful over the SDF. Affected horses resent palpation of the area. In racehorses, however, the inciting cause may be more chronic (e.g., chronic exercise), and abnormalities can be detected at times as an increase in the sensitivity of the tendon to palpation before the onset of obvious heat and swelling. The same is true for any athletic horse, in which mild signs may manifest early as mild swelling or pain on palpation.

35. What are the treatment options for tendinitis of the SDF tendon?

In the acute phase, antiinflammatory treatments are needed. They may be given systemically (e.g., NSAIDs and/or 5–10% DMSO in intravenous fluids) or locally under a bandage (e.g., topical DMSO). Cold hosing or icing is critical in the first 48 hours, as is bandaging to provide counterpressure and prevent edema formation. After swelling and pain subside (typically within days), controlled exercise (e.g., hand-walking) can be started, depending on the severity of the injury. If ultrasound evaluation reveals a core lesion, other measures, such as tendon splitting, beta-aminopropionitirile fumarate therapy, and superior check ligament desmotomy, can be performed.

JOINT DISEASE

36. What are the causes of septic arthritis in foals?

Bacteria that cause hematogenous septic arthritis in the joints of foals usually originate from remote sites such as the respiratory tract, gastrointestinal tract, or umbilicus. Consequently, the most commonly implicated bacteria include the Enterobacteriaceae, namely *Escherichia coli, Klebsiella pneumoniae,* and *Salmonella* species. *Actinobacillus* species also may be involved. Mycoplasmal and chlamydial species also have been associated with septic arthritis of foals. The "end-loop" capillary configurations of the arteries at the epiphyses of long bones allow sluggish blood flow and hence are a perfect medium for the establishment of infection. Therefore, bacteria establish themselves at the epiphyses and subsequently spread into the joint.

37. How is septic arthritis diagnosed?

The hallmark characteristics of septic arthritis are lameness, moderate-to-severe pain on palpation, and warmth and swelling of the joint. The best way to diagnose the disease is by arthrocentesis and cytologic evaluation of the fluid. White blood cell counts greater than 30,000/µl with predominant neutrophils are indicative of infection. Further bacterial evaluation of the fluid, namely culture and sensitivity procedures, is also essential for determining bacterial type and sensitivity to antimicrobials, although results are often negative despite suspected sepsis.

38. How can you determine that a small wound penetrated a joint?

Visual inspection of a joint often leads to misdiagnosis in cases of penetration of the joint cavity, especially if the wound is small, such as a puncture wound. Therefore, sterile infusion of 0.9% saline or lactated Ringer's solution (LRS) into the joint at a site remote to the wound and visual inspection of the wound for extrusion of fluid during infusion are essential to determine whether the wound communicates with the joint cavity. For instance, if a horse has a wound over the dorsum of its fetlock joint, sterile 0.9% saline or LRS can be infused into the palmar recess and the wound inspected for extrusion of fluid.

39. What treatment should be instituted for septic arthritis?

Treatment first should be aimed at eliminating the infection with aggressive systemic antimicrobial therapy as well as joint irrigation and local treatment with antimicrobials. Systemic antimicrobial therapy is necessary to get high levels of antimicrobials into the soft tissues of the joint, which harbor infection. The author uses potassium penicillin (22,000 IU/kg IV every 6 hours) and gentamicin (6.6 mg/kg IV every 24 hours). Joint lavage is essential for removing not only bacteria, but also inflammatory mediators (e.g., prostaglandins and interleukins) that can damage articular cartilage. Joint lavage also decompresses the accumulated joint fluid, thus providing pain relief. Lavage may be accomplished with solutions such as LRS or 0.9% saline. Antiinflammatory agents, such as DMSO (5–10% solution in 1 liter of fluid), and/or antimicrobial solutions, such as povidone-iodine solution (0.1%), also may be used. Local administration of antimicrobials into the joint has also proved helpful. The author routinely lavages the joint with 2–3 liters of 0.9% saline/LRS, then 1 liter of 10% DMSO, and places 1–2 ml of Amikacin (250 mg/ml) within the joint. More refractory cases can be treated with arthroscopic debridement of infected synovial tissues and arthrotomy to allow continuous drainage of infected synovial fluid. Other clinicians may prefer to place a continuous suction drain for constant evacuation of fluid.

40. What signs indicate joint pain in a horse?

The hallmark signs of joint pain in a horse are heat, pain, and swelling (synovial effusion). More subtle signs of pain include pain on flexion and increased lameness after flexion of a particular joint. Horses with joint pain also show reduced range of motion of the joint and differences in the use of the affected limb. For example, a horse with carpal pain may move "wide" at the knees to reduce the need to flex the carpus during jogging.

41. What structures within a joint may be the cause of pain?

Any structure within the joint may be the source of pain. However, it appears that joint distention caused by effusion is often the primary source of pain. Disruption or disease of the synovial membrane, joint capsule, ligaments, articular cartilage, or subchondral bone may be the inciting cause of the problem and thus the distention. However, articular cartilage damage itself may not be as painful as the synovitis and effusion that it causes.

42. Describe the treatment options for horses with osteoarthritis of a joint.

The primary form of treatment is to remove the inciting cause. For example, removal of osteochondral fragments or repair of intraarticular fractures is required to stop the inflammatory cascade responsible for causing synovial effusion and pain. The second priority is to decrease the inflammation already established within the joint. Methods include systemic NSAIDs (e.g., phenylbutazone: 2.2–4.4 mg/kg every 12–24 hours, depending on severity of the disease) and local infusion of antiinflammatory drugs such as corticosteroids (the dose depends on the particular joint). Finally, the normal balance of the joint must be restored. Use of chondroprotective agents, such as polysulfated glycosaminoglycans (e.g., 500 mg Adequan, intramuscularly once a week for 5 weeks) and hyaluronic acid (40 mg intravenously once a week for 3 weeks) may assist.

NONSTEROIDAL ANTIINFLAMMATORY DRUGS

43. Which NSAID preparation is said to work best for pain of the musculoskeletal system?

Although this impression is subjective, most clinicians believe that phenylbutazone works better on orthopedic pain than flunixin meglumine. Flunixin meglumine is believed to work better for soft tissue problems such as visceral pain. Yet some clinicians and some research have shown better results with flunixin meglumine or ketoprofen for relief of musculoskeletal pain. The point is controversial and depends on the prior experiences of the clinician. Phenylbutazone is significantly cheaper than flunixin meglumine or ketoprofen.

44. What are the signs of phenylbutazone toxicity in a young horse?

The signs of phenylbutazone toxicity include (1) gastrointestinal ulceration, which may occur even in the oral mucosa (typically gastric ulceration and right dorsal colitis are diagnosed); (2) renal papillary necrosis; (3) platelet dysfunction; and (4) neutropenia and toxic left shift, possibly due to suppression of granulopoiesis or, more likely, neutropenia due to margination (as in most cases of equine endotoxemia) or consumption. Young horses with a history of phenylbutazone overuse often have right dorsal colitis, resulting in loss of protein from this area. Affected horses often appear with chronic signs of weight loss, lethargy, and sometimes colic. Total serum protein levels are low.

45. What test can be performed to detect phenylbutazone toxicity?

Before development of signs, horses on high doses of phenylbutazone may start to show reduction in total protein levels. Therefore, if a horse is knowingly going to be placed on high levels of phenylbutazone for a prolonged period, it may be a good idea to get a baseline total protein level and follow-up periodically. Another precautionary test is to check the serum creatinine and blood urea nitrogen (BUN) before NSAID use. It may be prudent to check them intermittently and also to get a urine sample (e.g., free catch) and utilize a dipstick check for blood, which may indicate renal papillary necrosis if positive. After development of signs, a chemistry panel checking protein, creatinine, BUN, and electrolytes as well as a complete blood count (CBC) should be performed. Finally, techniques such as gastroscopy, abdominocentesis, and white cell-labeled scintigraphy may be performed.

OSTEOCHONDROSIS

46. What are the causes of osteochondrosis (OCD) in young horses?

Many of the causes of OCD in young horses are poorly understood. Trauma to the osteo-chondral area or to its blood supply has been hypothesized as a cause. Nutritional factors, such as overfeeding (especially of digestible energy), copper deficiency, and abnormal calcium-to-phosphorus ratio (especially too much phosphorus) have also been speculated as causes of OCD. Hereditary problems have been indicated as contributing factors, such as propensity for fast growth and conformation abnormalities.

McIlwraith CW, Trotter GW (eds): Joint Disease in the Horse. Philadelphia, W.B. Saunders, 1996.

47. What sites in the tarsocrural joints may be affected by OCD?

Most commonly the dorsal intermediate ridge of the tibia, the lateral trochlear ridge of the talus (tibiotarsus bone), the medial malleolus of the tibia, and the medial trochlear ridge of the talus are affected. Because any of these sites may be affected, a complete radiographic examination is needed for diagnosis. Even then subtle lesions may be missed.

48. What are the signs of OCD in young horses?

Young horses with OCD manifest signs in different ways. Mild lesions may not manifest clinically until the horse is put to strenuous work, although sometimes joint distention is noticed and the young horse may not move as readily as its peers. More severe lesions may manifest as synovial effusion without lameness at a young age. Some lesions, especially if severe, may manifest as severe lameness and synovial effusion.

ORTHOPEDIC FIRST AID

49. Should a horse with a fracture of the tibia face forward or backward in a trailer during transport?

Horses with hindlimb fractures should face forward in the trailer, and horses with forelimb fractures should face to the rear because the driver can more easily control acceleration than unforeseen braking. Thus, horses with hindlimb fractures have to place less sudden force on the fractured limb in case of a sudden stop.

50. How should a fracture of the second phalanx be treated for transport?

Ideally, the limb should be bandaged and suspended from the ground with a PVC splint placed dorsally from the carpus to the toe to align the third metacarpal bone, phalanges, and dorsal hoof wall in a single line. A Kimsey splint, which accomplishes the same goal, or a Farley compression boot also may be used. The idea is to align the lower limb for best support and to decrease the chances of worsening the fracture.

Nixon AJ (ed): Equine Fracture Repair. Philadelphia, W.B. Saunders, 1996.

51. Should a horse with a fracture of the third metacarpal bone be treated with a dose of NSAID before referral to a hospital?

Some clinicians argue that NSAID treatment of horses with a severe fracture makes them comfortable enough to place weight on the limb and thus worsen the fracture. Others argue that no dose of NSAIDs can accomplish that degree of pain relief and that proper splinting will alleviate the problems of potential weight-bearing. Horses that are allowed to be in pain, especially if they realize that the limb has no axial support, may become quite frantic, leading to severe sweating, dehydration, and shock. Therefore, most clinicians agree that the comfort of the horse is paramount to successful anesthesia and recovery from surgery and that institution of pain relief should be immediate to ensure a good anesthetic candidate for repair.

52. How should a horse that has lacerated its SDF tendon, deep digital flexor (DDF) tendon, and suspensory ligament be stabilized?

The wound should be thoroughly lavaged and cleaned, then placed within a sterile bandage. The clinician also must assess whether the tendon sheath has been invaded and may institute therapy as for joint penetration (described earlier). The horse should be placed into some sort of splint support. A Kimsey splint works well for such injuries, as does the dorsal PVC splint placed from the carpus to the toe to align the third metacarpal bone, the phalanges, and the dorsal hoof wall in a single line (see question 50). Antimicrobial and NSAID treatment also should be administered. Tetanus status should be determined, and tetanus vaccine should be given if the status is unknown. Horses with any distal limb injury also should be physically assessed for hydration, because excitement and fear may cause excessive sweating.

53. What medications should be administered to a horse with an open radius fracture?

Local wound care should be instituted and the horse placed on systemic antimicrobials and NSAIDs. The limb then should be bandaged and splinted properly. Tetanus status also should be determined and a tetanus toxoid administered if the status is unknown or if the most recent vaccination occurred more than 6 months previously.

PROGNOSIS

54. What resources are best for determining the prognosis for a specific injury to a horse?

Textbooks supply some basic information about the prognosis for a specific injury. More recent and detailed information can be obtained from retrospective studies in journals. However, there may be regional and athletic use differences between the patient and cases described in the literature. Sometimes the best resources are people in the same geographic area who commonly deal with equine injuries or specialists at referral hospitals in the area.

55. What factors play a role in determining the prognosis for a specific disease?

Both medical and nonmedical factors play a role in determining prognosis for a specific disease. Medical factors include accurate diagnosis and grading of the severity of the disease, duration of the disease, and response to treatment. Nonmedical factors include the expectations of the owners about the anticipated level of competition for the animal and the ability to treat the horse (perhaps over the long term) effectively and legally during competition, if this is desirable.

BIBLIOGRAPHY

1. American Association of Equine Practitioners: Definition and classification of lameness. In Guide for Veterinary Service and Judging of Equestrian Events. Lexington, KY, American Association of Equine Practitioners, 1991, p 19.
2. Bertone JJ (ed): Veterinary Clinics of North America—Emergency Treatment of the Adult Horse. Philadelphia, W.B. Saunders, 1994.
3. Hunt RJ: A retrospective evaluation of laminitis in horses. Equine Vet J 25:61–64, 1993.
4. Jackman BR, Baxter GM, Doran RE, et al: Palmar digital neurectomy in horses: 57 cases (1984–1990). Vet Surg 22:285–288, 1993.
5. McIlwraith CW, Trotter GW (eds): Joint Disease in the Horse. Philadelphia, W.B. Saunders, 1996.
6. Nixon AJ (ed): Equine Fracture Repair. Philadelphia, W.B. Saunders, 1996.
7. Riebold TW (ed): Veterinary Clinics of North America Equine Practice—Principles and Techniques of Equine Anesthesia. Philadelphia, W.B. Saunders, 1990.
8. Stashak TS (ed): Adams' Lameness in Horses, 4th ed. Philadelphia, Lea & Febiger, 1987.
9. Stick JA, Jalm HW, Scott EA, Robinson NE: Pedal bone rotation as a prognostic sign in laminitis of horses. J Am Vet Med Assoc 188:251–253, 1982.

14. NEUROLOGY

Stephen M. Reed, D.V.M., Dip. ACVIM, Richard J. Piercy, M.A., Vet. M.B., and Elias E. Perris, D.V.M.

1. What is the best way to evaluate horses with disease of the central nervous system (CNS)?

The approach to diseases of the CNS in horses begins with a review of basic neuroanatomy because the critical first step is localization of the lesion. In some cases, such as cerebellar abiotrophy, seizures, hyperkalemic periodic paralysis, and cervical vertebral stenotic myelopathy, the signalment (age, breed, sex, and use) may help to determine the disease process. However, in most horses the anatomic localization of the lesion helps to determine the etiology. The brain, spinal cord, and peripheral nerves have specialized functions. The various components of the nervous system contain neuronal cell bodies arranged in layers of laminae, nuclei, and columns of gray matter (polio); tracts, sheets, and pathways of dendrites (afferent) and axonal (efferent) processes of these cell bodies make up white matter (leuko). These tracts are covered with an insulating fatty layer known as myelin. The cerebrum and cerebellum have an outer cortex and an inner medulla. The brainstem consists of the thalamus, midbrain, pons, and medulla oblongata. Lesions in these specialized areas may result in specific clinical signs that allow localization of the lesion to a discrete or defined region.

2. What portions of the neuroanatomy are important for the clinician?

In most cases the specific identification of spinal tracts of brain pathways should be left for the neuroanatomist or clinical neurologic specialist. The clinician should be familiar with certain areas such as the cortical brain, cerebellum, vestibular region, and other specific portions of the brainstem; the spinal cord and spinal root; and peripheral nerve and neuromuscular junction as well as muscle. A working familiarity with the signs associated with disease of these structures aids in localization of lesions.

3. How are symptoms localized to the neuroanatomic regions?

The neuroanatomic localization of a lesion begins when you take the history. The owner typically describes specific clinical signs that may help to localize the area most likely affected. The history is a useful tool and should not be overlooked before starting the examination of the horse. The neurologic examination should be methodical and may be reliably performed by starting at the head and proceeding caudally to the tail and anus. At each portion of the examination it is important to observe carefully and record the clinical findings, as well as to ask additional historical questions of the owner or attendant to help explain the additional signs demonstrated by the horse.

4. What clinical features of brain disease can be elicited by the history and physical examination?

Horses presented with brain disease often have a history of abnormal or unusual behavior, such as aimless wandering, appearing blind, head pressing, seizures, dementia, or coma. Such clinical signs are typical, although brain disease is an infrequent problem in horses. In a few horses fine resting tremors of the lips and difficulty with prehension may be noted. These signs indicate a lesion in the region of the globus pallidus and substantia nigra and may be seen with yellow star thistle or Russian knapweed toxicity.

5. Which features of cerebellar brain disease can be elicited by the history and physical examination?

The cerebellum is important in the regulation of rate and range of motion. Cerebellar abiotrophy is seen occasionally in Arabian or mixed Arabian breeds and also has been observed in other breeds. The most important clinical features include lack of a menace response, failure to blink to bright light, and tremors of the head that worsen or become more obvious with intentional movements (intention tremors). Horses with cerebellar disease show good preservation of strength but profound evidence of spasticity and hypermetria. They are often base-wide with ataxic movements.

6. Name the 12 cranial nerves.

I	Olfactory nerve	VII	Facial nerve
II	Ophthalmic (optic) nerve	VIII	Vestibulocochlear nerve
III	Oculomotor nerve	IX	Glossopharyngeal nerve
IV	Trochlear nerve	X	Vagus nerve
V	Trigeminal nerve	XI	Accessory spinal nerve
VI	Abducens nerve	XII	Hypoglossal nerve

7. Which clinical features of brainstem disease can be elicited by the history and physical examination?

The 12 cranial nerves are located in the brainstem; therefore, careful questioning along with systematic examination can be helpful in this evaluation. The brainstem is the pathway for long tracts passing to and from the spinal cord. Therefore, many horses with brainstem disease show clinical signs similar to those of spinal cord disease. Localization is made possible by the associated cranial nerve deficits unless the neurologic disease is characterized by multiple discrete foci (e.g., spinal cord and peripheral nerves, as may happen in a horse with equine protozoal myeloencephalitis [EPM]). Deficits may be noted in any of the 12 cranial nerves (see question 6) but are least common in cranial nerves I, II, and XI. The signs may vary but often include weakness of the extraocular muscles of the eye (CN III, IV, VI), decreased sensation of the face and nasal passages (CN V) and facial paralysis (CN VII), head tilt and nystagmus (CN VIII), difficulty with swallowing and phonation (CN IX, X), and/or decreased motor function of the tongue (CN XII). The examination of horses with brainstem lesions often reveals ptosis of the eyelid, deviation of the muzzle, drooping of the ear, head tilt, nystagmus, and occasionally strabismus. In addition, the horse appears weak, ataxic, and spastic in both thoracic and pelvic limbs.

8. Which of the clinical features of spinal cord disease can be elicited from the history and physical examination?

Horses with spinal cord disease frequently present with neurologic disease characterized by loss of coordination and weakness in the limbs *caudal* to the site of the lesion. Some horses may show evidence of sensory deficits (unusual) or focal sweating. Focal sweating may be a sign of damage to the peripheral pre- or postganglionic sympathetic nervous system or evidence of tectotegmental spinal tract damage, which results in sweating along one side of the body.

9. What are the neurologic findings in horses with spinal cord disease?

The clinical signs of spinal cord disease in horses depend on the neuroanatomic location of the lesion. Horses that have cervical spinal cord involvement demonstrate signs of weakness, ataxia, and spasticity involving both thoracic and pelvic limbs. The presence of gait deficits in the pelvic limbs only indicates a lesion located caudal to T2. Proprioceptive pathways travel to the thalamus and cerebral proprioceptive centers, whereas unconscious proprioceptive pathways, such as the spinocerebellar tracts, ascend directly to the cerebellum. A spinal cord lesion located at either the brachial or lumbosacral intumescence and involving local reflex arcs for the muscles of the limbs results in flaccid paralysis of those muscles. Lesions cranial to a reflex arc result in loss of upper motor neuron (UMN) inhibition and lead to spastic paralysis. An UMN lesion usually involves concurrent damage to the proprioceptive and nociceptive pathways, resulting in ataxia and sometimes hypoalgesia. This scenario, however, is sometimes difficult to ascertain in horses.

10. How frequently do horses with spinal cord disease demonstrate signs of a radiculopathy ("root signs")?

It is unusual to identify signs of pain or focal neuroanatomic lesions suggestive of a radiculopathy in horses. In some horses, however, the clinical signs are confined to one region and may include apparent neck pain, muscle atrophy, and sometimes fasciculations. According to recent reports, cervical vertebral pain and stiffness with or without neurologic gait deficits may be caused by degenerative vertebral joint disease of the articular facets or outpouching of the joint capsule.

11. Which clinical features of peripheral neuropathy can be elicited by the history and physical examination?

Peripheral neuropathies are characterized by regional loss of motor function and sometimes accompanied by sensory deficits. If a horse is presented with the peripheral nerve injury characterized by Sweeney, it is helpful to ask whether other horses are affected. The disorder may develop when two horses hit shoulder to shoulder while running or playing. Horses with peripheral nerve injuries show evidence of muscle atrophy and profound weakness that usually involves only one limb or a regional part of the body. Diffuse muscle wasting, despite a ravenous appetite, in a horse with signs of weakness and trembling that stands with all four limbs together and the head hung low may be early evidence of equine motor neuron disease (EMND). This condition appears to be a model of aymotrophic lateral sclerosis (Lou Gehrig's disease) in humans and to be associated with some form of oxidative injury to the ventral horn cells of the spinal cord. It may be associated with a deficiency of vitamin E.

12. Which clinical features of muscle and neuromuscular junction disease can be elicited by the history and physical examination?

Primary muscle disease is not unusual in horses. Conditions such as exertional rhabdomyolysis, myotonia, and hyperkalemic periodic paralysis (HYPP) have been reported. Horses that suffer from generalized weakness characterized by trembling, dysphagia, or recumbency may be suffering from diffuse neuromuscular junction disease, such as botulism. Poor muscle tone, weakness, and difficulty with swallowing may be early signs of botulism.

13. What are the clinical features of spinal cord compression in horses?

The most common cause of spinal cord compression in horses is cervical vertebral stenotic myelopathy (CVM). This condition has been observed in all breeds but appears most prevalent in Thoroughbreds. The problem appears to have a multifactorial and poorly defined etiology. The clinical signs are most often observed in horses younger than 2 years, although spinal cord compression due to caudal cervical degenerative osteoarthritis has been reported in older horses. The disorder results in compression of the spinal cord in the cervical region and leads to weakness, ataxia, and spasticity in the thoracic and pelvic limbs. The signs are frequently about one grade more severe in the pelvic limbs. Some affected horses demonstrate cervical vertebral pain or stiffness when the head and neck are moved to the left and right or in a dorsal-to-ventral direction.

14. What are the most useful diagnostic tests for evaluation of horses with cervical vertebral stenotic myelopathy (CVM)?

The diagnosis of CVM can be predicted by use of standing lateral radiographs of the cervical vertebrae. Radiographs should be performed with the neck as straight as possible to facilitate measurement of the vertebral canal width as well as to evaluate vertebral facet alignment and/or degenerative changes of the vertebral bodies and facets. A myelogram is required for definitive diagnosis of CVM.

15. How is spinal cord compression best managed?

In horses with stenosis of the vertebral canal, the management of spinal cord compression may involve stall rest or other confinement along with antiinflammatory medications. If the diagnosis is made in a suckling or weanling foal, one management technique includes strict stall confinement to prevent trauma to the spinal cord within the vertebral canal and dietary restriction to slow the development of malformed or malaligned vertebrae. In older animals that are mildly to moderately affected, stall rest and antiinflammatory medications such as corticosteroids or dimethyl sulfoxide may be helpful. Surgical intervention is indicated when compression is associated with malaligned or deformed vertebrae that cause moderate-to-severe clinical signs. Early surgical intervention is preferable. The goals of vertebral surgery are to stabilize adjacent vertebrae, to stop trauma to the spinal cord, and to decompress the spinal cord within the vertebral canal. Ventral stabilization, the most commonly used technique, involves fusion of the vertebrae by use of a metal Bagby basket and a bone graft. Dorsal laminectomy is an alternative technique used occasionally in stenotic lesions. Both procedures are technically difficult to perform and usually provide improvement of only one grade.

16. What is the most common cause of multifocal disease of the CNS in horses?

Equine protozoal myeloencephalitis (EPM) is a serious and sometimes fatal neurologic disease of horses. The classic presentation includes signs of asymmetric involvement of the brain, brainstem, cranial nerves, and/or spinal cord. The disease may affect both white and gray matter and sometimes leads to profound muscle atrophy as a result of lower motor neuron damage. EPM is caused by *Sarcocystis neurona*, a protozoan parasite in the order Apicomplexa and family Sarcocystidae. Serologic surveys have shown that approximately 50% of horses in the United States have been exposed, although the greatest number of exposed horses appears to be in the South and Midwest. Other Sarcocystidae parasites known to infect the nervous system include *Toxoplasma* and *Neospora* species. In horses, *S. neurona* is found only in the asexual stage of the life cycle. The organism is found principally in neurons, often in association with a mixed inflammatory response. Various stages of the life cycle, such as schizonts or merozoites, are sometimes found in phagocytic cells, giant cells, and inflammatory macrophages. In some horses the organism may be detected in intravascular neutrophils and eosinophils as well as capillary endothelial cells. Although the exact life cycle, including the intermediate hosts, is not known for *S. neurona*, other *Sarcocystis* species have an obligatory predator-prey life cycle. Sarcocysts are usually found embedded in the skeletal muscle of the intermediate host (i.e., prey animals, usually birds). The definitive host appears to be the opossum, which is the site for the sexual stage of the life cycle. The resultant oocysts of *S. neurona* are passed in the feces of the definitive host and are the source of infection for the intermediate host as well as aberrant dead-end hosts, such as the horse. There is no evidence of patent infections in horses; hence direct horse-to-horse transmission does *not* occur (i.e., the disease is not contagious).

17. How is EPM diagnosed?

Definitive diagnosis of EPM is often difficult and cannot be made by clinical signs alone, although it should be suspected in horses that present with multifocal neurologic disease. In horses that die of EPM, characteristic inflammatory lesions may be observed, and in some cases the causative organism may be identified within the spinal cord. The best antemortem diagnostic test for EPM is made by recognition of clinical signs combined with a positive immunoblot (Western blot) for detection of antibodies against the causative organism found in the cerebrospinal fluid (CSF) of the horse. The most typical bands recognized on SDS-gel electrophoretograms are 22.5, 13, and 10.5 kDa. False-positive tests may result from serum or blood contamination during the collection of CSF. Use of albumin quotient (AQ) to detect the presence of serum albumin in the sample *and* IgG index to determine the presence or absence of intrathecal production of immunoglobulins may be useful to identify whether a specific test result is to be believed:

$$AQ = albumin_{CSF}/albumin_{SERUM} \times 100$$
$$IgG\ index = IgG_{CSF}/IgG_{SERUM} \times albumin_{SERUM}/albumin_{CSF}$$

Increasing evidence indicates that false-positive tests may be common. The nested polymerase chain reaction (PCR) technique has been used to amplify the small subunit ribosomal RNA gene of *S. neurona* primarily for the purpose of phylogenetic classification of the organism. It does not appear to be useful as a clinical tool because the organism is rarely found free in the CSF.

18. What treatments are most useful in horses with EPM?

Current treatment most typically involves oral formulations combining pyrimethamine (Daraprim, Burroughs-Wellcome) and a sulfonamide, usually sulfadiazine or sulfamethoxazole. These drugs are synergistic and act by inhibition of sequential steps in the synthesis of protozoal tetrahydrofolate. The usual dosage is 1 mg/kg of pyrimethamine daily and 25–30 mg/kg once or twice daily for the sulfonamide. At present affected horses usually are treated for 5 months or longer. Prolonged treatment involves the potential for toxicity, such as anemia, neutropenia, and thrombocytopenia, because of inhibition of the dihyrofolate reductase and folic acid deficiency. Administration of folic acid in an attempt to prevent these side effects is not indicated; in fact, it may worsen the clinical response. It is important to monitor the response to treatment as well as to look for evidence of toxicity. Complete blood counts (CBC) and serum folate concentrations should be monitored, and treatment should be stopped if unwanted side effects arise. Plenty of green forage and supplementation with brewer's yeast lessen the chances of toxicity. Recent research to investigate the usefulness of other coccidiostatic agents, such as diclazuril or toltrazuril, is under way. These benzeneacetonitrile agents are used in the prophylaxis of coccidiosis in poultry. They appear to be selectively toxic for apicomplexans because of the presence of a chlorplast-related binding site conserved in the parasites but believed to be absent in mammals.

19. What cause of spinal ataxia in horses is characterized by hypometria and spasticity?

Young horses with signs of symmetric ataxia and incoordination without concurrent evidence of spinal canal stenosis are often affected with equine degenerative myeloencephalopathy (EDM). EDM has been recognized in all equine species, including horses, asses, and zebras. It appears to have a familial predisposition in some breeds, and a heritable relationship has been demonstrated in Appaloosa, Standardbred, and Morgan horses. The time of onset is usually before 1 year of age, although EDM has been observed in horses older than 10 years. The clinical signs are sometimes self-limiting, and affected horses live with permanent neurologic deficits. In such cases the cause of the neurologic disease may never be determined or may be identified only by recognition of characteristic postmortem lesions.

20. What factors have been associated with EDM in horses?

The exact cause of EDM is not known. However, familial tendency, vitamin E deficiency, exposure to wood preservatives, and copper deficiency have been implicated. The most popular theory appears to be related to either a deficiency of vitamin E or an abnormality in vitamin E metabolism. The characteristic lesions of axonal and dentritic swelling, neuronal depletion, and accumulation of lipofuscin-like pigment within brainstem nuclei (most often in cuneatus and gracilus nuclei and nucleus thoracicus) and throughout the spinal cord are characteristic of oxidant type injury. A deficiency of an important antioxidant such as vitamin E may be expected to result in such lesions. Antioxidants limit the deleterious effects of oxidant free radical species, thereby sparing lipid membranes, cellular DNA, and proteins.

21. What is the usefulness of CSF evaluation in the diagnosis of neurologic diseases in horses?

CSF analysis may be useful in the evaluation of horses with neurologic disease. In horses with equine herpesvirus 1 (EHV1) myeloencephalopathy, the CSF is often xanthochromic, contains an elevated protein concentration (100–500 mg/dl), and has a high albumin quotient, indicating leakage of protein from the vascular space (presumably because the virus results in vasculitis). The CSF cytology of horses with EHV1 myeloencephalopathy is usually within normal limits. The CSF of horses affected with EDM is within normal limits in protein concentration, cytology, and enzyme concentration, whereas horses affected with EPM or an aberrant parasite migration may have mild-to-moderate increases in protein concentration (> 70 mg/dl) and normal to slightly increased white blood cell counts (> 6 cells/µl) in the CSF. Neoplastic cells are seen rarely in equine CSF.

22. What is the best way to diagnose EHV1 myeloencephalopathy?

EHV1 should be included in the list of differential diagnoses for a horse with acute onset of neurologic signs involving any part of the nervous system, especially when more than one horse on a farm is affected. The most common signs are pelvic limb ataxia, weakness, and urinary incontinence, although other signs, including cranial nerve or other peripheral nerve deficits, may be present concurrently or independently. The history often reveals previous fever, abortion, or viral respiratory disease on the farm. The diagnosis is confirmed by identification of the virus in the CSF. A diagnosis is also likely if virus is isolated from the buffy coat or respiratory tract in a horse with compatible clinical signs. A fourfold or greater increase in serum antibody titers is further evidence of recent EHV1 infection. Indirect fluorescent antibody (IFA) and polymerase chain reaction (PCR) techniques help to establish the diagnosis at postmortem examination.

23. What are the most important causes of a diffuse distribution of lesions affecting the CNS of horses?

The list of differential diagnoses for diffuse distribution of lesions in the CNS of horses should include EPM, spinal cord trauma, polyneuritis equi (neuritis of the cauda equina), rabies, aberrant parasite migration, EDM, togaviral infection, plant toxicity, and other neurotropic toxins and chemicals.

24. Which conditions should be considered in horses presented for head tossing, difficulty with chewing, head tilt, circling, and for ipsilateral weakness?

In horses that demonstrate head tossing, difficulty with chewing, and/or abnormal behavior the differential diagnoses should include inner ear disease, external ear disease (e.g., ectoparasitism), dental disease, guttural pouch infection or mycosis, stylohyoid osteitis (seen within the guttural pouch), and eye or sinus disease. If the principal signs include head tilt, nystagmus, ipsilateral weakness, and difficulty with ambulating and chewing, one should consider infection of the inner ear, otitis externa, aberrant parasite migration, head trauma involving the basisphenoid, basioccipital, and stylohyoid bones, or osteitis or osteomyelitis of the temporohyoid apparatus. The vesticulocochlear nerve carries fibers involved in hearing and balance. Fibers course from the inner ear through the petrous temporal bone into the lateral medulla oblongata; a few fibers pass to a small portion of the cerebellum, which is part of the vestibular system. Vestibulocochlear nerve damage results in ipsilateral head tilt and nystagmus with the fast phase away from the side of the lesion. With peripheral vestibular disease the nystagmus is usually horizontal, whereas with central lesions in the medulla oblongata the nystagmus may be horizontal, vertical, or rotary. Horses with vestibular lesions accommodate within a few days by proprioceptive and visual mechanisms.

25. What is the innervation of the pupil and the origin of the pupillary light response?

The diameter of the pupil is controlled by the constrictor muscles of the pupil (constrictor pupillae), which are innervated by the parasympathetic fibers in the oculomotor nerve, and by the dilator muscles of the pupil, which are controlled by the sympathetic fibers of the cranial cervical ganglion. The oculomotor nerve (i.e., parasympathetic portion of the autonomic nervous system) responds to light, whereas the cranial cervical ganglion (i.e., sympathetic portion) responds to fear and excitement. For a normal pupillary light response the stimulus travels through the optic nerve and optic chiasm, laterally and dorsally to the thalamus, and then ventral to the midbrain. Crossover occurs and interconnections to the parasympathetic oculomotor nuclei occur in the midbrain. The motor response is from these nuclei to the ciliary ganglia and constrictor muscles of the pupil.

26. What is the pathway for sympathetic nervous control of the head and neck?

Nuclei in the brain that control sympathetic motor function are located in the hypothalamus, midbrain, pons, and medulla. First-order neurons descend through the midbrain, medulla, and cervical spinal cord and synapse on cell bodies on the lateral intermediate gray columns in the thoracolumbar spinal cord. The axons of preganglionic, second-order sympathetic cell bodies in the T1–T3 region ascend in the cervical sympathetic trunk adjacent to the vagus and pass to the cranial cervical ganglion under the atlas. In horses this ganglion is beneath the lining of the caudal dorsal wall of the medial compartment of the guttural pouch. Postganglionic, third-generation sympathetic fibers leave the cranial cervical ganglion and supply the glands, smooth muscle, and blood vessels of the eye, head, and cranial cervical area.

27. What causes Horner's syndrome? What are the clinical signs? Where are lesions likely to be found in horses?

Horner's syndrome is caused by damage to the sympathetic innervation of the eye. The clinical features of Horner's syndrome include ptosis (i.e., drooping of the upper eyelid), miosis, protrusion of the third eyelid, and enophthalmos. Loss of tone in the eyelid muscle results in decreased size of the palpebral fissure or ptosis; lack of pupillary dilation in response to painful stimuli or stress causes the pupil to be smaller than the normal opposite pupil at rest; and lack of retraction of the third eyelid makes it protrude. Loss of sympathetic innervation results in lack of tone of the periorbital smooth muscle so that the eyeball retracts slightly, producing enophthalmos. Vision and pupillary light responses are unaffected. In horses ocular signs are often accompanied by sweating of the face, dilation of facial blood vessels, and hyperemia of the nasal and conjunctival mucosa. If the lesion is preganglionic, the sweating is along the side of the face and to the level of the axis. Sweating is seen to the level of the atlas with postganglionic lesions. Large lesions of the brainstem or cervical spinal cord that involve the sympathetic pathways, particularly the tectotegmental spinal tract, may result in Horner's syndrome along with sweating along the entire side of the body. Focal lesions in spinal cord segments from T1–T3 result in focal sweating and Horner's syndrome.

28. What portions of the CNS are likely to be affected in horses that have difficulty with swallowing and phonation and sometimes have exercise intolerance?

Difficulty with swallowing and upper airway function may result from damage to the glossopharyngeal (CN IX), vagus (CN X) or accessory spinal (CN XI) nerves, which innervate the pharynx and larynx. The glossopharyngeal and vagus nerves contain both sensory and motor fibers. Major control centers are the nucleus ambiguus and nucleus solitaire in the caudal medulla oblongata. Damage to these nerves or their nuclei may result in dysphagia and/or abnormal respiratory noise (and thus exercise intolerance).

29. What diseases in horses result in profound weakness and recumbency, sometimes associated with muscle atrophy?

The most common neurologic causes of recumbency in horses are EHV1 myeloencephalopathy, EMND, spinal cord trauma, and botulism.

EHV1 is a neuroendothelial trophic virus that results in vasculitis and often manifests in horses with pelvic limb weakness along with poor tail and anal tone and urinary incontinence. This problem may occur in several horses on a farm concurrently.

When a single horse is affected with profound weakness accompanied by severe generalized muscle atrophy and muscle fasciculation, EMND should be considered. It is a sporadic disease of older horses that often have a history of maintenance on dry lots with little or no access to grass. EMND appears to be an acquired neurodegenerative disease and is assumed to result from oxidant damage to the nervous system. It affects all breeds but has been observed most often in Quarter Horses, possibly as a result of how they are managed. The EMND primarily affects cell bodies of ventral motor neurons of the brainstem and spinal cord and has been likened to sporadic cases of Lou Gehrig's disease in humans. The diagnosis is aided by recognition of typical clinical signs along with presence of a pigmented retinopathy due to ceroid-like (lipofuschin) deposits observed in vitamin E deficiency in animals. Changes consistent with degenerative disease are observed in muscle biopsies along with neurodegenerative lesions in the motor nerves and ventral horn cells. Accessory nerve biopsy has been used as an aid to diagnose EMND.

Weakness associated with botulism in horses may result from ingestion of preformed toxin in feed material due to decaying vegetative matter (generally type B botulism) or decaying animal carcasses (often type C botulism) or from contamination or infection of a wound. The onset of clinical signs is variable and depends on the concentration or dose of toxin absorbed from the gastrointestinal tract or wound. In Shaker foal syndrome the bacteria in the intestine actually produce toxin and result in clinical signs. Horses with botulism may have a subtle-to-acute onset of weakness that sometimes progresses quickly to recumbency and even death. They often have difficulty with prehension, chewing, and swallowing of feed material. Eyelid tone and pupillary light responses are often slow and weak, the tongue may protrude from the mouth, and tail and anal tone may be weak.

30. How common is trauma to the CNS of horses?

Trauma to the CNS of horses is not uncommon in veterinary practice; the incidence may be higher than thought. Often traumatic episodes go unrecognized or unobserved by owners; consequently, the onset of acute neurologic signs in a horse may go undiagnosed. Common causes of CNS trauma include halter-breaking accidents in young horses, athletic injuries sustained during racing or jumping, trailer or road traffic accidents, falls, kicks, and gunshot wounds. Rare causes include ruptured intervertebral discs (in older horses) and pathologic fractures of vertebrae following muscular spasms in horses with tetanus or horses with nutritional secondary hyperparathyroidism. Horses with underlying developmental or structural malformations of the spine are more prone to spinal cord trauma. Frequently such trauma is seen in the neck, presumably associated with its relative mobility and its lack of protection from surrounding tissue. Horses with cervical vertebral malformation (CVM) may present with spinal cord trauma after a traumatic episode, as may young horses with an occipito-atlanto-axial malformation that allows vertebral subluxation.

31. Where are the common sites of injury of the equine CNS? What are the clinical signs?

The clinical signs associated with CNS trauma depend on the location of the injury and the severity of the underlying lesion. Neurologic signs may progress or change as the lesion develops. Penetrating injury to the head may result in direct exposure of areas of the brain (predominantly the cerebrum). Blunt trauma also frequently affects the forebrain. Clinical signs vary from mild depression, circling, or head pressing to stupor or coma. Seizures are sometimes recognized. Uncontrolled edema may result in various other signs because cerebral swelling causes other parts of the brain to be affected. Signs may include cranial nerve dysfunction and respiratory center or reticular formation abnormalities with compression of the brainstem. Tentorial or foramen magnum herniation may result in sudden death in an animal that has suffered previous head injury. Penetrating injury may result in severe focal necrosis and/or bacterial infection.

Young horses that rear over backward and hit the poll during halter-breaking accidents appear predisposed to injuries involving the caudal brainstem and its associated cranial nerves. Commonly they fracture the basisphenoid or basioccipital bones during such an episode, allowing displacement of the bones toward the brainstem. Vestibular disease, manifested by pathologic nystagmus, head tilt, and ataxia, is frequently seen along with clinical signs due to damage of other closely associated structures (e.g., facial nerve paralysis). Affected horses may present with epistaxis after hemorrhage into the guttural pouch from a rectus capitis muscle rupture or may bleed from the ear.

Spinal cord trauma results in signs associated with the site of injury. Commonly, a neck trauma results in pain and varying degrees of ataxia and weakness in all four limbs with predominantly hindlimb involvement (i.e., approximately one grade worse in the hindlimbs). Clinical signs vary from mild to severe, resulting in recumbency. Horses may be presented with signs that progress over several hours to days. Initially they may demonstrate hindlimb ataxia, followed by gradual involvement of all four legs, dog sitting, sternal recumbency, and finally lateral recumbency. The changing clinical signs reflect the gradual involvement of predominantly white matter tracts in the cervical spinal cord as the lesion develops. Thoracolumbar injury caudal to T2 causes signs in the hindlimbs without forelimb involvement. Gray matter involvement at either the brachial or lumbosacral plexus also may result in lower motor neuron (LMN) signs in the muscles of the legs.

Sacral fractures occur relatively commonly in horses after falling or rearing backward onto the rump. Signs involve the sacral spinal cord and cauda equina, such as urinary and fecal incontinence, loss of perineal sensation, and tail paralysis.

32. How can brain or spinal cord trauma be diagnosed?

Clearly, a history of a traumatic episode or direct evidence of penetrating injury negates the necessity of confirming a diagnosis by other means in a horse with neurologic dysfunction. Unfortunately, horses may be found recumbent, stuporous, ataxic, or weak with no such evidence of traumatic injury. Consequently, the clinician is left with a large number of differential diagnoses after an extensive physical and neurologic examination. The physical size of the horse precludes many tests used routinely in the evaluation of human and small animal trauma. Nonetheless, a number of tests are available and may be performed reliably either in the practice setting or at a referral institution. CSF collection, either at the atlantooccipital (AO) or lumbosacral (LS) space, can be useful. CSF collection may help to differentiate other potential diagnoses. After acute trauma CSF may be normal or hemorrhagic. The repeatable collection of blood-tinged CSF is highly suggestive of trauma and subarachnoid hemorrhage. However, care should be taken to distinguish this scenario from an iatrogenic, traumatic collection. In the latter case, the CSF usually clears after several minutes. Careful judgment should be used in deciding to perform AO centesis because of the risk of brain herniation, particularly in horses with signs of brain or brainstem dysfunction. In other cases, cytologic evaluation of the fluid may show evidence of erythrophagocytosis by macrophages and a mildly elevated total protein. Blood introduced during traumatic collection may result in similar cytologic changes, if the CSF is not examined quickly after the procedure. Xanthochromia may be seen in CSF from horses with longer-standing injury or EHV1 myeloencephalopathy.

Radiography may be diagnostic in cases of skull and cervical fractures and often is useful in the thoracolumbar regions of foals and ponies. Standing, plain cervical radiographs may help to diagnose underlying CVM. Myelography may be necessary to diagnose spinal cord compression. Care should be used in manipulating the neck of an anesthetized horse for fear of worsening an unstable fracture. Sacral fractures sometimes can be seen radiographically in small horses (e.g., miniature horses, ponies, foals) or may be palpated rectally in larger animals. Endoscopy of the guttural pouches is indicated in horses with injuries of the head and cranial nerve signs, to visualize localized trauma close to the brainstem. Other ancillary tests used with increasing frequency are computed tomography (CT) and magnetic resonance imaging (MRI). At present, unless the horse is small, only the head and neck may be examined by CT and MRI.

33. What is the pathophysiology of CNS trauma?

A complex cascade of events follows traumatic injury to the CNS, including local ischemia, edema formation, necrosis and extension of the lesion. These events are evident at the tissue, cellular, and molecular levels. Release of the excitatory neurotransmitter, glutamate, immediately after trauma results in rapid movement of calcium ions into neurons from the extracellular space. These events initiate the pathophysiologic cascade. Various events, principally calcium-mediated, result in protease enzyme induction and production of arachidonic acid metabolites such as vasoactive leukotrienes and prostaglandins, which cause localized ischemia and thrombus formation. After reperfusion, free radical production results in lipid membrane peroxidation, enzyme dysfunction, and DNA oxidative damage. Neurologic dysfunction results from edema formation, followed by cell necrosis and apoptosis. The location of the brain within the cranium usually confers a significant degree of protection; however, elevations in intracranial pressure after edema formation as a result of trauma may result in further damage. The anatomic arrangement of the spinal cord—tightly packed white matter tracts surrounding a central core of relatively loosely bound gray matter— allows edema to form initially within the gray matter. In addition, the arterial blood supply to the whole of the gray matter is predominantly from a ventrally located spinous artery and differs from that of the white matter, which receives blood from an anastomosing network of radiating arteries. As a consequence, thrombosis within the ventral artery or its major branches results in localized gray matter ischemia and subsequent necrosis. The central core of necrosis may extend over time to involve the surrounding white matter tracts, causing significant motor or proprioceptive dysfunction.

34. What is the prognosis of horses that have suffered CNS trauma? How should they be treated?

The prognosis of horses suffering from CNS trauma involving the brainstem or spinal cord is guarded to poor for return to athletic use, depending on the severity of the injury. The prognosis of horses with cerebral lesions varies from guarded to good, depending, in part, on the timing of treatment. Regeneration within the CNS is limited; hence, treatment attempts should be made early during lesion development to improve outcome. A large variety of treatment modalities is used clinically in CNS trauma in small animals and humans, and an even greater variety of therapeutic intervention has been used experimentally. Unfortunately, the conflicting evidence of the efficacy of many treatments, together with the lack and difficulty of objective studies in horses and the cost associated with using drugs at doses extrapolated from other animals, frequently precludes their use in horses. Nevertheless, treatment should be aimed at (1) minimizing further injury and providing immediate first aid, (2) blocking the biochemical cascade in early lesion development, (3) scavenging free radicals, (4) reducing edema formation or preventing its detrimental effects, and (5) providing adequate nursing care.

Horses that are in pain or disoriented or severely ataxic after CNS trauma may require analgesic nonsteroidal antiinflammatory drugs or sedation and housing in a safe, well-bedded environment. Seizuring horses may require head protection (e.g., padded head mask) and medication with diazepam in the acute stages or phenobarbital over the longer term. Calcium channel blockers, opiate antagonists, thyrotropin-releasing hormone, and specific neurotransmitter agonists and antagonists have been used experimentally to limit the cascade following trauma. They are not routinely used in horses. Methylprednisolone, given early in the course of disease, promotes free radical scavenging in humans and small animals. The cost of this drug and the lack of studies in horses addressing the concerns of laminitis have prevented its use in horses. Traditionally (although with conflicting experimental efficacy studies), dimethyl sulfoxide (DMSO) has been used as a free radical scavenger and antiinflammatory agent in horses with CNS trauma. Subjective evidence suggests that it may be beneficial. DMSO has the advantages of being cheap and well tolerated by horses when used at the correct dose and concentration. Vitamin E, a fat-soluble, dietary antioxidant, possesses free radical scavenging properties but probably takes too long to reach adequate tissue concentrations to have much, if any, effect in trauma cases. It has the advantages, however, of being cheap and safe, even at high doses. Glucocorticoids are generally no longer administered to humans with head trauma because of a number of prospective and blinded studies that indicate lack of efficacy. Edema formation is managed by early surgical intervention (craniotomy), mannitol therapy, or hyperventilation. Mannitol may be useful in the management of head trauma in horses, although the risk of exacerbating hemorrhage has been a concern. Dexamethasone is frequently used as an antiinflammatory in horses with head or spinal cord trauma; despite significant clinical improvement, experimental studies in other species suggest that long-term steroid use may be contraindicated. In severe cases of head or spinal cord injury in horses, early aggressive treatment is indicated.

Response to treatment during the first 48 hours may be helpful in establishing the long-term prognosis. Recumbent horses that are refractory to treatment after this interval are candidates for euthanasia. Decisions about the future athletic use of the horse in cases that initially responded to treatment should be delayed for 6 months to 1 year after injury or for the period beyond which no further improvement has been noted. Significant neurologic improvement may be seen through compensation during this period.

35. What is the most common cause of meningitis in horses? What are the clinical signs?

The most common cause of meningitis in horses is bacterial, usually *Streptococcus* species, although viral and fungal causes also have been reported. The clinical signs of meningitis include fever, anorexia, hyperaesthesia, and a stiff or painful neck. In severe cases, horses progress to recumbency, seizures, and death. Definitive diagnosis is made by CSF analysis, which reveals a marked increase in white blood cell count and an elevated protein concentration. The CSF may appear turbid, cloudy, or opaque. Although identification of a positive culture is not always possible, affected horses should be treated with broad-spectrum antimicrobial agents with good CNS penetration. Sulfonamides, potentiated-sulfonamides, and third-generation cephalosporins may be used. Treatment with antiinflammatory agents such as DMSO or flunixin meglumine may be initiated and may improve clinical signs. Diazepam may be helpful if seizures are present.

36. What additional causes of brain, brainstem, or spinal cord disease should be considered in horses?

Neurologic deficits are a common problem in horses, but their cause cannot always be ascertained. Verminous encephalomyelitis; fungal toxins; viral, bacterial, and fungal infections; and degenerative or granulomatous diseases also may result in neurologic signs in horses.

Currently *Halicephalobus delitrix* is considered the most important cause of verminous encephalitis in horses. The route of infection is unclear, but the most likely source is decaying vegetative matter in the environment. The clinical signs are variable and may progress at a rapid or slow rate. The presence of peripheral eosinophilia or a finding of eosinophils in the CSF is suggestive of parasitic involvement. Treatment of verminous encephalitis is quite difficult and should include anthelmintics such as ivermectin, fenbendazole, levamisole, and possibly diethylcarbamazine. Horses also should be placed on low-dose systemic corticosteroids to reduce the inflammation that may be associated with killing of the parasites.

Leukoencephalomalacia caused by exposure to fumonisins has been observed in horses. Fumonisins are mycotoxins produced by *Fusarium* species found on contaminated corn. The clinical signs are compatible with multifocal neurologic disease and usually affect more than one horse in the herd. The condition most often results in death, but supportive care and use of antiinflammatory agents may help to save some animals.

Although many horses are vaccinated against togaviral infections, Eastern, Western, and Venezuelan encephalomyelitis have been observed in horses in various regions of the world. These viral infections are transmitted by insect vectors and may result in serious, often life-threatening disease. Horses usually show signs of fever, aimless wandering, stupor, seizures, and eventually coma and death. The diseases have the potential to affect more than one horse in the herd, although in most cases it appears to be sporadic, presumably because of vector transmission.

An important differential consideration for encephalitis in horses is rabies, a sporadic zoonosis that likely persists in a wildlife reservoir. Rabies virus is a rhabdovirus that affects all warm-blooded animal species with the possible exception of the opposum. Although infection is unusual, the horse is a susceptible species. Infection results from the bite of an infected animal, and the presence of bite wounds followed by onset of neurologic signs should prompt inclusion of rabies on the differential diagnostic list. The diagnosis is confirmed at postmortem examination by immunofluorescent antibody tests and occasionally (in horses that have lived for sufficient time) by the finding of negri bodies (intracytoplasmic inclusions of viral protein) in the hippocampus and Purkinje cells of the cerebellum.

An unusual disorder that results in frequent loss of tail tone, muscle atrophy, urinary and fecal incontinence, and sensory deficits around the tail and anus is neuritis of the cauda equina or polyneuritis equi. The exact mechanism is not fully understood, but the disorder probably results from antibodies directed against the P2 protein of myelin. Affected horses often show ascending paralysis, and the condition may be difficult to distinguish from EHV1 encephalomyelitis or rabies. There appears to be no effective long-term treatment.

BIBLIOGRAPHY

1. Beech J, Haskins ML: Genetic studies of neuraxonal dystrophy in the Morgan. Am J Vet Res 48(1): 109–113, 1987.

2. Blythe LL, Watrous BJ, Schmitz JA, et al: Vestibular syndrome associated with temporohyoid joint fusion and temporal bone fracture in three horses. J Am Vet Met Assoc 185:775–782, 1984.
3. Critchley MR: A comparison of human and animal botulism: A review. J R Soc Med 84:295–298, 1991.
4. Cummings JF, de Lahunta A, George C, et al: Equine motor neuron disease: A preliminary report. Cornell Vet 80:357–379, 1990.
5. Dill SG, Correa MT, Erb HT, et al: Factors associated with the development of equine degenerative myeloencephalopathy. Am J Vet Res 51(8):1300–1305, 1990.
6. Dubey JP, Davis SW, Speer CA, et al: *Sarcocystis neurona* n. sp (Protozoa: Apicomplexa), the etiological agent of equine protozoal myeloencephalitis. J Parasitol 77:212, 1991.
7. Granstrom DE: Equine protozoal encephalomyelitis: Antigen analysis of cultured *Sarcocystis neurona* merozoites. J Vet Diag Invest 5:88, 1993.
8. Green SL, Smith LL, Vernau W, et al: Rabies in horses: 21 cases (1970–1990). J Am Vet Med Assoc 200:1133, 1996.
9. Mayhew IG: Equine herpesvirus 1 (rhinopneumonitis) myeloencephalitis. In Mayhew IG (ed): Large Animal Neurology. Philadelphia, Lea and Febiger, 1989, p 272.
10. Mayhew IG: Large Animal Neurology: A Handbook for Veterinary Clinicians. Philadelphia, Lea & Febiger, 1989.
11. Moore BR, Reed SM, Biller DE, et al: Accuracy of cervical vertebral radiographs in the assessment of vertebral canal diameter. Am J Vet Res 1:5–12, 1996.
12. Reed SM: Neurological examination of horses. In Reed WM, Bayly WM (eds): Textbook of Equine Internal Medicine. Philadelphia, W.B. Saunders, 1997.
13. Santschi EM, Foreman JH: Equine bacterial meningitis, Part 1. Comp Cont Ed 11(4), 1989.
14. Slater JD, Borchers K, Thackray AM, Field HJ: The trigeminal ganglion is a location for equine herpesvirus 1 latency and reactivation in the horse. J Gen Virol 75:2007, 1994.
15. Uhlinger CH: Leukoencephalomalacia. Vet Clin North Am Equine Pract 13(1):13–20, 1997.

15. NEONATOLOGY

Guy Lester, B.V.M.S., Ph.D., Dip. ACVIM

NORMAL PHYSIOLOGY

1. What is the average gestational length in the Thoroughbred?

Gestational length is variable in the Thoroughbred, ranging from 320–365 days with a mean length of 341 days. Normal-appearing foals have been born to mares that have had gestational periods as short as 305 days and as long as 400 days. Mares that foal in late winter or early spring have a longer gestational period (by up to 10 days) than those that foal in late spring or summer. Colts also may have a 2–3 day longer gestation than fillies.

Howell CE, Rollins WC: Environmental sources of variation in the gestation length of the horse. J Animal Sci 10:789, 1951.

Roipha RT, et al: The duration of pregnancy in Thoroughbred mares. Vet Rec 84:552, 1969.

2. How much milk is a healthy newborn 45-kg foal expected to consume over 24 hours?

The healthy foal may consume as much as 25% of its body weight daily in milk. Therefore, a 45-kg foal may consume over 11 liters of milk per day.

3. When does peak lactation occur in mares?

The average light-breed mare produces around 16 kg of milk daily during the first 7 days of lactation (approximately 25% of the foal's body weight). Lactation peaks around 5–6 weeks at around 18 kg of milk daily (approximately 18% of the 6-week-old foal's body weight daily). Quarter Horses produce less milk than Thoroughbreds, and heavy breeds, as expected, produce more than Thoroughbreds. Heavy breeds produce a similar volume based on body weight. The record in milk production of 29 kg per day was recorded for a 724-kg Soviet draft mare.

Oftedal OT, et al: Lactation in the horse: Milk composition and intake by foals. J Nutr 113:2096, 1983.

4. What is the normal or expected rate of growth for a light-breed neonatal fold?

The average weight gain is around 1.5 kg per day with a range from 1.0–2.2 kg per day for the first few weeks of life. In sick foals weight is influenced by various factors other than true gain (deposition of new tissue of normal composition). Such factors include water accumulation or losses, bandages, splints, and scale variability. In sick foals daily weight gain of 1.0 kg is considered excellent.

5. The blood chemistry profile in young foals needs to be interpreted with a knowledge of normal deviations from values in adults. What elements of the profile may differ? Why?

Variables that May Differ in Young Foals and Adult Horses

VARIABLE	DIFFERENCE FROM ADULT	POSSIBLE CAUSE OF DIFFERENCE
Phosphorus	Values at birth (4.7 ± 1.6 mg/dl) mimic those of adults, increase-significantly during first 2 mo (7.4 ± 1.4 mg/dl), then slowly de-cline to adult values (4.5 ± 1.4 mg/dl)	Related to changes in chemical composition and metabolism of bone, although no such changes are seen in calcium or magnesium concentrations
Glucose	Increased in foal	Frequent sucking of milk during first month of life

Table continued on following page

Variables that May Differ in Young Foals and Adult Horses (Continued)

VARIABLE	DIFFERENCE FROM ADULT	POSSIBLE CAUSE OF DIFFERENCE
Serum alkaline phosphatase (SAP)	Large elevations (up to 3000 IU/L) during first 48 hr of age; smaller-increases during first few months of life	Initial elevations best explained by intestinal pinocytosis; later increases related to osteoblastic activity and hepatic maturation
Aspartate amino-transferase (AST)	Slight increase after 7 days of age	Related to increased muscle activity
Gammaglutamyl transferase (GGT)	Transiently elevated between 5 and 14 days of age	Due to "overshoot" phenomenon associated with hepatic enzyme induction; not believed to be from colostral ingestion (as in calves)

From Bauer JE: Normal blood chemistry. In Koterba AM, et al (eds): Equine Clinical Neonatology. Philadelphia, Lea & Febiger, 1990, pp 602–614.

6. What are the differences between neonatal foals and adult horses with respect to total body water and the relative contributions of intracellular fluid (ICF) and extracellular fluid (ECF) compartments?

The total body weight of an adult horse is composed of around 60% water, of which approximately 67% is located in the intracellular spaces and 33% is extracellular (i.e., approximately 20% [0.33 × 60] of body weight is ECF). In contrast, in newborn foals almost 80% (70–79%) of body weight is water, with an estimated 44% in the ICF and 56% in the ECF (i.e., approximately 45% [0.56 × 80] of body weight is ECF). Therefore, the contribution of ICF to total body weight remains relatively constant independent of age, whereas both ECF and total body water contract with age. A clinical example of this difference can be seen in dehydration. From a distance, the dehydrated adult horse may look normal, but the fluid-deprived foal falsely appears malnourished and emaciated.

SEPSIS AND PASSIVE IMMUNITY

7. What bacterial organisms are most commonly isolated from neonatal foals with sepsis?

The enteric gram-negative bacteria are most frequently isolated from diseased foals; *Escherichia coli* is the most common example. Others include *Klebsiella pneumoniae*, *Enterobacter* species, *Salmonella* species, and *Serratia marcescens*. Common nonenteric gram-negative organisms include *Actinobacillus equuli* and *Pasteurella* species. An *Actinobacillus suis*-like organism has been reported in newborn foals from California. Of the gram-positive agents, *Streptococcus* species and, less commonly, *Staphylococcus* species are also causes of severe sepsis. Various anaerobic agents, including *Clostridium* species, have been isolated from the blood of foals with hemorrhagic diarrhea.

8. What is a sepsis score?

The sepsis score was developed as a tool to help predict sepsis and thus to guide therapy before the return of blood culture results. The score is calculated using a combination of historical information, physical findings, and laboratory data. Sensitivity and specificity were originally reported as 93% and 88%, respectively, based on a positive score of 11 or greater. Premature foals often are falsely reported as positive. False negatives are uncommon but, when present, were reported more frequently in older neonatal foals.

Brewer BD, Koterba AM: The development of a scoring system for the early diagnosis of equine neonatal sepsis. Equine Vet J 20:18–23, 1988.

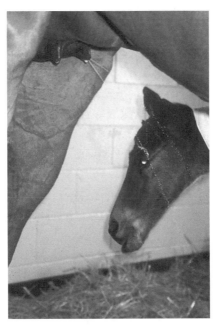

Septic foal.

9. Discuss antimicrobial selection for a foal with a positive sepsis score when blood culture results are pending.

A broad-spectrum approach must be used, but specific drug selection is based on knowledge of common organisms and resistance patterns in the geographic region as well as consideration of drug costs, interactions with other medication, and potential toxicity. Initial therapy can be altered when blood cultures and sensitivity data become available. Given the predominance of enteric gram-negative organisms in neonatal sepsis, aminoglycosides or third-generation cephalosporins are often used in conjunction with either penicillin or ampicillin. The latter two agents are required for effective control of gram-positive bacteria. Amikacin and gentamicin are the most commonly used aminoglycosides in neonatal practice. Both appear to be equally efficacious against common isolates; amikacin is the superior choice to treat nosocomial infections. The true third-generation cephalosporins, ceftazidime and cefotaxime, are expensive and generally reserved for bacterial meningitis and unresponsive pneumonia. Ceftiofur is more cost-effective, but efficacy data are lacking. Metronidazole is frequently added to the treatment schedule in neonatal folds with diarrhea, particularly if clostridial infection is suspected.

10. Systemic hypotension may occur in foals with sepsis or prematurity or foals that have been exposed to hypoxia and/or ischemia. Without intervention many develop multiple organ dysfunction and die. Discuss their medical management.

Maintenance of mean blood pressure (> 65 mmHg) appears to be critical in the prevention of cardiopulmonary collapse and secondary organ failure. Management of the failing cardiovascular system can be quite challenging. The initial approach to treatment commonly involves restoration of plasma volume with fluid therapy. If hypotension continues after dehydration has been corrected, intravenous plasma can be used, followed by dopamine infusion at 3–5 µg/kg/min. If this approach is ineffective, dobutamine infusion (5–20 µg/kg/min) is added. Preservation of renal function is critical, and the foal should be monitored closely for urine production; subcutaneous tissues should be inspected for edema; and the foal should be weighed frequently when possible.

11. What factors influence the passive transfer of maternal immunoglobulins to the foal?

Maternal factors that influence passive transfer include age (colostral quality declines with age), mammary development and milk letdown before parturition (as may occur with placental infection), premature labor, and maternal illness. Foal factors include the age at which sucking begins, strength, presence and vigor of suckle reflex, and conditions of stress that may be responsible for closure of specialized enterocytes.

12. What volume of colostrum does a mare typically produce?

The average broodmare produces between 1.8 and 2.8 liters of good-quality colostrum at the beginning of each lactation.

LeBlanc MM, et al: Factors that influence passive transfer of immunoglobulins in foals. J Am Vet Med Assoc 220:179–183, 1992.

13. What methods are used to rapidly assess colostral quality?

Colostrum can be assessed subjectively by evaluating its appearance. Good-quality colostrum is thick and sticky with a yellow-to-tan color. A more objective measurement can be made using a Colostrometer (Jorgensen Laboratories, Loveland, CO). This simple device determines the specific gravity of colostrum. Good-quality colostrum should have an immunoglobulin G (IgG) content > 3000 mg/dl, as reflected by a colostral specific gravity > 1.060.

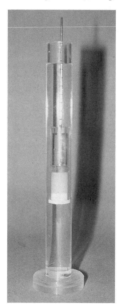

Colostrometer.

14. What quantitative or semiquantitative methods are used to determine the adequacy of passive transfer of maternal immunoglobulin?

Various commercial tests are available to measure blood IgG levels in newborn foals. Selection of tests is based on a range of factors, including sensitivity, speed of result, difficulty of use, and availability. Radial immunodiffusion (RID) is considered to be the gold standard but takes 18–24 hours to yield a result. The zinc sulfate turbidity test, hemagglutination inhibition test, Latex agglutination test, glutaraldehyde coagulation, and membrane enzyme-linked immunosorbent assay (ELISA) are commercially available and yield a rapid, semiquantitative or quantitative assessment of foal IgG.

15. What IgG measurement in foals is consistent with a diagnosis of failure of passive transfer?

Investigators disagree about the significance of specific IgG values or IgG ranges with respect to susceptibility to disease. Factors other than foal IgG concentration are involved in whether an individual animal succumbs to pathogen challenge. A serum IgG ≤ 200 mg/dl is considered to reflect complete failure of passive transfer. A value > 200 but ≤ 800 mg/dl is classified as partial failure of passive transfer. Foals with a serum IgG concentration < 400 mg/dl generally require intervention with colostrum or a commercial oral IgG product if less than 18 hours of age or with intravenous plasma thereafter. Foals with a serum IgG between 400 and 800 mg/dl should receive intervention if other factors may predispose to disease, such as prematurity, dysmaturity, overcrowding, other diseased foals on the farm, or early signs of sepsis.

16. What volume of plasma should be administered to foals with partial or total failure of passive transfer?

A minimum of 2 liters of good-quality plasma is recommended for foals with complete failure of passive transfer (40 ml/kg or 400 mg/kg of IgG). Generally 1 liter of plasma is sufficient for treatment of partial failure of passive transfer (20 mg/kg body weight or 200 mg/kg IgG). Foals with active infection may benefit from a greater volume. Good-quality donor plasma should have at least 1200 mg/dl of IgG. A whole blood filter should always be used for plasma administration.

17. Foals are highly susceptible to hypoglycemia. Describe an effective treatment strategy for reversal of hypoglycemia and a maintenance approach for prevention in the foal that is not receiving milk.

Hypoglycemia is managed acutely by rapid infusion of 20 ml/kg of a 10% dextrose solution over several minutes, followed by a constant infusion at about 4–6 mg/kg/minute (approximately 200–300 ml/hour of a 5% dextrose solution to a 30–40 kg foal). Rapid infusion of 50% dextrose is not required and results in rebound hypoglycemia if a maintenance protocol is not continued.

18. Detail a plan to provide calories to a neonatal foal that will not tolerate enteral feeding.

A small percentage of foals will not tolerate enteral feeding and develop clinical signs that may include abdominal distention, colic, gastric reflux, and diarrhea. Milk intolerance is commonly observed in neonatal foals with birth-associated asphyxia, prematurity, sepsis, and enterocolitis. Ideally such foals are given intravenous nutrition either alone (total parenteral nutrition [TPN]) or in conjunction with reduced enteral feeding (partial parenteral nutrition [PPN]). The aim is to provide enough nutrients to prevent further catabolism of energy stores and to enhance immunity and wound healing. Normal foals consume 140–160 kcal/kg/day based on a milk caloric density of 0.60 kcal/ml milk. Significant benefit can be gained by providing a fraction of this amount to diseased foals intravenously (50–100 kcal/kg/day). The three primary components of a TPN solution are glucose or dextrose, amino acids, and lipids. Carbohydrate is commonly used in the form of 50% dextrose and provides 3.4 kcal/gm dextrose. Lipid emulsions contain long-chain triglycerides that are derived from either safflower or soybean oil and glycerol with egg phospholipid as an emulsifier. The lipid/glycerol combination provides approximately 11 kcal/gm. Commercial amino acid solutions vary in protein concentration from 3.0–10% and are supplied with or without electrolytes. The caloric value of protein is approximated at 4.0 kcal/gm. A commonly used simplified formula includes:

- 1000 ml 50% dextrose
- 2000 ml 8.5% amino acid solution with electrolytes
- 500 ml 20% lipid emulsion
- 500 ml saline (0.9%)
- 90 mEq potassium chloride (KCl)
- 0.8 ml of MTE-6, a trace mineral supplement

The ingredients are placed in a 4-L TPN bag and infused over 24 hours. The formulation provides in excess of 50 kcal/kg/day to most foals. A central vein should be used, because the solution is hypertonic. Strict adherence to aseptic technique is necessary.

Hansen TO: Nutritional support: Parenteral feeding. In Koterba AM, et al (eds): Equine Clinical Neonatology. Philadelphia, Lea & Febiger, 1990, pp 747–762.

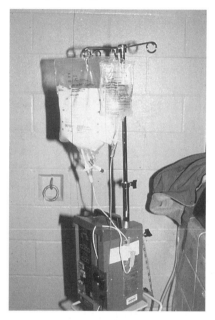

TPN solution.

19. What complications are associated with the use of TPN?

Complications of dextrose infusion include hyperglycemia and glucosuria. Metabolic carbon dioxide production is increased with carbohydrate loading and may be of concern in foals with respiratory disease. Hyperglycemia can be treated with insulin therapy or replacement of glucose calories with fat calories. Hypertriglyceridemia and lipemia may occur with fat infusion but rarely to a degree that evokes concern. Lipids are theoretically contraindicated in foals with hyperbilirubinemia because they may contribute to the deposition of unconjugated bilirubin in the brain (kernicterus). Premature or septic foals may have decreased abilities to clear lipids. Intolerance to or excessive use of amino acids may cause elevations in blood urea nitrogen and ammonia, but they are rarely of clinical relevance. Infection may occur with inappropriate mixing, storage, or administration of TPN solutions.

PREMATURITY

20. What is the difference between prematurity and dysmaturity?

Various terms have been used to describe foals with physical characteristics of immaturity. Prematurity has been defined as a gestational age of ≤ 320 days; although this definition may hold true for many foals, it is inadequate for others. The use of defined ages can be misleading; for example, a 340-day-old fetus may possess many characteristics of immaturity if its normal or expected gestational length is 360 days. Dysmaturity is generally used to describe foals in which physical maturity is inappropriate for gestational age.

Koterba AM: Definitions of equine perinatal disorders: Problems and solutions. Equine Vet Educ 5:271, 1993.

21. What physical characteristics are typically seen in the premature or dysmature foal?

The physical characteristics of prematurity include low birth weight, weakness, a short and silky hair coat, an increased range of joint motion, rear limb flexural laxity, "floppy" ears, and incomplete skeletal ossification (as assessed radiographically). Premature foals often take longer than normal to stand (> 60 minutes) and nurse from the mare (> 120 minutes). The suckle reflex may lack vigor. A prominent or domed forehead is commonly seen in foals that have been exposed to intrauterine growth retardation (e.g, twins).

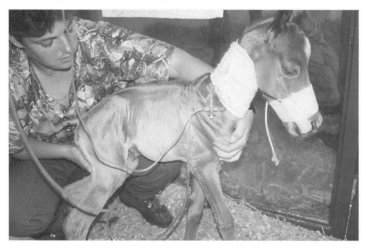

Foal with the physical attributes of prematurity.

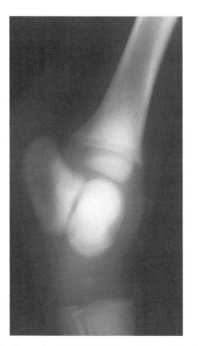
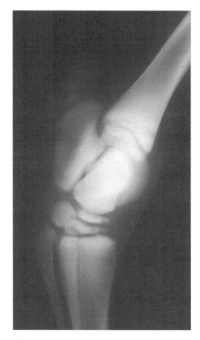

Left, Radiograph of a foal with incomplete ossification of tarsal bones. *Right,* Early radiographic changes consistent with tarsal bone collapse.

22. What laboratory features are commonly seen in premature foals? How can they help to formulate a prognosis for survival?

Premature foals that have a low total white blood cell (WBC) count (< 5000 cells/μl) and low-to-normal fibrinogen level (100–300 mg/dl) are likely to experience difficulties in the neonatal period. Such foals typically have a low neutrophil-to-lymphocyte ratio and low blood cortisol and fail to produce an adequate rise in cortisol when challenged with adrenocorticotropic hormone (0.125 mg intramuscularly) during the first 24 hours after birth. A low WBC count or lack of fibrinogen elevation by day 2 is an additional poor prognostic sign. It is important to determine whether sepsis is present, because neutropenia is a common hematologic findings associated with infection. Evidence of shifting toward immature cell types and neutrophil toxicity should point the clinician toward primary sepsis or prematurity complicated by sepsis. Premature foals without septicemia often return a positive sepsis score because they often share clinical and laboratory features of septicemic neonates, including neutropenia, hypoglycemia, and systemic weakness.

Premature foals with elevations in total WBC count and fibrinogen often have a better chance of survival because of precocious maturation in utero. The most common basis for this stress is placental infection. Such foals, however, are often infected and are at risk for musculoskeletal problems inherent in any physically immature animal.

Cottrill CM: Maturation of the cardiopulmonary system. Equine Vet J 14(Suppl):26–30, 1993.

Koterba AM: Prematurity. In Koterba AM, et al (eds): Equine Clinical Neonatology. Philadelphia, Lea & Febiger, 1990, pp 55–70.

Thorburn GD: A speculative review of parturition in the mare. Equine Vet J 14(Suppl):41–49, 1993.

UMBILICAL AND RENAL DISORDERS

23. How is hydration most easily monitored in neonatal foals?

Urine specific gravity provides an excellent method of approximating hydration and fluid intake and is easily measured with a refractometer. Healthy foals produce a large amount of dilute urine, typically around 150 ml/kg/day (7.5 L/day), with a specific gravity between 1.000 and 1.007. Packed cell volume varies widely in neonates, and plasma protein values are strongly influenced by colostral transfer, limiting their value in single-point assessment of hydration.

24. What is the average period between birth and passage of first urine in healthy foals?

The mean time to first urination is 6 hours in colts and nearly 11 hours in fillies.

25. What are the typical laboratory findings associated with uroperitoneum in foals?

Foals receiving a milk diet develop hyperkalemia, hyponatremia, hypochloremia, and an elevated serum creatinine. The concentration of creatinine in the peritoneal fluid is usually twice that in the serum. If the foal has not been on a milk-based diet, as when concurrent illness is present, classic electrolyte abnormalities may not develop in the face of uroperitoneum.

26. Describe the medical management of a foal with severe hyperkalemia secondary to uroperitoneum.

The most life-threatening consequence of hyperkalemia is fatal arrhythmia. Electrocardiographic (EKG) changes include widening of the QRS complex, P-wave obliteration, atrioventricular block, and ventricular fibrillation. These changes are best prevented by infusion of calcium-containing fluids (10% solution of calcium chloride, 0.2 ml/kg body weight; 10% solution of calcium gluconate, 1 ml/kg body weight); dextrose infusion with or without insulin treatment (0.1 units of regular insulin/kg body weight); or sodium bicarbonate (5% solution infused at a rate of 2 mEq/kg over 60 minutes). Each of these therapies has hazardous side effects that require continual close monitoring of the patient. Intravenous infusion of sodium chloride and peritoneal dialysis are indicated for the foal with uroperitoneum. Additional therapies such as diuretics and cation exchange resins are indicated in the management of chronic hyperkalemia, as may occur in cases of renal failure.

27. What factors commonly contribute to an elevated serum creatinine level in newborn foals?

Primary renal dysfunction in the first day of life is rare. Factors that contribute to elevations in creatinine in adult horses, including dehydration, toxemia, and circulatory collapse, produce similar increases in neonatal foals. Uroperitoneum and specific drug toxicities also cause elevations in plasma or serum creatinine. Large increases in creatinine (up to 32 mg/dl) have been reported in foals and most likely reflect placental disease or dysfunction rather than neonatal renal disease. Dysmature foals or foals with hypoxic ischemic encephalopathy (HIE, formerly known as neonatal maladjustment syndrome) frequently have an elevated serum creatinine level. If a normal glomerular filtration rate is preserved, creatinine levels will fall rapidly to normal during the first 72–96 hours of life.

28. Describe the options for management of a patent urachus.

A urachus that reopens (becomes patent) without ultrasonographic evidence of umbilical remnant infection usually resolves within several days with medical therapy. Various treatments have been suggested, but use of silver nitrate sticks is probably the preferred method. The applicator sticks can be used 3 times daily for several days and are inserted into the external opening of the urachus. Care should be used not to insert too far into the urachal lumen (usually 1–2 cm is sufficient). Injection of procaine penicillin G or application of 2% iodine solution also has been suggested. Stronger iodine solutions should be avoided because subsequent tissue necrosis may increase the risk of infection. If resolution has not occurred within 1 week of patency, surgical closure is recommended.

GASTROINTESTINAL DISORDERS

29. What are the most common infectious causes of diarrhea during the neonatal period?

Common bacterial agents include *Salmonella* species and *Clostridium* species (most commonly *C. difficile* or *C. perfringens* type A or C). *C. perfringens* type B has been isolated from the feces of older foals. *Rhodococcus equi* may cause an ulcerative typhlocolitis in 1–5-month-old foals. The most commonly observed viral agent is rotavirus, but the disease is more common in older foals (1–3 months of age). Both coronavirus and parvovirus have been isolated from foals with diarrhea, but their significance is not known. Cryptosporidium and Giardia species also have been reported as causes of diarrhea but have been observed more commonly outside the neonatal period. Parasitic causes of diarrhea in newborn foals are rare. *Strongyloides westeri* may cause mild enteritis when present in large numbers.

Cohen ND: Diarrheal diseases of foals. In Robinson NE (ed): Current Therapy in Equine Medicine, 4th ed. Philadelphia, W.B. Saunders, 1997, pp 631–636.

30. What is foal heat diarrhea? What is its most likely cause?

The syndrome of foal heat diarrhea describes a nondebilitating diarrhea that typically occurs between days 6 and 12 of life. The diarrhea often coincides with the return to estrus of the dam after parturition; hence the term foal heat diarrhea. The syndrome most like reflects the establishment of normal flora within the large intestine and frequently follows coprophagy of maternal feces by the foal. It probably has nothing to do with the hormonal status of the dam or *S. westeri* infestation (see figue at top of following page).

31. What is the most appropriate method for establishing a diagnosis of rotaviral diarrhea?

Rotaviral diarrhea is most easily diagnosed by fecal immunoassay (enzyme-linked immunosorbent assay). The test should be used in conjunction with signalment, history, and clinical signs because healthy foals and foals with other enteric pathogens also may shed the virus. Electron microscopy is an additional excellent diagnostic tool.

32. Rotavirus is a highly contagious cause of diarrhea in young foals. What management procedures should be used to limit spread through a facility?

Foals with diarrhea should be isolated from other foals and adult horses. Attendants should wear protective clothing and footwear that can be scrubbed and disinfected. Hands should be

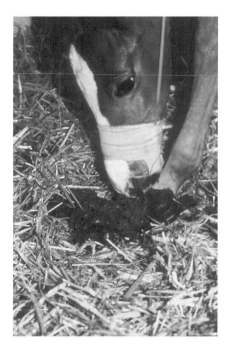

Foal demonstrating coprophagy of maternal feces.

washed thoroughly for a minimum of 30 seconds with an effective disinfecting soap after handling foals with diarrhea. Contaminated clothing should not be worn from stall to stall. Footbaths should be commonplace and should contain a disinfectant that kills rotavirus. The ideal agents are the phenolic compounds. Quarternary ammonium compounds and bleach do not kill rotavirus and are inactivated by organic matter.

33. What is lethal white foal syndrome?
The lethal white foal syndrome is seen in Overo or Tovero Paint horse crosses. The foals are fully white, or almost all white, and normal at birth but develop signs related to intestinal obstruction during the first 24 hours of life. The condition primarily involves aganglionosis of the intestinal tract (ileum, cecum, and/or large colon) but also may include various atresias or anatomic strictures of the intestine. The condition is fatal.

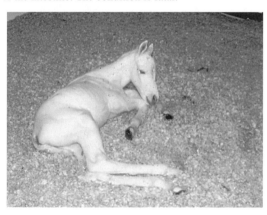

Lethal white foal syndrome.

34. Can the newborn foal produce gastric acid?

Yes. The neonatal foal actively secretes gastric acid. Measurement of intragastric pH in healthy foals frequently identifies periods in which the pH is less than 1.0. Milk ingestion acts as an effective buffer.

Sanchez LC, et al: The effect of ranitidine on intragastric pH in clinically normal neonatal foals. J Am Vet Med Assoc 212:1407–1412, 1998.

35. Can sick neonatal foals develop gastric ulcers?

Although the condition is uncommon, sick foals can develop gastric ulcers in the glandular region of the stomach. In contrast to adult horses and older foals with gastroduodenal ulcer disease (GDUD), neonatal foals may not express overt signs of disease and may be asymptomatic even to the point of rupture. The difficulty in diagnosis has led to the widespread practice of ulcer prophylaxis. The most commonly used drugs include ranitidine (2.0 mg/kg body weight IV 3 times daily or 6.6 mg/kg body weight orally 2–3 times daily), cimetidine (4.0 mg/kg body weight IV 4 times daily or 15–22 mg/kg orally 4 times daily), or omeprazole (2.0–4.0 mg/kg body weight orally once daily). Sucralfate (20–40 mg/kg body weight orally 4 times daily) also has been commonly used in this age group, but concerns about dose rate and efficacy in the prevention of ulceration have led to a decline in its use over recent years.

36. The administration of sodium bicarbonate may worsen acidemia in some foals. Why?

The administration of sodium bicarbonate is ideally limited to acidemic foals with obvious electrolyte losses. The most common loss is through the intestinal tract (diarrhea) or in the urine (renal tubular acidosis in older animals). The binding of bicarbonate ions with hydrogen ions ultimately leads to the production of water and carbon dioxide. The carbon dioxide is easily eliminated through ventilation in animals without pulmonary disease. If a foal is unable to increase its ventilation, hypercapnia and respiratory acidemia may follow.

37. Why is cow's milk a poor substitute for mare's milk in supplementing a newborn foal?

Cow's milk frequently causes diarrhea and, on rare occasions, abdominal discomfort in foals. Mare's milk has a lower fat content and higher sugar content (lactose). Protein content and mineral composition appear to be similar in both species. Dilution of cow's milk with water (2 parts whole milk to 1 part water) with the addition of dextrose (20 gm/L) is reportedly well tolerated by most foals.

Lewis LD: Growing horse feeding and care. In Lewis LD (ed): Equine Clinical Nutrition. Baltimore, Williams & Wilkins, 1995, pp 334–349.

NEUROLOGIC DISORDERS

38. What is a barker foal?

The term is often used to describe newborn foals with nonseptic neurologic disease. Rarely, affected foals demonstrate abnormal vocalization; hence the name barker foals. Other descriptive terms include wanderers or dummy foals. The syndrome is probably best known as neonatal maladjustment syndrome, but recently the term hypoxic ischemic encephalopathy (HIE) has been suggested. Although doubt surrounds the pathophysiology of HIE, it is likely that peripartum central nervous system (CNS) hypoxia and/or ischemia plays an important role. Typically, affected foals behave normally in the first hours of life but then develop a range of neurologic deficits that vary from mild depression through grand mal seizure (see figure at top of following page).

39. What treatment strategies have been advocated in the management of HIE in newborn foals?

The doubt about the pathophysiology HIE has led to a wide variety of suggested treatment strategies. It is also likely that no common mechanism is involved in all foals with clinical signs consistent with HIE. Probably the most important therapeutic aspect is maintenance of hydration,

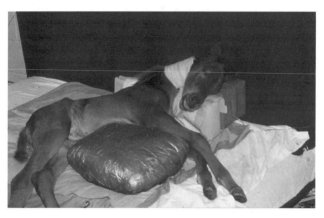

Foal with hypoxic ischemic encephalopathy.

adequate nutritional support, and management of seizures. The following treatments have been used singly or in combination at many practices:

1. **Dimethyl sulfoxide (DMSO).** DMSO has a variety of properties that may benefit foals with HIE. The delay in clinical signs may suggest a role for reperfusion injury mediated through the formation of oxygen radicals. DMSO is a putative hydroxyl radical scavenger.

2. **Magnesium supplementation.** Increasing the extracellular concentration of magnesium may inhibit neuronal cell electrolyte influx caused by glutamate-induced depolarization of N-methyl-D-aspartate (NMDA) receptors. Calcium channel-blocking agents have been used in experimental models of hypoxic ischemic brain damage.

3. **Mannitol infusion.** Mannitol is a potent diuretic that may limit neuronal edema formation in HIE; it also has some antioxidant properties.

4. **Naloxone hydrochloride.** Naloxone has been used with apparent success in a small number of foals. The theoretical basis involves reversal of an endorphin-induced sleep state.

40. What is the prognosis for short- and long-term survival of neonatal foals with uncomplicated HIE?

Formulation of a prognosis is based not necessarily on the severity of neurologic signs but rather on history and onset of abnormal behavior. For example, foals that are obviously affected at the time of birth, as in cases of dystocia, have a poor chance of short-term survival (< 25%), regardless of what facilities are available. In contrast, foals with classic HIE, in which development of signs is often delayed until 12–24 hours of age, have a good short-term survival rate (> 80%) with appropriate care and support. Data indicate that surviving foals perform as well as their siblings in adulthood.

41. What is shaker foal syndrome?

The disease referred to as shaker foal syndrome is caused by an exotoxin of *Clostridium botulinum*. The toxin interferes with the release of acetylcholine from neuromuscular junctions. Typically, botulism in adult horses occurs through ingestion of preformed toxin, whereas in foals the toxin is usually produced in the intestine and absorbed across the intestinal wall (toxicoinfectious form). Of the eight types of *C. botulinum*, type B is considered to be the most important. A third form is wound botulism, in which the bacteria colonize and elaborate toxin in open wounds. The mortality rate in cases of untreated botulism approaches 90%, but use of type B botulinum antitoxin (200 ml IV) has reduced the mortality rate in foals to around 20%. Most affected foals are between 3 and 12 weeks of age. The clinical signs of botulism include generalized weakness, dysphagia, tremor, sweating, flaccid paralysis, ileus, and respiratory failure. Dysphagia may lead to milk aspiration. Additional treatment includes intravenous sodium penicillin G and metronidazole.

The spectrum of antimicrobial coverage should be broadened if aspiration pneumonia is suspected. Procaine penicillin G, tetracyclines, and aminoglycosides are contraindicated because of theoretical potentiation of neuromuscular blockade. Mechanical ventilation is necessary if significant hypoventilation ensues.

42. Describe the strategy used for prevention of botulism in foals.
Prevention is achieved through vaccination of the dam with toxoid (Bot Tox B, Neogen Biologics Corporation, Lexington, KY; 1-800-477-8201 within U.S.). Initial immunization involves 3 vaccines given 1 month apart, starting at 2 months of age, or in the pregnant mare 3, 2, and 1 months before expected parturition. A booster is suggested 30 days before foaling.

CARDIOPULMONARY DISORDERS

43. What is the relative importance of oxygen and carbon dioxide to respiratory drive in sick newborn foals?
In many foals hypoxic drive is more important than hypercapnic drive. Premature foals and newborns with HIE frequently demonstrate hypoventilation in the face of significant hypercapnia (hypercarbia). This "insensitivity" to carbon dioxide is also seen in other disease states, including pneumonia. Reversal of the hypoxic state through oxygen therapy often results in decreased minute ventilation and further carbon dioxide retention.
Lester GD: Neonatal pulmonary disease. In Robinson NE (ed): Current Therapy in Equine Medicine, 4th ed. Philadelphia, W.B. Saunders, 1997, pp 604–609.

44. What oxygen flow rate is commonly used to supplement foals through nasal insufflation in the absence of blood gas data?
The selection of an oxygen flow rate is ideally based on arterial blood gas data. A good starting flow rate is 5 L/minute. In normal foals a flow of 10 L/minute is probably close to an inspired oxygen concentration (FiO_2) of 1.0 or 100%.

45. What is idiopathic or transient tachypnea?
The syndrome of idiopathic tachypnea involves an elevation in both respiratory rate and rectal temperature. Clydesdale foals are commonly affected, but the syndrome also has been seen in other breeds, including Thoroughbreds and Arabians. Important environmental factors include both heat and humidity. Routine diagnostic investigation, including complete blood count, fibrinogen concentration estimation, arterial blood gas analyses, blood culture, and chest radiographs, produce no evidence of infection or inflammation. The onset of signs is within days of birth; spontaneous resolution occurs, sometimes after several weeks of life.

46. Describe the medical management of transient tachypnea.
The hyperthermia associated with this syndrome is typically unresponsive to nonsteroidal antiinflammatory therapy. A rapid reduction in both rectal temperature and respiratory rate frequently occurs after body clipping and/or alcohol baths. The difficulty in differentiating this syndrome from pneumonia usually results in the administration of broad-spectrum antibiotic therapy.

47. Explain why a newborn foal tolerates hypoxemia better than an older foal or adult horse.
Foals often appear to be bright and active with mild-to-moderate hypoxemia. This phenomenon likely reflects lingering adaptation to the in utero environment, in which the foal is exposed to partial pressures of oxygen around 30 mmHg. The increased affinity of fetal hemoglobin for oxygen compared with adult hemoglobin is an adaptive response to the in utero environment. Although equine fetal hemoglobin appears to be structurally identical to adult hemoglobin, it is accompanied by reduced levels of 2,3-DPG in the fetal erythrocyte. Membrane cyanosis does not usually occur in newborn foals until the arterial pressure of oxygen is very low (< 40 mmHg).
Silver M, Comline RS: Transfer of gases and metabolites in the equine placenta: A comparison with other species. J Reprod Fertil 23(Suppl):589–594, 1975.

48. Grunting and paradoxical chest wall motion may occur in foals with respiratory disease. Explain the basis of these signs.

In an attempt to maintain adequate lung volumes, the foal with respiratory disease may have a prolonged expiratory phase against a partially closed glottis, which may coincide with an audible expiratory grunt. Paradoxical chest wall motion occurs when the chest wall moves inward during inspiration, a warning sign of impending respiratory failure.

49. What is the most common congenital cardiac defect in foals?

Ventricular septal defect (VSD) is the most common congenital anomaly reported in newborn foals.

Crowe M, Swerczek TW: Equine congenital cardiac defects. Am J Vet Res 46:353, 1984.

MUSCULOSKELETAL DISORDERS

50. Describe the management of a newborn foal with bilateral congenital flexural deformity of the carpi and distal forelimb joints.

Mild contracture requires little intervention. Limb splints are needed for foals that are unable to stand or that have difficulty in ambulating. If the contracture is restricted to the distal limb, good success can be achieved using a dorsal polyvinylchloride (PVC) splint over a layer of padding that extends from beneath the carpus to the base of the hoof. Carpal contracture can be treated using a variety of splint types, depending on the severity of the deformity. Splints should be changed every 24 hours to prevent the formation of pressure sores. Oxytetracycline (2–3 gm as an intravenous infusion) is commonly used with splinting for moderate-to-severe cases of flexural deformity. Nonsteroidal antiinflammatory drugs are also indicated for many foals.

51. What is the most likely cause of soft, fluctuant swelling over the dorsolateral aspect of the carpus in a young foal?

Rupture of the common digital extensor tendon. Dorsal splinting and stall confinement may be necessary if the leg knuckles forward. Prognosis is generally good.

MISCELLANEOUS DISORDERS

52. What is lavender foal syndrome?

In this poorly described syndrome seen in Egyptian or half-Egyptian Arabians, affected foals have a diluted coat color (lavender) and are unable to stand or walk. The prognosis is apparently hopeless. The major finding on histologic examination of tissues is neuronal cell vacuolization.

Madigan JE: Manual of Equine Neonatal Care, 3rd ed. Woodland, CA, Live Oak Publishing, 1997, pp 210–211.

53. What is combined immunodeficiency (CID) syndrome? How is it diagnosed before death?

CID is a primary immunodeficiency that occurs almost exclusively in Arabian or part-Arabian foals. The lethal characteristic is transferred as an autosomal recessive trait and result in failure to produce functional B- and T-lymphocytes. The defect is in the maturation of lymphoid stem cells. Other components of the immune system, such as neutrophils and macrophages, are unaffected. CID can be diagnosed in presuckle foals by demonstration of lymphopenia and absence of serum IgM. In postsuckle foals the diagnosis is more difficult but involves demonstration of persistent lymphopenia (< 1000 cells/μl) and low levels of IgM and IgG by 4–6 weeks of age. Whole blood, blood in acid-citrate-dextrose, and mucosal cells may be sent to the VetGen LLC (Ann Arbor, MI, 1-800-4-VETGEN) for DNA testing. The DNA test shows whether the gene is present in the tested horse, whether the horse is a carrier, or whether the horse is affected.

54. Contrast the clinical signs of corneal ulceration in neonates and adult horses.

In contrast to adults, neonatal foals rarely develop photophobia, blepharospasm, and increased tearing in response to corneal ulceration. Consequently, the sick foal should be monitored daily for ulceration using a fluorescein dye.

Brooks DE, Clark CK: Ocular problems in the foal. In Robinson NE (ed): Current Therapy in Equine Medicine, 4th ed. Philadelphia, W.B. Saunders, 1997, pp 636–643.

55. Describe the management of entropion in newborn foals.

Entropion occurs commonly in newborn foals secondary to dehydration, prematurity/dysmaturity, trauma, or poor nutrition. Primary entropion is rare. The management of secondary eyelid inversion involves correction of the primary problem and eversion of the lid with nonabsorbable sutures or surgical staples. Sutures are placed using a vertical mattress pattern. Some clinicians advocate the use of subcutaneous procaine penicillin G as a method to cause lid eversion. Surgical procedures are rarely indicated.

BIBLIOGRAPHY

1. Bauer JE: Normal blood chemistry. In Koterba AM, et al (eds): Equine Clinical Neonatology. Philadelphia, Lea & Febiger, 1990, pp 602–614.
2. Brewer BD, Koterba AM: The development of a scoring system for the early diagnosis of equine neonatal sepsis. Equine Vet J 20:18–23, 1988.
3. Brooks DE, Clark CK: Ocular problems in the foal. In Robinson NE (ed): Current Therapy in Equine Medicine, 4th ed. Philadelphia, W.B. Saunders, 1997, pp 636–643.
4. Cohen ND: Diarrheal diseases of foals. In Robinson NE (ed): Current Therapy in Equine Medicine, 4th ed. Philadelphia, W.B. Saunders, 1997, pp 631–636.
5. Cottrill CM: Maturation of the cardiopulmonary system. Equine Vet J 14(Suppl):26–30, 1993.
6. Crowe M, Swerczek TW: Equine congenital defects. Am J Vet Res 46:353, 1984.
7. Hansen TO: Nutritional support: Parenteral feeding. In Koterba AM, et al (eds): Equine Clinical Neonatology. Philadelphia, Lea & Febiger, 1990, pp 747–762.
8. Howell CE, Rollins WC: Environmental sources of variation in the gestation length of the horse. J Animal Sci 10:789, 1951.
9. Koterba AM: Prematurity. In Koterba AM, et al (eds): Equine Clinical Neonatology. Philadelphia, Lea & Febiger, 1990, pp 55–70.
10. Koterba AM: Definitions of equine perinatal disorders: Problems and solutions. Equine Vet Educ 5:271, 1993.
11. LeBlanc MM, et al: Factors that influence passive transfer of immunoglobulins in foals. J Am Vet Med Assoc 220:179–183, 1992.
12. Lester GD: Neonatal pulmonary disease. In Robinson NE (ed): Current Therapy in Equine Medicine, 4th ed. Philadelphia, W.B. Saunders, 1997, pp 604–609.
13. Lewis LD: Growing horse feeding and care. In Lewis LD (ed): Equine Clinical Nutrition. Baltimore, Williams & Wilkins, 1995, pp 334–349.
14. Madigan JE: Manual of Equine Neonatal Care, 3rd ed. Woodland, CA, Live Oak Publishing, 1997, pp 210–211.
15. Oftedal OT, et al: Lactation in the horse: Milk composition and intake by foals. J Nutr 113:2096, 1983.
16. Roipha RT, et al: The duration of pregnancy in Thoroughbred mares. Vet Rec 84:552, 1969.
17. Sanchez LC, et al: The effect of ranitidine on intragastric pH in clinically normal neonatal foals. J Am Vet Med Assoc 212:1407–1412, 1998.
18. Silver M, Comline RS: Transfer of gases and metabolites in the equine placenta: A comparison with other species. J Reprod Fertil 23(Suppl):589–594, 1975.
19. Thorburn GD: A speculative review of parturition in the mare. Equine Vet J 14(Suppl):41–49, 1993.

16. REPRODUCTION IN MARES AND STALLIONS

William B. Ley, D.V.M., M.S., Dip. ACT

If I have seen further than others, it is by standing upon the shoulders of giants.

Isaac Newton (1642–1727)

1. You are asked to evaluate a 4-year-old Thoroughbred mare retiring from the racetrack for prepurchase breeding soundness. Outline your diagnostic plan.

The appropriate breeding soundness examination includes a thorough history; complete physical examination; external conformation evaluation of the perineum; both digital and visual vaginal examinations; thorough rectal palpation of both ovaries, the uterus, and cervix; ultrasonography of the internal genitalia; endometrial cytologic examination; and serologic analysis for equine infectious anemia and equine viral arteritis.

2. What is Pascoe's Caslick index?

The effective length of the vulva (cm) and the angle (°) of declination of the vulva are used to derive this value. The effective length (l) is from the level of the pelvic brim to the dorsal commissure of the vulva (cm); the angle of declination (a) is the angle of difference between vertical (90°) and the anatomic angle of the vulva, when the mare's head (anterior) is 180° and the mare's tail (posterior) is 0°. These measurements are best obtained when the mare is in estrus. The product of $l \times a$ is equal to the Caslick index (CI). Normal mares should have an index of < 100. Mares with CI > 150 are at risk of pneumovagina and therefore would benefit from a Caslick vulvoplasty. A CI > 150 suggests a greater angle of declination, which is abnormal, and/or a greater effective length.

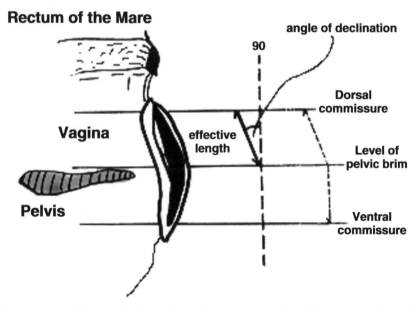

Perineal anatomy of the mare showing landmarks for measurement of the effective length of the vulva and the angle of declination. (Redrawn from Pascoe RR: Observations on the effective length and angle of declination of the vulva and its relation to fertility in the mare. J Reprod Fertil Suppl 27:299–305, 1979.)

3. What are the landmarks of the normal clitoral anatomy of the mare?

The glans clitoris is a circular, wrinkled structure that lies within the fossa clitoridis and is located within the ventral vulval commissure. The dorsal border of the fossa is a transverse band, also called the transverse frenular fold, that attaches the central dorsal region of the clitoris to the lateral walls of the fossa. The recesses of the fossa are deep, especially ventral and lateral to the glans. Within the dorsal glans is a central median sinus that is bordered by two shallow lateral sinuses. It is often necessary to elevate the transverse frenular fold to visualize the opening of the sinuses.

4. What physical barriers of defense prevent endometrial infection of the mare's uterus?

The symmetry, position, angle, and tone of the vulval lips and the effective mucous membrane apposition created by these characteristics of the vulva are the first physical barriers that prevent ascending bacterial contamination of the more cranial reproductive tract. Additional anatomic barriers against ascending bacterial invasion of the uterus include the vestibulovaginal seal and cervix.

5. What is the clinical significance of endometrial biopsy classification grades?

The clinical significance of the biopsy score is related to the prognosis for the mare to carry the pregnancy to term once she conceives. Various methods of endometrial histomorphologic classification have been proposed. They are named after the authors that described their use: Kenney, Doig, Gordon-Sartin, and Ricketts, to name a few. Interpretation is based on the pathologist's estimate of the number and distribution of endometrial glandular structures and the frequency and distribution of inflammation and fibrosis throughout the biopsy samples. Classifications are generally based on a grading scale of one to three or four. Category I includes mares that have minimal or no pathologic changes in endometrial architecture and have a > 70% chance of carrying their pregnancy to term. Category II (or IIA) indicates that endometrial changes are predominantly inflammatory with minimal periglandular fibrosis; such mares have a 50–70% chance of carrying their pregnancy to term. Category III (IIB) endometria have changes that show moderate-to-severe inflammation and a greater degree of fibrosis of periglandular submucosal areas; such mares have a 30–50% chance for maintenance of pregnancy. Category IV (III) endometrial biopsy specimens exhibit widespread fibrosis, widespread and severe inflammation, severe lymphatic stasis, or endometrial glandular atrophy; such mares have a < 10% chance for maintenance of pregnancy. The assigned score is important but must not be interpreted alone. Further consideration must be given to the individual mare's age, past breeding history, other medical history, number of years barren, and response to therapy as well as to quality of breeding management.

6. What are the advantages to performing endometrial cytology simultaneously with collection of a sample for endometrial culture?

Cytologic interpretation of the endometrial smear supports the clinical significance of bacterial or fungal isolates recovered from an endometrial culture. More than 1–2 polymorphonuclear (PMN) leukocytes (neutrophils) per 5 microscopic fields (i.e., × 400 magnification) indicate an active inflammatory response. Since slide preparations vary considerably in density of cell number, the number of neutrophils per high-powered field is a less consistent interpretive guide than an estimation of neutrophil-to-endometrial cell ratio. In acute uterine infections, the ratio of neutrophils to endometrial cells exceeds 40 : 1. The absence of inflammatory cells on the endometrial cytologic smear indicates that any bacterial isolates recovered on endometrial culture are contaminants of the sampling technique. A predominance of lymphocytes, eosinophils, and macrophages on the endometrial cytologic smear indicates chronic uterine infection. Correlation between inflammatory endometrial cytologic smears and the recovery of pathogenic bacteria from endometrial culture ranges from 76–88%. Similarly, correlation between acute inflammation observed in endometrial histopathologic samples and the culture of uterine pathogens has ranged from 70–75%. Endometrial cytology is equally acceptable as endometrial biopsy in the determination of acute inflammatory responses associated with bacterial endometritis. Cytology, however, is not as indicative of chronic inflammatory or fibrotic changes of the endometrium as endometrial biopsy.

7. How is the diagnosis of fungal endometritis confirmed?

An inflammatory endometrial smear pattern (i.e., PMN leukocytes, neutrophils) associated with the presence of fungal elements or vegetative yeast forms on cytology or identified by endometrial culture must be demonstrated to confirm the diagnosis of fungal endometritis. Yeast forms are often detected on endometrial cytology using the Dif-Quik stain (Harleco Division, American Hospital Supply Corp., Gibbstown, NJ 08027), but the presence of significant fungal hyphae may be overlooked. Cytologic smears should be prepared with Trichrome or silver stains when nonyeast fungal elements are suspected. It is also advisable to repeat the culture to verify the initial fungal recovery and identification.

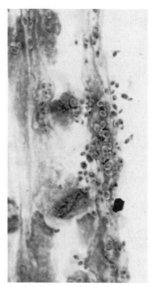

Yeast on endometrial cytology
($\times$ 400, Dif-Quik stain).

8. Is a single endometrial biopsy sample representative of the entire endometrium?

A single endometrial biopsy was initially thought to be adequate for the diagnosis and prognosis of equine uterine disease. This belief was substantiated by Waelchli and Winder (1989), who demonstrated that multiple (n = 5) uterine biopsies, obtained at slaughter from 110 mares, were in good agreement 73.6% of the time within the same mare and that only 2.7% were in poor agreement within the same mare. Disagreements were most often due to variation in the distribution of fibrotic periglandular lesions. A more recent study by Dybdal et al. (1991) involved endometrial samples recovered during the postmortem examination of 88 mares. The investigators reported that agreement between biopsy classification grades for samples obtained from the left uterine horn, right uterine horn, and uterine body in the same mare was only 29%. Fifty-five percent of the mares examined were rated as differing by 1 biopsy grade from at least 2 of the 3 uterine locations sampled. Assessment of the true histomorphologic character of the equine endometrium, therefore, may need to be based on multiple (> 3) biopsy samples at different locations within the uterus. Multiple samples, however, do not guarantee a correct diagnosis.

Dybdal NO, Daels PF, Cuoto MA, et al: Investigation of the reliability of a single endometrial biopsy sample, with a note on the correlation between uterine cysts on biopsy grade. J Reprod Fertil Suppl 44:697, 1991.

Waelchi RO, Winder NC: Distribution of histological lesions in the equine endometrium. Vet Rec 124:274–276, 1989.

9. What further information can be obtained by hysteroscopic examination of the mare?

Typical abnormal hysteroscopic findings include cystic structures, intraluminal adhesions, fluid accumulation in one or both horns, and textural and color changes of the endometrium. Endometrial glandular cysts are usually small (i.e., < 1-mm diameter), smooth on the surface, round, firm, embedded in the endometrial tissue, and of the same color as the endometrial surface. Lymphatic cysts are larger, ranging in diameter from 1 to > 20 mm. They range from individual small, pedunculated sacs filled with yellow-colored watery fluid to much larger, flattened multilobulated structures with a tough, fibrous outer surface lining. Some are also reported to be round-to-elongated, thin-walled, and occasionally rough in surface appearance. Lymphatic cysts are freely movable in any direction with forceps. Most cysts are located at the base of one uterine horn or at the uterine horn bifurcation. Intraluminal adhesions may be central, transverse, or marginal. Endometrial tissue adhesions appear similar in color to the surrounding endometrium and are relatively fragile; connective tissue adhesions have a glossy, white surface appearance and are much more resistant to disruption or excision. Exudates within the uterine lumen may range from serous to serosanguinous or mucoid to mucopurulent (with or without clumps of inspissated debris) and vary considerably in quantity. Textural and color changes range from small, localized areas of roughening, thickening, and pallor (e.g., fibrosis) to large, diffuse areas of hyperemia. Ulceration may be associated with areas of fibrosis. Acute inflammation of the endometrium is observed as areas of intense hyperemia and irregular edema. Atrophy of endometrial folds is noted as marked decrease in size, contour, consistency, and symmetry when observed during physiologic estrus and with the uterine cavity in the collapsed state.

10. What cystic congenital anomalies may be encountered in examining the mare for breeding soundness?

Adnexal structures that may be occasionally found in or near the internal genital tract of the mare are often fluid-filled embryonic vestiges. Fimbrial cysts (hydatids of Morgagni) are common in mares. They frequently are pedunculated and histologically are lined with ciliated columnar epithelium, indicating that they are of müllerian duct origin. Fossal cysts also may be found in the region of the ovulation fossa. They are similar to fimbrial cysts, and their impact on fertility of the mare is open to question. Large cysts or multiple small cysts may obstruct the normal ovulatory function of infundibulum and ovulation fossa. Tubal cysts are remnants of the mesonephric duct system. They may be found in the mesosalpinx or mesovarium and range from 2–50 mm in diameter. Cysts forming in the cranial group of mesonephric tubules are epoophoron; those forming more caudally are paroophoron.

11. Should oviductal function be considered in performing a breeding soundness examination of the mare?

Oviductal dysfunction is a little understood area in equine reproduction. The oviduct in the mare has been considered well protected from uterine pathologic conditions by the strong muscular papillae at the uterotubal junction and its dorsal position in the abdominal cavity. An oviductal dysfunction or blockage cannot be diagnosed through rectal palpation, ultrasound, or laparoscopic examination unless a grossly obvious condition exists. Mares that cycle and ovulate normally, that fail to conceive despite good breeding practice, and that possess otherwise normal or acceptable uterine, cervical, and vulvovaginal health may be suspected of having oviductal dysfunction. A report of a study to evaluate sperm transport in the equine oviduct found pathologic changes by scanning electron microscopy (SEM) in the caudal isthmic epithelium of four subfertile mares with confirmed susceptibility to chronic uterine infection. In contrast, the isthmic epithelium of the four normal mares in the same study appeared healthy. The authors concluded that sperm transport patterns for subfertile mares was significantly different from normal mares and that the oviductal region in which differences were most striking was the caudal isthmus. This finding does not imply oviductal occlusion or obstruction but supports oviductal dysfunction. The oviducts of mares can be evaluated grossly by laparoscopic examination.

12. What is the starch granule test for evaluation of oviductal patency?

Evaluation of uterine tubal patency, as described in 1979 by Allen, is relatively simple and requires little in the way of advanced technology or training. A solution of starch granules is deposited onto the ovarian surface by a transabdominal approach with a long needle; 24 hours later the uterus and os cervix are lavaged for sample collection by a vaginal approach. The recovered fluid is stained with 2% Lugol's iodine and examined microscopically for the presence of any starch granules that may have been transported to the uterine environment via the uterine tubes. The test must be repeated to evaluate left vs. right uterine tubal patency, one side per procedure. A minimum interval of 10 days between procedures is appropriate. This technique is used clinically with good result, however, the drawback of having to perform the procedure twice (first for the left and then for the right uterine tube) makes it time-consuming and stressful to the mare. In the original study starch granules from 6–56 μm in diameter were transported in all mares with patent oviducts, as recovered at 24 hours after deposition. Starch granules were transported in all mares, regardless of the stage of the estrous cycle, with one noted exception: when starch granules were deposited on an ovary that ovulated the same day, starch granule transport could not be demonstrated until 4–7 days later.

Allen WE, Noakes DE: Evaluation of uterine tube function in pony mares. Vet Rec 105:364–366, 1979.

13. Why are superovulation protocols not as successful in mares as in other domestic large animals?

Development of a superovulation technique that is successful, safe, and commercially available would revolutionize the equine breeding industry. In reality, however, ovulation rates for mares after existing superovulatory treatment are much lower than for cattle. This dichotomy has been attributed to the relatively limited area available in the ovulation fossa and the large size of the equine preovulatory follicle. In addition, the number of ovulations in mares may be limited physiologically by the size of the follicular cohort rescued by administration of gonadotropins. Clearly, additional research is necessary to optimize superovulation regimens in mares.

14. What is deslorelin? How successful is it in inducing ovulation in estrous mares?

Deslorelin, a nonapeptide, is a gonadtropin-releasing hormone (GnRH) agonist. Its efficacy and safety, when it is administered subcutaneously (2.2 mg) as a short-term implant, was evaluated in a recent placebo-controlled clinical trial in normally cycling mares in estrus with a dominant ovarian follicle > 30 mm in diameter. Treatment with deslorelin reduced the mean time to ovulation from 84–88 hours to 50–54 hours. The percentage of mares ovulating within 48 hours increased from 26–37% in control mares to 81–86% in treated mares. The duration of estrus in the deslorelin-treated mares was reduced from 6.1 days to 4.3 days, and the number of matings or artificial inseminations was reduced from 2.5 to 1.7. The deslorelin treatments did not cause systemic side effects, and local reactions at the implantation sites were slight and of short duration.

Meyers PJ, Bowman T, Blodgett G, et al: Use of the GnRH analogue, deslorelin acetate, in a slow-release implant to accelerate ovulation in oestrous mares. Vet Rec 140:249–252, 1997.

15. What are the most common reasons for a mare's failure to exhibit estrous behavior?

Season of the year is most commonly associated with failure to exhibit estrous behavior. Pregnancy is the second most common reason. The mare's age, infectious conditions of the uterus, lactation, social dominance, and pseudopregnancy (i.e., prolonged maintenance of a corpus luteum) play less important roles.

16. Are artificial lighting programs a successful means of manipulating the mare's pattern of reproductive cyclicity once she has entered the physiologic breeding season?

When applied correctly for at least 60 days, artificial lighting programs work well in anestrous mares to stimulate an earlier return to estrous activity. Once the mare has entered the transitional phase between the anestrous and physiologic breeding seasons, artificial lights are unlikely to have further benefit in altering estrous behavior.

17. What is the best means of artificially advancing the breeding season in anestrous mares?

Increasing perceived daylength with artificial lighting a total of 16 hours per day remains the most effective means.

18. What ultrasonographic changes are observed in the uterus of mares during the estrous cycle?

The prominence of endometrial folds varies with the stage of the estrous cycle. Prominent endometrial folds, often highlighted by intervening areas of decreased echogenicity (i.e., endometrial edema) and sometimes accompanied by small amounts of free intraluminal fluid, are observed when the mare is in early estrus. As estrus progresses, the degree of endometrial edema and the prominence of endometrial folds decrease. In diestrus, the endometrial folds are often indistinguishable.

19. What are the advantages of ultrasonographic examination of the mare's ovarian structures?

Ultrasonic examination of the ovaries is relatively rapid, noninvasive, and objective. It allows visualization of ovarian structures that may not be detectable by simple rectal palpation, such as the corpus luteum (CL), corpus hemorrhagicum (CH), follicles developing within the ovary (but not distorting the ovarian surface), ovarian hematoma, and ovarian tumor. Follicles greater than 3 mm can usually be detected. Detection of characteristic changes of the preovulatory follicle allows greater accuracy in prediction of ovulation. Within the first 24 hours after ovulation the CH appears as a strongly echogenic, circumscribed mass of tissue. Its echogenicity decreases as it develops into a functional CL.

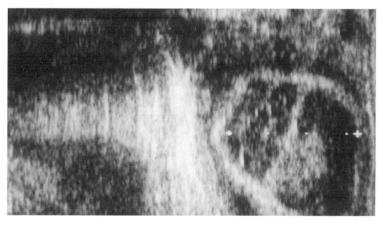

Ultrasonogram of an equine ovary with a newly forming corpus hemorrhagicum.

The CL usually can be visualized throughout its functional life span; in one study, the mean duration of time that a CL was visible by transrectal ultrasonographic observation was 17 days. The CL increases in echodensity just before its regression. Prolonged maintenance of a CL (pseudopregnancy) is easily diagnosed by ultrasonography in the mare that fails to exhibit estrous cyclicity. The differential diagnoses for large fluid-filled structures detected on palpation can be narrowed by ultrasonography, which detects whether the structure is singular or has multiple portions and characterizes the echogenic quality of its internal compartment(s): (1) follicular fluid is anechogenic; (2) hematomata, when organized, have strands of hyperechoic structures in a honeycombed pattern; and (3) granulosa cell tumors usually are mutlicompartmented with anechoic-to-hypoechoic centers, although they vary greatly (see chapter 17). Paraovarian cysts, although infrequent in mares, may be confused with anovulatory follicles. In the author's experience, paraovarian cysts can be confirmed by ultrasonography, which shows them as separate from the ovary proper.

20. Why is the ovulation fossa of the ovary distinct in mares?

The histologic structure and embryogenesis of the equine ovary are unique among domestic animals. The mature ovary has a peripheral vascular zone (or medulla) of collagenous connective tissue that surrounds a central parenchymatous zone (or cortex). The central zone contains developing and atretic ovarian follicles, corpora lutea, corpora hemorrhagica, and corpora albicantia. The germinal epithelium of the horse is confined to the ovulation fossa of the adult ovary. The parenchymatous zone emerges at the ovarian fossa; during folliculogenesis, Graafian (maturing) follicles move toward the fossa, where ovulation occurs in all cases.

21. How many waves of follicle development occur during the mare's estrous cycle?

Mares have one or two major episodes or waves of follicle development during the estrous cycle.

22. What is known about inhibin activity in mares?

The relationship of inhibin and follicle-stimulating hormone (FSH) has been investigated during the estrous cycle of mares. Plasma levels of inhibin in ovariectomized mares were undetectable. Concentrations of FSH, estradiol, and inhibin change during the estrous cycle. Inhibin levels are the highest on the day of ovulation, decline rapidly after ovulation, and reach a low on about day 7 after ovulation. Plasma inhibin and estradiol concentrations follow a similar profile, whereas inhibin and FSH levels have an inverse relationship throughout the estrous cycle. The mare's ovaries appear to be the source of bioactive and immunoreactive inhibin, as observed in other species. Inhibin concentrations may be the most useful hormonal assay in determining whether a mare has a granulosa cell tumor. In one study, the concentration of inhibin was increased in the majority of affected mares.

Roser JF, McCue PM, Hoye E: Inhibin activity in the mare and stallion. Domest Animal Endocrinol 11:87–100,1994.

23. What is meant by a retained or prolonged corpus luteum in mares?

Prolonged luteal activity is one of the most formidable taxonomic challenges in mare reproductive biology. Prolonged luteal activity may result from persistence of an individual corpus luteum or sequential development of luteal glands, each of which may have a normal life span. Luteal tissue may originate from an unovulated follicle or from an ovulation occurring during either follicular or luteal dominance. These complexities, together with ambiguous and inconsistent terminology, have resulted in confusion about conditions that can be grouped broadly under the term prolonged luteal activity. Persistence of an individual corpus luteum may occur in association with severe damage to the endometrium, resulting in loss of the uterine luteolytic mechanism. Spontaneous (no known uterine pathology) persistence of the corpus luteum from follicular-phase ovulation has not been documented adequately as a clinical entity. The occurrence of ovulation toward the end of diestrus may cause confusion about the origin of prolonged luteal activity. Such immature diestrous corpora lutea may not respond to the release of uterine luteolysin, thereby leading to prolonged luteal activity, even though the original corpus luteum regressed at the normal time. In the absence of critical monitoring of the corpus luteum (e.g., by ultrasonographic evaluation), the prolonged activity may be attributed erroneously to persistence of the corpus luteum from follicular-phase ovulation. Pseudopregnancy is another term that is sometimes used to describe persistence of the corpus luteum, especially when it is caused by embryonic loss after the embryo has blocked the uterine luteolytic mechanism.

Ginther OJ: Prolonged luteal activity in mares—a semantic quagmire. Equine Vet J 22(3):152–156, 1990.

24. Does treatment of the mare with altrenogest alter the reproductive performance of her female offspring?

Maternal treatment with altrenogest alters gonadotrophin secretion before puberty but has no effect on functional reproductive performance in fillies. Puberty was studied using 15 fillies of

Quarter Horse phenotype. Fillies were from dams treated daily from days 20–325 of gestation with (1) 2 ml neobee oil per 44.5 kg body weight (controls) or (2) 2 ml altrenogest (2.2 mg/ml) per 44.5 kg body weight. Prenatal altrenogest treatment caused clitoral enlargement (p < 0.05) and increased serum concentrations of LH from 1–7 months of age. The median age at puberty was 90 weeks. Durations of estrus, diestrus, and the estrous cycle were not different between groups and were similar to those for adult mares. First-cycle pregnancy rates and overall rates were 100% and 82% and 100% and 91.7% for control and treated fillies, respectively (p > 0.05).

Naden J, Squires EL, Nett TM: Effect of maternal treatment with altrenogest on age at puberty, hormone concentrations, pituitary response to exogenous GnRH, estrous cycle characteristics and fertility of fillies. J Reprod Fertil 88:185–195, 1990.

25. What is the risk of abortion for mares presenting with colic signs in late gestation?

One study reviewed the medical records of pregnant mares over a 3-year period. In all cases, persistent pain or progressive abdominal distention was the main reason for referral. The overall survival rate for the 115 mares treated for colic was 73.9% (85 cases). The abortion rate was 20.5% in surgical patients (34 cases), 40% for mares with uterine torsion (5 cases), and 10.8% after medical treatment (46 cases). The total abortion rate was 16.4%. Clinical evidence of endotoxemia was present in all but one of the aborting mares after colic treatment. Anesthesia did not appear to be a problem because abortion occurred in 5 of 46 medically treated cases as well as in 9 of 39 mares treated surgically. Mares with uterine torsions received anesthesia and were included in the "surgical" category. Abortion occurred in 3 mares that suffered intraoperative hypoxia, but fasting for > 30 hours did not seem to cause prolonged hypoglycemia and subsequent abortion. Clenbuterol hydrochloride was used as a tocolytic agent in 9 mares with uterine displacement, abortus imminens, and postoperative uterine torsion; 3 mares aborted during treatment.

Boening KJ, Leendertse IP: Review of 115 cases of colic in the pregnant mare. Equine Vet J 25:518–521, 1993.

26. What are the differences in the use of isoflurane and halothane inhalant anesthesia in pregnant mares?

Despite minor differences, clinically neither appears to have an advantage over the other as long as the mare is well ventilated during the anesthetic period. Physical signs of postanesthetic myopathy or vital-organ dysfunction are not associated with either agent.

Daunt DA, Steffey EP, Pascoe JR, et al: Actions of isoflurane and halothane in pregnant mares. J Am Vet Med Assoc 201:1367–1374, 1992.

27. Can ovariectomized mares be used as recipients in an embryo transfer program?

Yes. Pregnancy has been established and maintained after embryo transfer in ovariectomized mares treated with progesterone only. Progesterone in oil (300 mg/day by intramuscular injection) is given starting 5 days before transfer of a 7-day embryo. If the mare is pregnant at 20 days, progesterone treatment is continued to 100 days of gestation. Pregnant, ovariectomized recipient mares carry to term and deliver live foals with normal parturition, lactation, and maternal behavior.

28. Is hydramnios (i.e., hydroamnion) life-threatening in mares?

Yes. One case report described an 18-year-old mare at around 285 days' gestation who was presented for apparent abdominal pain of 8 hours' duration. A large volume of sanguinous fluid was obtained on abdominocentesis, and digital vaginal examination revealed a dilated cervix and blood in the uterus. Abdominal palpation per rectum revealed the uterus to be large and distended with fluid. Ultrasonography revealed a fetus devoid of movement or heartbeat on the floor of the cranial portion of the abdomen. Elective euthanasia was performed because of the poor prognosis. Postmortem examination confirmed that the uterus had ruptured and that the fetus, within its chorioallantois, was in the abdomen. The amniotic sac contained approximately 96 L of amniotic fluid. Hydramnios was diagnosed on the basis of the excessive amniotic fluid and was believed to be the cause of the uterine rupture.

Honnas CM, Spensley MS, Laverty S, Blanchard PC: Hydramnios causing uterine rupture in a mare. J Am Vet Med Assoc 193:334–336, 1988.

29. A 16-year-old mare that is 9 months pregnant is presented with a complaint of muco-purulent discharge from the vulva. What should the differential diagnosis include?

The appropriate differential diagnoses include (1) urethritis, (2) cystitis, (3) cervicitis, (4) vulvovaginitis, (5) endometritis, and (6) placentitis.

30. A 30-month-old Arabian filly of unknown breeding history appears to have an abnormally large udder. The filly may be pregnant, but you are hesitant to perform a rectal examination because of concerns of rupturing the filly's rectum or small colon. How do you confirm pregnancy?

One option is to collect a venous blood sample for an endocrine test for estrone sulfate. If the observed udder enlargement is potentially related to late gestation, the test for equine chorionic gonadotrophin (eCG, PMSG) would be invalid. eCG is not detectable after days 120–150 of gestation. Transabdominal ultrasonography is the other appropriate choice for diagnosis of pregnancy in later stages of gestation.

31. Describe the findings of rectal palpation and ultrasonography in a mare that is 17–19 days pregnant with bicornuate twin embryos.

Rectal palpation may reveal excellent tone in both uterine horns with a gap or loss in tone at the base of each uterine horn; a long, tightly-closed, cigar-shaped cervix; some follicular activity; and no significant structure identifiable as a corpus luteum on either ovary. Ultrasonography reveals two anechogenic structures, one in each uterine horn, that are spherical in shape and measure 14–18 mm in vertical diameter.

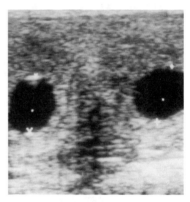

Ultrasonogram of a mare's uterus with bicornuate twin pregnancy at or near 17 days after ovulation.

32. Of the many methods of pregnancy diagnosis in mares, which can be performed at the earliest day with respect to the last day of breeding?

Transrectal B-mode ultrasonography using a 5–7-MHz linear array transducer around days 11–13 is the earliest and most accurate method for pregnancy diagnosis in mares. However, rectal palpation of uterine horn content for size and tone and palpation of the cervix for shape and tone can be performed reliably around days 17–19 after breeding.

33. Endometrial cups in the mare are active during which days of gestation?

Endometrial cups form around days 35–40 of gestation and continue to function through days 85–100 of gestation. Their endocrine product (eCG) is usually detectable in serum samples from days 40–150 of gestation.

34. What happens if pregnant mares are maintained under an extended photoperiod similar to the artificial lighting program used for anestrous nonpregnant mares?

Over a 2-year period, mares (n = 32) of predominantly Quarter Horse breeding and their foals were used to study the effects of photoperiod on reproduction during the periparturient period. Specific objectives of the study were (1) to evaluate the effects of an extended photoperiod regimen (16 hours of light) on gestation length, foal development, and postpartum reproductive performance and (2) to measure changes in plasma progesterone concentrations during the last trimester of gestation and plasma luteinizing hormone (LH) concentrations after foaling until ovulation. Mares in the extended daylength treatment group had shorter (10 days) mean gestation length (p < 0.01) than control mares (exposed to normal daylight hours). Although foals of mares exposed to a long photoperiod were carried for a shorter term, they tended to have heavier birth weights than foals from control mares, but the difference was not statistically significant. Foal size, as determined by body measurements, was not affected by the photoperiod. Neither interval from parturition to first ovulation nor interval from onset of estrus to ovulation was significantly affected by the extended photoperiod.

Hodge SL, Kreider JL, Potter GD, et al: Influence of photoperiod on the pregnant and postpartum mare. Am J Vet Res 43:1752–1755, 1982.

35. What pathologic changes are observed and what bacteria are isolated from cases of equine placentitis?

In a study of placentas from 954 aborted, stillborn, and premature foals during the 1988 and 1989 foaling seasons, placentitis was found in 236 (24.7%). Microorganisms associated with placentitis were isolated or demonstrated from 162 of the 236 (68.6%) cases. Major pathogens identified, in decreasing order, were *Streptococcus zooepidemicus, Leptospira* species, *Escherichia coli,* a nocardioform actinomycete, fungi, *Pseudomonas aeruginosa, Streptococcus equisimilis, Enterobacter agglomerans, Klebsiella pneumoniae,* and alpha-hemolytic streptococci. *Leptospira* species and the nocardioform actinomycete are important, newly emerging bacteria associated with equine placentitis.

Pathogens were not recovered in 64 cases (27.1%), and overgrowth by saprophytic bacteria was recorded in 10 cases (4.2%). Twenty-seven cases (16.6%) had mixed bacterial growth, and in 93 cases (57.4%) bacteria were cultured from both placenta and fetal organs. Most cases of placentitis caused by bacteria, with the exception of *Leptospira* species and the nocardioform actinomycete, occurred in two forms. The first form was acute, focal or diffuse; had an infiltration of neutrophils in the intervillous spaces or necrosis of chorionic villi; was associated with bacteremia; and frequently occurred in the placenta from fetuses expelled before or at mid-gestation. The other form was observed from foals expelled at late gestation, was mostly chronic and focal or focally extensive, and occurred mostly at the cervical star area. Chronic placentitis was characterized by the presence of one or a combination of the following lesions: (1) necrosis of chorionic villi, (2) presence of eosinophilic amorphous material on the chorion, and (3) infiltration of mononuclear inflammatory cells in the intervillous spaces, villous stroma, chorionic stroma, vascular layer, and allantois.

Hong CB, Donahue JM, Giles RC Jr, et al: Etiology and pathology of equine placentitis. J Vet Diagn Invest 5:56–63, 1993.

36. What are the main types of fetal malposition associated with mares referred for management of dystocia?

Severe dystocia is often multifactorial. Most cases involve malposture and over one-half of these involve more than one extremity. Head and/or neck deviation is a major reason for dystocia referral. In about one-third of cases malposition is a factor, and abnormal presentation is involved in about one-quarter of referrals. A recent retrospective investigation determined the population characteristics of horses presented for dystocia at two equine referral hospitals and the types of fetal maldispositions. The study population consisted of a similar number of Thoroughbreds (25%), Standardbreds (24%) and draft horses (22%). Eighteen percent of the draft mare dystocias (6 of 33) were transverse presentations, whereas only 8% (6 of 73) of the two major light breeds (Thoroughbred, n = 3; Standardbred, n = 3) had transverse presentation dystocias. Despite the significant breed differences between the two populations (p < 0.001), the prevalence of all other fetal maldispositions was not different from previous reports.

Frazer GS, Perkins NR, Blanchard TL, et al: Prevalence of fetal maldispositions in equine referral hospital dystocias. Equine Vet J 29:111–116, 1997.

37. How long is stage 2 of parturition in mares?

Stage 2 of labor should last only 20–30 minutes; rarely does it exceed 1 hour. On the average most mares are in the active portion of stage 2 for around 17 minutes.

38. What is the normal or expected duration of stage 3 of parturition in mares?

Placental passage (dehiscence) should be expected within 1 hour of delivery of the foal after an otherwise normal parturition. The events include continued myometrial contractions, which assist the diffuse chorionic microcotyledons to detach or separate from their endometrial glandular sites. Tension by the externalized umbilical cord and amnion assist the slow exteriorization of the entire placental unit. In most circumstances the placenta is delivered "inside-out." The smooth, grayish surface of the allantois is on the outer surface, and the velvety red-to- brown surface of the chorion is situated inside.

39. What should be done for mares presented within 1 hour of foaling with evidence of a third-degree perineal laceration?

The mare should be given a thorough physical examination to ensure that she is not suffering from other parturient complications such as intramural or uterine arterial hemorrhage. If she is not, the extent of the perineal injury should be assessed, and the cervix and uterus should be palpated under aseptic conditions to rule out more proximal reproductive tract tearing or injury. In general, if the mare has suffered no other detectable pathology or injury and the foaling injury is less than 3 hours' duration, immediate repair may be attempted. However, the extent of bruising and edema that may develop after injury usually prevents successful healing when primary closure is attempted. Repair of such injuries is most often delayed for a period of 6–8 weeks after foaling. Two of the more commonly performed perineal reconstruction techniques are the Aanes and Goetze techniques.

Moll HD, Slone DE: Perineal lacerations and rectovestibular fistulas. In Wolfe DF, Moll HD (eds): Large Animal Urogenital Surgery, 2nd ed. Baltimore, Williams and Wilkins, 1998, pp 103–108.

40. What is the significance of an orange-brown discoloration of amniotic fluid with similar staining of the white portions of delivered or aborted foals?

The amniotic fluid has been discolored by the excretion of meconium in utero. Meconium is a sterile concretion of intestinal cells and debris that forms during gestation in the foal's distal intestinal tract. Its presence in amniotic fluid usually is associated with some type of in utero stress to the foal. Its clinical significance relates to the stress experienced by the foal as well as the likelihood that the foal may have aspirated some of the meconium. Aspiration may result in obstruction or plugging of the smaller airways and act as a nidus for sterile inflammation as well as bacterial infection. Prophylactic antimicrobial and oxygen therapy should be considered.

41. A large bloody structure with a roughened surface is hanging from the vulva of a mare 4 hours after foaling. What are the appropriate differential diagnoses?

The differential diagnostic list includes (1) placenta (chorionic surface); (2) prolapsed uterus; (3) urinary bladder; (4) small intestine or small colon; (5) vaginal prolapse with bruising and hemorrhage within its wall; and (6) rectal prolapse.

42. What is the cervical star?

The cervical star is the area of the chorioallantois that is typically star-shaped. It is present on every placenta and corresponds to the area that has an absence or diminished number of chorionic villi and juxtaposes the internal cervical os uterus. The chorioallantois normally ruptures at this site during parturition.

43. What methods are used to induce foaling in mares?

The protocols for induction of parturition vary in mode of action and time of onset to delivery of the foal. The three main agents are oxytocin, prostaglandin F_2-alpha, and dexamethasone.

44. How do the agents used to induce parturition have their effect?

Understanding the action of these drugs requires an explanation of the hormonal events during late gestation. Cortisol gradually rises in late gestation, which tends to be a sign of fetal maturity. This rise causes a decrease in progesterone and an increase in maternal estradiol-17ß. Cortisol acts on the fetal gonads, which produce pregnenolone. The pregnenolone changes to the androgen dehydroepiandrosterone (DHEA), which circulates back to the placenta and aromatizes to estrogen. Estrogen has a positive inotropic effect on the myometrium. The estrogen also stimulates prostaglandin production, causes myometrial gap junction formation, and decreases the threshold of sensitivity of oxytocin receptor sites in the myometrium. Oxytocin is secreted normally in a pulsatile fashion secondary to a neuroendocrine reflex known as Ferguson's reflex. Stretching of the cervix and vagina stimulates this reflex to release maternal oxytocin. Oxytocin activity depends on extracellular calcium. Oxytocin binds to sites in the sarcolemmal membrane of myometrial cells and causes an influx of calcium, which in turn inhibits the sarcolemmal calcium extrusion pump and produces myometrial contractions.

Prostaglandin metabolism increases during the last two weeks of gestation and peaks before delivery. The fetoplacental unit is the primary site of prostaglandin synthesis, and the rise in prostaglandin concentration relates to fetal maturity. Prostaglandin also has a direct inotropic effect on myometrial contractions. It increases intracellular calcium mobilization from sarcolemmal stores just like oxytocin. Some sources say that prostaglandins mediate oxytocin release, and others say that oxytocin mediates release of prostaglandins. No matter which is released first, they work hand in hand and are important in the mediation of parturition.

45. How does one select the best agent to use for induction of foaling?

Considering the number of induction protocols described for mares, the choice depends on practitioner experience. It is imperative to determine fetal readiness for birth to the fullest extent possible in every circumstance of elective induction of foaling. Caution should favor a conservative judgment and give the benefit of doubt to the mare. Unless there are definite indications that the fetus is suffering in utero stress that may be life-threatening or that the mare has a life-threatening disorder, it is best to let the mare and foal decide the time of delivery. No induction method can be guaranteed to be safe and effective in every mare and every circumstance. More foaling complications tend to be seen as the number of inductions increases.

46. Which agent is most commonly used for induction of parturition in mares?

Oxytocin is generally considered the drug of choice for inducing parturition in mares. It is associated with a rapid effect; foaling usually occurs within 15–90 minutes of administration. Various dosages and routes of administration have been used to induce parturition. An intramuscular dose of 20 IU results in slower progression toward delivery, whereas a dose of 100 IU initiates a rapid delivery response. Oxytocin also may be given intravenously either as a small bolus dose of 2.5–10 IU every 15–20 minutes or as 60–120 IU in 1 L of saline administered by gravity infusion (1 IU/min) to effect initiation of stage 2 of labor. Pluriparous mares tend to progress to stage 2 of labor more rapidly than primiparous mares. One disadvantage of oxytocin is that it may override the physiologic events responsible for normal parturition without considering fetal maturity. High doses of oxytocin may increase the incidence of perineal tears, cause uterine rupture, elicit a fetal cerebrovascular accident, or cause premature placental separation.

47. How does one select which dose of oxytocin to use when so many options exist?

A recent trial compared methods of oxytocin induction in 16 mares using 3 treatment groups: (1) one intramuscular dose of 75 IU; (2) intramuscular doses of 15 IU at 15-minute intervals for a maximal dose of 75 IU; and (3) 75 IU in 1 L saline given intravenously at the rate of 1 IU/minute. The overall incidence of premature placental separation (PPS) in the 16 mares was 38%; the incidence of dystocia (D) was 25%. Time from administration of oxytocin to rupture of the chorioallantois (initiation of stage 2 labor) was shortest for the IV drip group and longest for the group receiving 15 IU at 15-minute intervals. One factor that affected neonatal outcome was whether the mare's cervix was dilated before initiation of the induction protocol. All mares that had intrapartum diffi-culties (PPS, D) had a nondilated cervix. Mares with a dilated cervix before induction did not deliver abnormal foals. The method of oxytocin-induced parturition did not affect neonatal outcome. The interval from induction until parturition, degree of cervical dilatation, and intrapartum complications influenced the success of the induction process. Although oxytocin is reliable and effective, if fetal membranes or feet are not readily observed externally within 30 minutes of initiation of stage 2 of labor, a manual vaginal examination must be performed to investigate fetal posture and presentation.

Macpherson ML, Chaffin MK, Carroll GL, et al: Three methods of oxytocin-induced parturition and their effects on foals. J Am Vet Med Assoc 210:799–803, 1997.

48. What criteria should be used in deciding to induce parturition in mares?

Timing for selection of candidates for induction of foaling can be determined by using several criteria that minimize complications. For example, one should wait at least until day 330 of gesta-tion; an accurate breeding date must therefore be known. The birth of weak, nonviable foals is more common if the mare is induced before day 330. Other significant signs are udder development and engorgement with milk, relaxation of the sacrosciatic ligaments, cervical softening or dilation, and electrolyte changes in the milk. A good indicator of in utero fetal maturity is prefoaling mammary secretion of calcium carbonate ($CaCO_3$) levels $\geq$ 200 ppm. Prefoaling mammary secretion of $CaCO_3$ can be measured with one of several commercially available tests (FoalWatch, CHEMetrics Inc., Calverton, VA; Predict-A-Foal, Animal Health Care Products, Vernon, CA). Fetal maturity can be assessed by using these parameters, which increase the likelihood of a positive outcome.

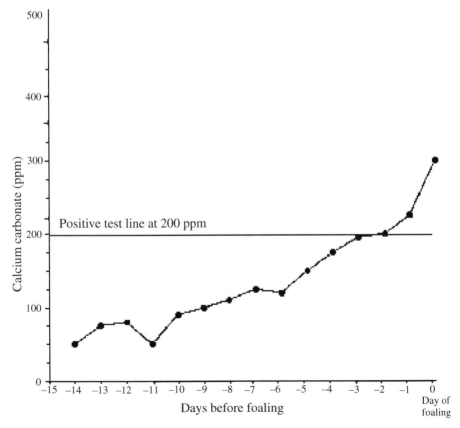

One mare's prepartum mammary secretion of $CaCO_3$ (ppm) as measured by the FoalWatch test from 14 days before foaling (–14) to the day of foaling (0).

Predictive Value of a Positive Test (PVPT)* for the Measurement of Prefoaling Mammary Secretion of Calcium Carbonate

PVPT	FOALING WITHIN FOLLOWING PERIOD
51%	24 hours
84%	48 hours
98%	72 hours

* The first occasion on which prefoaling mammary secretion of calcium carbonate exceeds 200 ppm (FoalWatch test).
From Ley WB, Bowen JM, Purswell BJ, et al: The sensitivity, specificity and predictive value of measuring carbon carbonate in mares' prepartum mammary secretions. Theriogenology 40:189–198, 1993.

Predictive Value of a Negative Test (PVNT)* for the Measurement of Prefoaling Mammary Secretion of Calcium Carbonate

PVNT	NOT FOALING WITHIN FOLLOWING PERIOD
99%	24 hours
92%	48 hours
82%	72 hours

* The prefoaling mammary secretion of calcium carbonate remains less than 200 ppm (FoalWatch test).
From Ley WB, Bowen JM, Purswell BJ, et al: The sensitivity, specificity and predictive value of measuring calcium carbonate in mares' prepartum mammary secretions. Theriogenology 40:189–198, 1993.

49. What significance does the aromatase P-450 enzyme play in the expression of behavioral changes in mares with granulosa thecal cell tumors of the ovary?

Aromatase P-450 (P-450arom) is a crucial regulatory enzyme that is necessary for conversion of androgens to estrogens. Immunoreactivity for P-450arom is confined to the granulosa layer of nonatretic follicles > 5 mm in diameter and to corpora lutea at all stages of the estrous cycle and during pregnancy. Aromatization of androgens occurs within the granulosa cells of the preovulatory follicle of the mare, and the corpus luteum of the mare has the capacity for estrogen production if adequate androgen substrate is available. Granulosa cells in ovarian tissue from mares with granulosa cell tumors show little staining for P-450arom, which suggests that the tumors have little aromatizing capacity. Since androgen substrates are not effectively aromatized to estrogens, more than 50% of mares with granulosa theca cell tumor of the ovary exhibit masculine behavior.

50. What is the preferred approach for ovariectomy of granulosa cell tumors in mares?

A diagonal paramedian approach for unilateral ovariectomy is preferred for the removal of the mare's granulosa cell tumor. Only minimal complications are detected postoperatively when the diagonal paramedian approach is used, regardless of the preferred technique for ovarian pedicle ligation or incisional closure and use of pre- and postoperative medications. The diagonal paramedian approach is advantageous for ovarian tumor removal because the ovary is immediately adjacent to the body wall at a portion of the incision site. Size of the ovary is not a limitation because muscle tissues at the edges of the incision are flexible and easily retractable. All of these factors improve exposure, decrease traction on the ovary, increase ability to observe the vasculature, and decrease postoperative morbidity. Laparoscopic removal also may be performed if the neoplastic ovary does not exceed 12–15 cm in size.

51. Which is more beneficial in the removal of intrauterine fluid accumulation in nonpregnant mares: systemic administration of oxytocin or intrauterine infusion of broad-spectrum antibiotics?

The effects on pregnancy rate of three different treatments to remove intrauterine fluid were assessed in 1,267 mares. The mares were allocated, in strict rotation, to four treatment groups: (1) untreated, (2) intrauterine infusion of broad-spectrum antibiotic in saline solution,

(3) intravenous injection of oxytocin, and (4) intravenous injection of oxytocin followed by intrauterine antibiotics as in treatment 2. In the estrous period that followed treatment, the mares were mated by natural service to a fertile stallion. The pregnancy status of the mares was determined 13–15 days and 27–30 days after ovulation by transrectal ultrasonography. The pregnancy rate of group 4 (72%) was higher than that of group 2 (64%, p < 0.01) or group 3 (63%, p < 0.01). The pregnancy rates of groups 2 and 3 were higher than that of group 1 (56%, p < 0.01). Treatment with intrauterine antibiotics and oxytocin (group 4) appeared to have an additive beneficial effect, which suggests two different modes of action of the combination treatment—namely antibacterial activity and fluid drainage. In untreated mares more fluid accumulated in the uterine lumen after mating; this accumulation was the most likely reason for the lower pregnancy rate.

Pycock JF, Newcombe JR: Assessment of the effect of three treatments to remove intrauterine fluid on pregnancy rate in the mare. Vet Rec 138: 320–323, 1996.

52. Are mares more susceptible to equine herpesvirus type 1 infection in early or late gestation?

In a recent study, 4 mares at 3 months and 1 mare at 5 months of gestation were inoculated intranasally with equine herpesvirus-1 (EHV-1: Ab4 isolate). All five mares became infected, but no cases of posterior paresis or abortion occurred. On postinfection days 8, 9, 11, 12 (3-month–pregnant mares), and 13 (5-month–pregnant mare), the pregnant uterus was examined in detail. Small numbers of vascular lesions with EHV-1 antigen expression in endothelial cells were present in the uteri of the 3-month–pregnant mares; thrombi were rare and foci of thromboischemic damage were not seen. Six other mares previously inoculated with the EHV-1 Ab4 isolate at 9 months of gestation had a significantly greater degree of vascular abnormality than the 4 mares infected at 3 months of gestation, but the degree of EHV-1 antigen expression and thrombosis in the uterus was similar to that in the single mare infected when 5 months pregnant.

Smith KC, Mumford JA, Lakhani K: A comparison of equid herpesvirus-1 (EHV-1) vascular lesions in the early versus late pregnant equine uterus. J Comp Pathol 114:231–247, 1996.

53. Can transabdominal ultrasound-guided amniocentesis be used for detection of EHV-1–induced fetal infection in utero?

Yes. Transabdominal ultrasound-guided amniocentesis may have a clinical role in the specific identification and isolation of mares carrying virus-infected fetuses during EHV-1 epizootics.

Smith KC, McGladdery AJ, Binns MM, Mumford, JA: Use of transabdominal ultrasound-guided amniocentesis for detection of equid herpesvirus 1-induced fetal infection in utero. Am J Vet Res 58:997–1002, 1997.

54. A nonpregnant mare has obvious vulval and cervical mucopurulent discharge. What is the appropriate therapeutic approach?

A good option is uterine lavage with sterile saline (2–5 L/day at 37–45° C), pending endometrial culture results for antimicrobial sensitivity pattern and selection of appropriate intrauterine or systemic antimicrobial therapy. The volume for infusion varies with the uterus; typically, however, 1–3 L are used for each lavage cycle. Lavage is repeated until the infusion comes out of the uterus as a clear solution.

55. A newborn filly at 12 hours of age appears to have a peculiar growth from the ventral commissure of her vulva. Your diagnosis is an enlarged clitoris. What should you recommend to provide a prognosis for the filly's future breeding ability?

Obtain a venous blood sample using aseptic technique in a sterile evacuated blood tube containing acid-citrated dextrose as an anticoagulant, and submit the sample for karyotype analysis. Karyotyping can be performed from peripheral blood lymphocytes isolated from a blood sample that has been sent to the laboratory by rapid courier. Lymphocytes are cultured for 3 days under conditions that stimulate them to divide, then harvested, stained, and photographed. The procedure generally takes 3–5 weeks to complete. Banding techniques may be applied to the sample to confirm the diagnosis of a detected abnormality. Three types of banding (CBG, GTG, or RBG) may be used to increase resolution, but the sample processing time is prolonged. A normal karyotype (64,XX) would rule out pseudohermaphroditism as the cause of clitoral enlargement.

56. Routine palpation of a 20-year-old mare reveals that the left ovary measures 100 × 150 × 125 mm. The entire ovarian surface is fluctuant. On the contralateral ovary, which measures 45 × 55 × 55 mm, you palpate one suspected follicle. The mare exhibited estrual behavior last week; it is now late summer. What should you recommend?

Recheck the mare next week to determine whether the size or consistency of the left ovary has changed. This finding may be simply a large corpus hemorrhagicum.

57. What is meant by endometrosis in mares?

Endometrosis describes the wide range of degenerative histomorphologic characteristics of the endometrium of older mares. The condition denotes degeneration, and the characteristic changes specifically lack signs of active inflammation. Infiltrates of lymphocytes, plasmacytes, and macrophages are the predominant cellular types observed in submucosal periglandular endometrial tissues of affected mares. The term is consistent with previous descriptions of chronic degenerative endometritis. Such mares have a history of (1) failure to conceive over successive seasons or estrous cycles, (2) chronic uterine infections based on uterine cultures, and perhaps (3) failure to maintain pregnancy beyond 60 days of gestation once they do conceive.

58. "Wind-sucking" is an unusual term. What does it mean in reference to broodmares?

Wind-sucking results from failure of the vulva and vulvovaginal constriction to seal properly the more proximal reproductive tract from aspiration of air during events that create increased negative pressure within the abdomen (e.g., normal or increased respiration).

59. What are the most common causes of bacterial endometritis in mares?

The predominant bacterial isolates from endometrial culture samples of the mare are *Escherichia coli*, B-hemolytic *Streptococcus* species, *Staphylococcus albus*, nonhemolytic *Streptococcus* species, *Staphylococcus aureus*, *Corynebacterium* species, other coliform bacteria, *Klebsiella pneumoniae*, *Taylorella equigenitalis*, and *Pseudomonas aeruginosa*.

60. What are the most common fungal isolates from the equine uterus?

Mares determined to have fungus-induced endometritis often—but not always—have a history of repeated intrauterine antimicrobial therapy. Organisms causing equine fungal endometritis include *Aspergillus fumigatus, Coccidioides immitis, Monosporium apiospermum, Candida albicans*, other *Candida* species, *Hansenulla polymorpha*, and *Mucor, Nocardia*, and *Trichosporum* species.

61. What choices are available for treatment of uterine infection with fungal species?

The choice of antimycotic agent to treat mares with fungal or yeast infections of the endometrium is not based on antimicrobial sensitivity testing. The cost-effectiveness and availability of the drug are considerations that must be addressed in every case. The more commonly chosen agents include nystatin, amphotericin B, povidone-iodine solution, clotrimazole, and griseofulvin. Uterine lavage should be a part of the treatment in every case, either alone or in combination with an antimycotic agent. Clinical success also depends on age of the mare, perineal conformation, and breeding management after the treatment period.

Antimycotic Agents Used for Equine Fungal Endometritis

DRUG	DOSAGE	ROUTE	COMMENTS
Nystatin	0.5–2.5 M units	IUI	Reconstitute in sterile water, volume 100–250 ml 4 times/day for 7 days
Clotrimazole	600 mg	IUI	Dissolve in 500 ml sterile saline; apply every other day for 7 treatments

Table continued on facing page

Antimycotic Agents Used for Equine Fungal Endometritis (Continued)

DRUG	DOSAGE	ROUTE	COMMENTS
Griseofulvin	2.5 gm	PO	Adjunct therapy given every 24 hr for 3 days during estrus
Amphotericin B	200 mg	IUI	Reconstitute in sterile water, volume 100–250 ml 4 times/day for 7–14 days
Amphotericin B	0.3 mg/kg	IV	Dissolved in 5% dextrose, every other day for 5 treatments
Povidone-iodine	0.5–2.0%	IUI	Dilution of stock solution on a volume-to-volume basis; 250–500 ml 4 times/day for 7–10 days

IUI = intrauterine infusion, PO = orally, IV = intravenously.

62. What are endometrial cysts?

A cyst is a normal or abnormal sac that contains a liquid or semisolid material and projects outward or away from the surface of surrounding tissue. Endometrial cysts are a frequent finding in older mares and are most commonly located at the base of the uterine horn. Cyst formation is thought to be due to one of several mechanisms: (1) constricting effect produced by periglandular fibrosis, (2) decreased myometrial tone and peristaltic activity associated with either prolonged anestrus or age-related changes, and (3) epithelial hypertrophy in response to periglandular fibrosis. The cysts may be of lymphatic or glandular tissue origin, single or multiple; when viewed by hysteroscopy, they are spheroidal or cylindrical structures that may be sessile or pedunculated.

63. Are all uterine cysts the same?

No. There are two distinct types: (1) endometrial or glandular and (2) lymphatic (see questions 9 and 10).

64. What is the significance of uterine cysts with respect to fertility?

The relationship between endometrial cysts and fertility in mares is not clear. Some authors state that cysts result in infertility, whereas others disagree. A negative correlation between number of endometrial cysts and foaling rate has been reported when the number of cysts exceeds five. However, mares have delivered live foals when both singular and diffuse endometrial cysts are present. It is not only the presence of cyst(s) that affects reproductive performance in the mare, but also their size, number, and distribution.

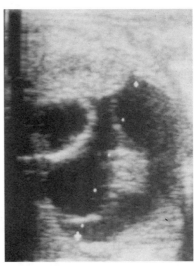

Ultrasonogram of a pregnant mare at 38 days after ovulation. The embryonic vesicle is located next to an endometrial cyst. (Cyst upper left; embryo lower right.)

65. What is the most common congenital anomaly of the mare's reproductive tract?

Persistent hymen is the most commonly observed congenital anomaly of the mare's reproductive tract. Maiden mares should be examined digitally in the area of the hymen for the presence of tissue remnants. The bands of tissue, if extensive, may contribute to rectovaginal perforation at foaling. Whether persistence is complete or incomplete or whether only remnants of tissue are encountered, it is relatively simple to open the hymen, and/or excise the tissue bands with scissors.

Since such findings are usually encountered during prebreeding or prepurchase examinations, the mare is prepared as for vaginoscopic examination. A blunt-end scissors is carried by sterile gloved hand into the vestibule, and the tissues are transected without direct visualization. Where a more directed excision is desired, a sterile spoon-billed Thoroughbred speculum is inserted partly into the vestibule to expose the tissues of interest. Long-handled thumb forceps are used to identify and stabilize tissues for excision, whereas long-handled scissors are used for transection under direct observation. The sterile 1-meter endoscope also may be used to visualize tissues.

66. Does estrous cycle activity aid the physical clearance of bacteria or other foreign materials by the uterus?

Yes. Relaxation of the cervix; increased fluid secretion from the endometrium, cervix, and vagina; and increased myometrial activity of the uterus during estrus contribute to the physical expulsion of uterine content to the exterior. Young, reproductively normal mares that were in estrus and challenged by intrauterine inoculation with live cultures of *Streptococcus zooepidemicus* were able to clear the uterus spontaneously of the challenge bacteria within 7 days. Similarly, the uterus of mares inoculated during anestrus were free of the challenge bacteria within 14 days. When uterine inoculation was performed during diestrus, the mares remained infected for up to 5 weeks. The diestrous period, during which progesterone is the main endocrine influence on the reproductive tract, is associated with suppression of physical clearance of uterine contents and polymorphonuclear leukocyte phagocytosis of intrauterine debris and infectious agents.

The physical clearance of uterine luminal contents appears to be a significant underlying problem associated with chronic or recurrent endometritis. One study documented significant delay in the clearance of nonantigenic markers from the uterine lumen of mares considered to be susceptible to chronic endometrial infection in comparison with mares considered to be resistant to chronic or recurrent infections. Although further work is necessary to document that a lack of effective physical clearance of the uterus in mares with chronic recurrent endometritis is a substantial problem, clinical evidence associated with the efficacy of uterine lavage with saline as a single treatment to promote clearance adds validity to this hypothesis.

67. In performing ultrasonography of the mare's uterus, what is the significance of apparent free fluid accumulations in the uterine lumen?

Positive correlation between the observation of intrauterine luminal fluid by ultrasonography, the recovery of inflammatory cells on endometrial cytology, and the isolation of pathogenic bacteria from endometrial culture has been demonstrated to be clinically useful. Ultrasonic characteristics of uterine fluid vary with the source of the fluid, the degree of accompanying inflammation, and the amount of debris. Purulent intraluminal fluid appears to be variably echogenic to nonechogenic, with a sprinkling of nonhomogeneous, hyperechoic dots (debris) that float within the field of view. Intrauterine saline appears for the most part to be nonechogenic, with homogeneous hyperechoic dots (air bubbles) swirling within the field of view. Intrauterine foreign bodies (e.g., retained fetal membrane remnants, tips of endometrial culture swabs) can be detected if their size and structure lend themselves to echogenicity. (See figure at top of facing page.)

68. What is the basis for systemic antimicrobial therapy in mares with endometritis?

The basis for systemic therapy is empirical. Practitioners have reported the use of dosages recommended for other systemic infections with the following drugs: procaine penicillin G,

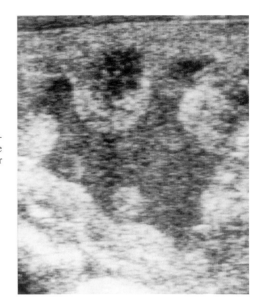

Ultrasonogram of a mare's uterus with a moderate amount of free fluid within the lumen. The fluid has variable echodensity and was later identified as urine.

gentamicin sulfate, amikacin sulfate, sodium ampicillin, and trimethoprim-sulfadiazine. Controlled clinical trials in mares for the treatment of endometritis with systemic antibiotics are few. The primary advantage of systemic treatment is avoidance of reproductive tract contamination by multiple intrauterine infusions. The disadvantages include increased drug costs, inconvenience of frequent administration, and variable acceptance by mares of the injectable or oral medications. Dosage recommendations are included in the tabled below:

Antimicrobials Used Systemically to Treat Endometritis in Mares

DRUG	DOSAGE	ROUTE	FREQUENCY
Amikacin sulfate*	14–18 mg/kg	IM or IV	Every 24 hours
Ampicillin sodium	10–15 mg/kg	IM or IV	3–4 times/day
Ampicillin trihydrate	11–22 mg/kg	IM	2–3 times/day
Gentamicin sulfate	6.6 mg/kg	IM or IV	Every 24 hours
Procaine penicillin G	20,000–50,000 IU/kg	IM	Twice daily
Trimethoprim-sulfadiazine	15 mg/kg	IV	Twice daily
Trimethoprim-sulfadiazine	15–30 mg/kg	PO	Twice daily

IM = intramuscularly, IV = intravenously, PO = orally.
• Use therapeutic drug monitoring to monitor dose and interval if possible.

69. What is the minimal treatment duration for a case of endometritis?

Minimal treatment duration is generally accepted to be 3 days; the average is 5 days; and in some cases an extension to 7–10 days may be desired. Once-daily intrauterine infusions are adequate. However, in cases of severe, acute endometritis that is necrotizing or potentially life-threatening, more frequent intervals of treatment (e.g., every 4–12 hours) may be preferred. Combined intrauterine and systemic therapy is feasible and provides prolonged antimicrobial levels in endometrial tissue when desired for certain types of bacterial infection (e.g., *Klebsiella* species, *Pseudomonas* species, *Taylorella equigenitalis*).

70. Have disinfectant or antiseptic agents been used as treatments for equine endometritis?

Disinfectant and antiseptic agents have been used for broad-spectrum or nonspecific treatment of endometritis but some also may cause tissue toxicity and endometrial damage and inhibit uterine polymorphonuclear leukocyte phagocytosis. Antiseptics tend to improve uterine tone after intrauterine administration because of their irritant nature. They tend to cause a reduction in uterine horn diameter and to stimulate uterine luminal fluid expulsion. Povidone-iodine solutions at 0.5–2% (v:v) dilution of commercial stock (1% active iodine) are commonly infused at 250–500 ml while the mare is in estrus and the cervix is relaxed. The mare should be carefully inspected by vaginoscopy before each treatment because some mares are overly sensitive to the iodine. Edema and hyperemia of vaginal mucous membranes are an indication that therapy should be discontinued. Excessive reactions may lead to adhesions in uterine (intraluminal), cervical, or vaginal areas. Chlorhexidine diacetate and Lugol's iodine (i.e., > 2% concentration) are notorious for inducing such reactions.

71. What are the advantages of uterine lavage in the treatment of endometritis in mares?

Uterine lavage is the preferred means of nonspecific intrauterine therapy for routine cases of endometritis, as well as for mares with acute postparturient metritis. Its advantages are mechanical clearance of uterine contents, dilution of uterine luminal toxins, reduction of uterine bacterial numbers, stimulation of endometrial blood flow, stimulation of polymorphonuclear leukocyte influx, and a resultant increase in uterine tone. Large-volume (3–5 L), warmed (45–50°C), or hypertonic (7.5%) saline may be used. Infuse 1.0–1.5 L at a time, using a large-bore (15–20 mm) sterile nasogastric tube or a 24–30 French, 80–cm Foley catheter. Allow the initially infused volume to return by gravity flow, collect return fluid for inspection, and repeat 2–3 times until return fluid is nearly the same quality (e.g., clarity, color, translucency) as the originally infused fluid. Flushing the uterus before administration of an intrauterine antimicrobial reduces bacterial population, removes potentially inactivating cellular debris, adjusts the intraluminal uterine pH (through control of the pH of the lavage fluid), and decreases uterine lumen volume because of the stimulated myometrial contractions induced by treatment. In a majority of cases, uterine lavage alone resolves active cases of endometritis.

72. What are the venereal diseases of mares and stallions?

Equine coital exanthema (equine herpesvirus-3 [EHV-3]), contagious equine metritis (*Taylorella equigenitalis*), equine viral arteritis (EVA), and genital infections with *Pseudomonas aeruginosa* and *Klebsiella pneumoniae* are the main causes of venereal disease in horses in North America. With the exception of EHV-3, the stallion generally remains asymptomatic while transmitting infections to mares during breeding.

73. Does *Brucella abortus* cause reproductive problems in horses?

Based on the study by MacMillan and Cockrem, it appears that *B. abortus* does **not** interfere with reproductive efficiency in horses. Five mares and 1 stallion were studied from 3–30 months after experimental infection with *B. abortus* strain 544. The mares bred, conceived, maintained their pregnancies, and foaled normally. No *B. abortus* organisms were recovered from any of the horses or from pregnant Friesian heifer contacts pastured in the same environment as the infected horses. Titers of serum antibody in the antiglobulin (Coombs' test) and complement fixation tests fell more slowly than titers assessed by other tests. The serum of one foal yielded maternal antibody to *B. abortus*. An intradermal test was positive only in infected adults and negative in all foals.

MacMillan AP, Cockrem DS: Observations on the long term effects of *Brucella abortus* infection in the horse, including effects during pregnancy and lactation. Equine Vet J 18:388–390, 1986.

74. What are the clinical indications for clitoral sinusectomy?

Bacteria that have the potential for venereal transmission are often located within the smegma found in the clitoral fossa and sinuses (e.g., *Taylorella equigenitalis, Klebsiella pneumoniae, Pseudomonas aeruginosa*). It may not be possible to eradicate these organisms from the mare with antimicrobial treatments, regardless of method of delivery. Therefore, it sometimes has been necessary to ablate surgically the dorsal glans clitoris, including the sinuses. This technique has been used as a method to control international spread of venereal pathogens in horses, especially the contagious equine metritis organism (CEMO; *Taylorella equigenitalis*).

75. What is equine viral arteritis (EVA)?

EVA is a contagious viral disease of horses that has assumed increased veterinary medical and economic significance since the 1984 epidemic in Thoroughbreds in Kentucky. The most important consequences of this infection are abortion in mares and establishment of the carrier state in stallions. EVA becomes localized in the reproductive tract of a relatively high percentage of infected stallions, which serve as highly efficient transmitters of the infection through direct or indirect venereal contact with susceptible mares. The long-term persistently infected stallion appears to play a major epidemiologic role in the dissemination and perpetuation of the virus in horse populations throughout the world.

76. What is the clinical significance of the carrier state in EVA infection of stallions?

The carrier state has been confirmed by virus isolation in Thoroughbred and non-Thoroughbred stallions naturally infected with EVA. Short-term or convalescent and long-term carriers have been found. The frequency rate of the long-term carrier state in Thoroughbreds was high, averaging 33.9% among the three groups of stallions studied. Although the convalescent carrier state lasted only a few weeks after clinical recovery, in some stallions the long-term carrier state persisted for years. Evidence indicates, however, that not all long-term carriers remain persistently infected for life. Carrier stallions appear to shed EVA constantly in semen but not in respiratory tract secretions or urine. All carrier stallions have continued to maintain moderate-to-high neutralizing antibody titers to EVA in serum. Virus shedding is associated with the sperm-rich and not the presperm fraction of semen. There is relatively little variation in virus concentration between sequential ejaculates from the same stallion. Transmission of EVA infection by long-term carrier stallions appears to occur solely by the venereal route. Such carriers are thought to play an important epidemiologic role in the dissemination and perpetuation of the virus.

77. What is contagious equine metritis (CEM)?

CEM is a highly contagious venereal infection of equidae caused by *Taylorella equigenitalis*, a bacterium with fastidious growth requirements. A disease of major international concern, CEM may be the cause of short-term infertility and, very rarely, abortion in mares. Unlike mares, stallions exposed to *T. equigenitalis* do not develop clinical signs of disease. CEM is transmitted by direct or indirect venereal contact. The carrier state occurs in mares and stallions, and carrier animals are frequently the source of infection for new outbreaks of the disease. There are streptomycin-sensitive and streptomycin-resistant biotypes of *T. equigenitalis*. Diagnosis is based primarily on culture of the bacterium from its predilection sites in the reproductive tract of mares and stallions. Treatment is available for elimination of the carrier state. Prevention and control of CEM are achievable through a comprehensive program of breeding farm management that includes early detection and treatment of carrier mares and stallions.

Timoney PJ: Contagious equine metritis. Comp Immunol Microbial Infect Dis 19:199–204, 1996.

78. What management procedures should be used in dealing with a potential venereal infection with *Klebsiella pneumoniae*?

Mares have been shown to carry pathogenic types of *K. pneumoniae* in the vestibule, urethra, or clitoris without necessarily infecting the cervix or uterus. Cultures should be obtained from the urethra and cervix of any mare believed to be at risk from an infected stallion, and these sites should be cultured again if the mare returns to estrus. Antimicrobial resistance has been encountered with *K. pneumoniae* capsule type 1 organisms, necessitating comprehensive sensitivity testing before treatment is initiated. Topical application of antimicrobial cream to clitoris and clitoral sinuses may be necessary in addition to intrauterine and systemic antimicrobial treatment. If an infected mare has been covered naturally by a stallion, swabs for culture should be taken from the stallion's sheath, penile shaft, glans penis, urethra, and urethral fossa. If the cultures are negative, the stallion should be sexually rested, and cultures should be repeated 7–14 days later.

79. Can coital exanthema present with lesions at sites other than the external genitalia of mares or stallions?

The virus causing equine coital exanthema (EHV-3) was isolated from a lesion on the nostril of a 2-month-old foal. One week after the foal's dam had returned from a breeding farm, vesicular lesions developed on her vulva. They were diagnosed clinically as coital exanthema, and 5 days later a lesion developed on the nostril of her foal. This case is an example of horse-to-horse transmission of the coital exanthema virus without coitus. A laboratory diagnosis is necessary to differentiate viruses that cause vesicular lesions about the oral and nasal cavities of horses.

80. Do certain isolates of *Pseudomonas aeruginosa* have a greater likelihood of venereal origin?

Atherton and Pitt categorized *P. aeruginosa* isolates from equine clinical material according to serotype and phage type. Epidemiologic evidence showed that serotypes 02a, 03, 04, 06, 09, and 010 were the cause of genital and nongenital infections; somatic type 03 accounted for 50% of isolates. The laboratory tests used in the study were of **no value** in predicting whether a particular isolate was likely to be a venereal pathogen, but all serotypes encountered had the potential to be pathogenic, given a favorable environment in which to multiply.

Atherton JG, Pitt TL: Types of *Pseudomonas aeruginosa* isolated from horses. Equine Vet J 14:329–332, 1982.

81. What is the predominant type of *K. pneumoniae* associated with venereal disease in horses?

A survey of *K. pneumoniae* isolates was performed on cervical swabs, feces, and nasal swabs of mares and samples from the genital tract of stallions. Type K1 was the predominant type (79 of 88 [89.8%]) in cases of endometritis due to *K. pneumoniae* in mares of racing breeds. The same type was isolated from semen and swabs of the fossa glandis of 6 of 20 (30.0%) stallions of racing breeds. Heavily encapsulated and less heavily encapsulated K1 strains were isolated from the stallions. Mares bred to stallions carrying heavily encapsulated strains developed endometritis, whereas mares bred to stallions carrying less heavily encapsulated strains did not.

Type K39 was isolated from cervical swabs solely from endometritis-infected mares of draft breeds and not from any mares of the racing breeds examined. Untypable strains were isolated from cervical swabs in 7 of 88 (8.0%) cases of endometritis in mares of racing breeds and from semen in 7 of 19 (36.8%) stallions of racing breeds. They were predominant in feces (19 of 21 [90.5%]) and nasal swabs (3 of 4 [75.0%]) of healthy mares of racing breeds.

Kikuchi N, Iguchi I, Hiramune T: Capsule types of *Klebsiella pneumoniae* isolated from the genital tract of mares with metritis, extra-genital sites of healthy mares and the genital tract of stallions. Vet Microbiol 15:219–228, 1987.

82. What are the expected reproductive performance indices for Thoroughbred mares?

Bruck et al. analyzed the records of 1630 mare years from six Thoroughbred stud farms. Overall pregnancy and foaling rates were 83.9% and 69.3%, respectively. The pregnancy rate per served estrous cycle and foaling rate per served estrous cycle were 54.7% and 43.1%, respectively. Pregnancy and foaling rates were higher (p < 0.001) for mares 3–10 years of age than for older mares. There was no difference in the pregnancy rates of maiden, barren, and foaling mares. The foaling rate was significantly higher (p < 0.001) in mares that became pregnant during the first served estrous cycle (77.8%) than in mares that needed two served estrous cycles to become pregnant (65.4%). Of all diagnosed pregnancies, 19.5% failed to continue to full term of gestation. Pregnancy losses were lower (p < 0.05) in maiden (12.4%) than in barren (19.7%) or foaling (20.9%) mares. Twins were diagnosed in 7.8% of all pregnancies. If one conceptus was lost without iatrogenic influence, 84.1% of pregnancies continued to term. If one conceptus was manually crushed, 55.9% of pregnancies were maintained. If prostaglandin was used to terminate twin pregnancies, 60% of mares so treated produced foals the following year.

Bruck I, Anderson GA, Hyland JH: Reproductive performance of thoroughbred mares on six commercial stud farms. Aust Vet J 70:299–303, 1993.

83. What is the success of interbreeding within the equine genus?

Horses possess the unusual ability to interbreed freely among the phenotypically and karyo-typically diverse species of the genus to produce viable, but usually infertile, offspring. The mule (female horse with male donkey) was the first successful attempt at genetic engineering, and its clear expression of both parental phenotypes has contributed much to our understanding of genetic inheritance over the centuries. Even more surprising, mares and donkeys have carried to term a range of true xenogeneic extraspecies pregnancies created by embryo transfer, including Prezwalski's horse (*Equus prezwalskii*; 2n = 66)-in-horse (*E. caballus*; 2n = 64) and Grant's zebra (*E. burchelli*; 2n = 44)-in-horse pregnancies. Transfer of intact and bisected demimule embryos (*E. mulus*; 2n = 63) to Jenny donkeys (*E. asinus*; 2n = 62) showed convincingly that maternal uterine environment, probably mediated by intrauterine growth factor production, can exert an over-riding influence on chorionic girdle development and its invasion of the maternal endometrium. Transfer of donkey embryos (2n = 62) to horse mares (2n = 64) results in the development of an exceptionally small chorionic girdle that completely fails to invade the endometrium to form en-dometrial cups. Around 70% of such donkey-in-horse pregnancies are aborted between days 80 and 85 of gestation in conjunction with delayed and abnormal placental attachment combined with a vigorous maternal cell-mediated reaction against the xenogeneic donkey trophoblast. This model of pregnancy loss shows strong evidence of immune memory, and the rate of fetal death is reduced by immunization of the surrogate mare against donkey lymphocytes. The findings suggest an impor-tant role for the invasive trophoblast cells of the equine placenta in initiating and driving attachment and interdigitation of the noninvasive placenta for fetal sustenance and in modulating maternofetal immunologic interaction to enable survival of the genetically foreign fetus in the uterus.

Allen WR, Short RV: Interspecific and extraspecific pregnancies in equids: Anything goes. J Hered 88:384–392, 1997.

84. Can equine embryos be successfully produced by in vitro methodology?

The success of producing equine embryos in vitro is still extremely low. More than likely the conditions for in vitro oocyte maturation are not optimized. Equine oocytes obtained either by transvaginal ultrasound-guided follicular aspiration or from slaughterhouse ovaries can be ma-tured in vitro. Production of live foals from intracytoplasmic sperm injection of in vivo-matured equine oocytes has been successfully performed.

85. How is equine embryo viability assessed when assisted reproductive techniques are used?

An objective method of assessing viability of equine embryos before and/or after oocyte or embryo manipulation is desirable. However, techniques that involve the manipulation of oocytes and/or embryos may be detrimental to embryo viability and subsequent development. Morpho-logic evaluation is currently the most widely used method of determining the viability of equine embryos. Although morphologic assessment of embryo quality is not always predictive of the survival of individual embryos, it is useful for predicting the survival of groups of embryos.

Other tests that have been used to evaluate equine embryo viability include (1) development during culture in vitro; (2) quantitating metabolism of the fluorescent substrate fluorescein diac-etate; (3) quantitating uptake of the fluorescent stain diamidino-phenylindole (DAPI); and (4) quantitating embryo metabolism. Although these tests offer potential advantages over morpho-logic assessment alone, their current limitations prevent routine use for embryo evaluation. As improvements are made in these methods, they may be useful alone or in combination.

86. How important is exercise to the breeding management of stallions?

To avoid behavioral problems a routine exercise program on a daily basis should be part of every stallion's basic husbandry management.

87. What method of breeding management in horses is associated with the best overall foaling rate?

In general, pasture breeding has been associated with the best overall foaling rate in horses on a seasonal basis.

88. What are the advantages of an artificial insemination (AI) program?

1. AI is an effective means to control venereally transmitted diseases.

2. AI is a more efficient use of stallion resources because more mares may be inseminated from a single ejaculate.

3. AI allows transportation of semen across states or to different countries.

4. AI reduces risk of injury and illness for the mare (and her foal, if the mare is nursing at the time of breeding).

5. AI reduces risk of breeding-related injury to both mare and stallion.

6. AI allows better monitoring of semen quality and output.

89. What is a "teaser" or "jump" mare?

A teaser or jump mare is used to excite a stallion before natural service or semen collection with an artificial vagina. The mare should be in natural standing heat (i.e., estrus) or induced to be in behavioral estrus by exogenous hormonal therapy. She also should be of an adequate size with respect to the stallion, sturdy, placid, and free of contagious disease. To keep the mare placid enough to be used as a jump mare throughout the year or breeding season, an ovariectomy should be performed. In some ovariectomized mares it may be necessary to administer estradiol benzoate at 50 mg/week by intramuscular injection to induce behavior consistent with a mare in natural estrus.

90. What is an appropriate insemination dose for mares bred by an artificial method?

Mares should be inseminated with a minimum of 100 million morphologically normal, progressively motile spermatozoa. The optimal insemination dose is 500 million morphologically normal, progressively motile spermatozoa. Most equine practitioners use insemination doses somewhere between these limits. Exceeding the optimum is not detrimental to fertility because most normal stallions naturally inseminate 2–10 times this number during live cover.

91. What fertility rate can be expected with the use of frozen semen?

Fertility rates of frozen stallion spermatozoa are not equal to those of fresh semen, but with careful management of both stallion and mare fertility rates of 40–60% can be achieved for a single mare reproductive cycle. Fertility rates of 60–75% during the course of a breeding season can be expected for a number of stallions. Because pregnancy rates have increased and because many breed registries now condone the use of frozen stallion semen, more people in the equine industry are using frozen semen. The practitioner should be aware of the large variation in semen quality between stallions. Postthaw fertility of the spermatozoa of some stallions can be improved by altering a standard cryopreservation protocol, but semen from other stallions does not produce acceptable postthaw fertility, regardless of the methods used.

92. Can semen be collected from a stallion that is physically unable or unwilling to mount a mare or a phantom?

Yes. Ataxic breeding stallions have been trained to ejaculate with manual stimulation or into an artificial vagina while standing on the ground. Ejaculates obtained in this manner can yield fertile semen with morphologic and motility characteristics within the range for normal stallions. This method of semen collection can extend the breeding life of a stallion unable to mount a live mare or phantom. Physically normal stallions also have been trained to this method of semen collection.

93. What is an appropriate volume of the insemination dose for mares?

Large insemination volumes (50 ml) containing a low concentration of motile spermatozoa (5×10^6 sperm/ml) result in decreased embryo recovery rates in mares, despite the fact that a 50-ml volume provides an estimated 250×10^6 progressively motile sperm, which is within the suggested range for optimal chance of conception. An appropriate range is 10–50 ml/mare; extended semen should contain more than 25×10^6 progressively motile sperm/ml. The concentration of progressively motile sperm/ml is more important than the volume as long as the volume does not exceed 50 ml/mare.

94. What techniques can be used to improve the longevity or viability of stallion semen?

Some stallion semen does not preserve well for use in extended, cooled (5°C) transportation programs. Attempts to improve longevity and viability have included (1) dilution by extending semen samples at a ratio of 1 part semen to 4 parts extender, (2) centrifugation to eliminate or reduce the amount of seminal plasma present, and (3) column separation to separate dead sperm from the viable, motile population.

Centrifugation involves extending semen samples to a concentration of 50×10^6 sperm/ml, centrifuging at 400–$500 \times g$ for 9–18 minutes, decanting the supernate, and resuspending the sperm pellet in fresh extender. Column separation involves layering the fresh or extended semen sample over a chromatography column containing glass wool, Sephadex, glass beads, or a combination of any two of the three. One method for column separation on the farm is to use a 50-ml syringe barrel that has a small layer of Nylon wool in the bottom, then a 2-cm layer of 105–150-μm glass beads. After collection and filtering, the semen is extended 1:1 with a nonfat, dried, skim milk semen extender, and 50 ml aliquots are allowed to pass by gravity through the syringe column. The separated semen is then used for insemination or cooled for shipping.

Samper JC: The Swedish National Stud: Breeding management and stallion semen evaluation in a large scale operation. Proceedings of the Annual Meeting of the Society for Theriogenology, Toronto, Ontario, Canada, August, 1990, pp 178–186.

95. What postbreeding treatments have the potential to improve conception rate in mares?

Nonspermicidal antimicrobials in aqueous solution may be infused 4–6 hours after each breeding. A 4–5-day postovulation window of opportunity allows clean-up of the endometrial environment before embryo descent. Treatments that increase uterine tone, promote uterine clearance of residual debris after breeding, and have no potential to be embryocidal or residual and irritating to the endometrium are desirable. Within the first 24 hours after breeding, successive uterine lavages with saline (until the return fluid is clear) are helpful in chronically infected mares. Fertility is not reduced if lavage is used within 2 hours after breeding and through day 3 after ovulation. Antimicrobials, plasma, or a combination of the two can then be infused immediately after each lavage procedure. Treatments can be repeated daily during the postovulation period for up to 3 days, or they can be applied on intervening days between each breeding. Oxytocin (20 IU) also has been administered systemically at 1, 6, and 12 hours after breeding in an attempt to aid uterine clearance of postcoital debris; clinical reports indicate substantial benefit to this palliative therapy.

Antimicrobials Used for Postbreeding Intrauterine Infusion in Mares

ANTIMICROBIAL	DOSAGE
Potassium penicillin G	3–5 million units
Ampicillin sodium	3 gm
Ticarcillin	6 gm
Amikacin sulfate	2 gm
Chloramphenicol sodium succinate	3 gm

96. What is the reproductive efficiency of feral horses under natural conditions?

The reproductive and foal survival rates of the free-ranging ponies on Assateague Island National Seashore were studied for 8 years (1975–1982). Most (52%) of the 86 foals were born in May, 13% were born in April, 22.6% in June, 10.4% in July, and less than 1% in August and September. The mean foaling rate was $57.1 \pm 3.9\%$, and the survival rate was $88.3 \pm 3.6\%$. Mares less than 3 years old did not foal; the foaling rate of 3-year-old mares was only 23%; of 4-year-old mares, 46%; of 5-year-old mares, 53%; and of 6-year-old mares, 69%. The relatively poor reproduction rate was believed to be a consequence of the stress of lactating while carrying a foal when forage quality on the island was low.

Keiper R, Houpt K: Reproduction in feral horses: An eight-year study. Am J Vet Res 45:991–995, 1984.

97. Does timing of frozen semen insemination affect the resulting pregnancy rate in mares?

The optimal time for insemination with frozen-thawed stallion semen is immediately before ovulation. A limited number of large-scale breeding trials have documented the success of frozen semen inseminations at wider time interval ranges.

Katila T, Celebi M, Koskinen, E: Effect of timing of frozen semen insemination on pregnancy rate in mares. Acta Vet Scand 37:361–365, 1996.

98. What is a typical protocol for freezing and thawing of stallion semen?

A typical protocol for cryopreservation of stallion spermatozoa includes (1) centrifugation of the fresh seminal ejaculate at 400 g for 14–16 minutes; (2) extension at 23° C with skim milk, egg yolk, and glycerol to 400×10^6 spermatozoa/ml; (3) cooling to 5° C for 2.5 hours; (4) packaging in 0.5-ml straws at 5° C; (5) freezing in liquid nitrogen vapor at –160° C; and (6) thawing for 30 seconds in 37° C water.

99. In the breeding soundness examination of the stallion, what are the most reliable indicators of satisfactory reproductive performance?

Significant correlation has been demonstrated between mean values for fertility estimates in stallions and the following determinations from conventional semen analysis: (1) percentage of motile sperm (r = 0.92); (2) progressively motile sperm (r = 0.90); (3) progressive sperm per ejaculate (r = 0.74); and (4) percentage of morphologically normal sperm per ejaculate (r = 0.71).

100. What is the most common cause of infertility in stallions?

Breeding mismanagement that leads to overuse, especially in young stallions that are not yet sexually mature or older stallions that have entered the early stages of seminiferous tubule degeneration.

101. What is the normal color of a stallion's ejaculate?

The color of a normal ejaculate from the stallion ranges from watery gray to creamy white. The variation depends on spermatozoal concentration. Yellowish discoloration may be indicative of either urine contamination of the ejaculate or infection of the accessory sex glands. Red or pinkish discoloration may indicate contamination with blood.

102. What is an appropriate method for performing a spermatozoal morphologic examination in stallions?

One accepted approach is to take a small drop of thoroughly mixed, fresh, gel-free semen and place it on one end of a clean microscope slide. Then add a similar small drop of a well-mixed morphology stain next to, but not touching, the drop of semen. Morphology stains most commonly used are either eosin and analine-blue or eosin and nigrosin (Hancock's) stains. The two drops are then gently mixed with a clean, dry, wooden applicator stick. After 1 minute of staining time, the pool of stained semen is gently pulled across the slide by a second clean, dry microscope slide backed into the pool at a forward 45° angle. It is sometimes useful to vary the density of the smear by varying the rate of forward pulling by the second slide. The smear is then allowed to air-dry. The slide is examined at × 1,000 magnification using oil immersion. Eosin penetrates the membrane of nonviable sperm cells, causing a pinkish coloration to the postnuclear cap region of the sperm head. Viable sperm cells at the time of staining exclude the eosin dye, and the postnuclear cap region retains a white color. Use of such stain combinations allows the examiner to estimate the live-to-dead ratio of the sperm population and to assess sperm morphology. At least 200 sperm cells should be counted, using a standard reference chart to determine the percentage of normal spermatozoa within the population of cells. Only one sperm abnormality within each cell is counted; the most proximal abnormality is the one scored.

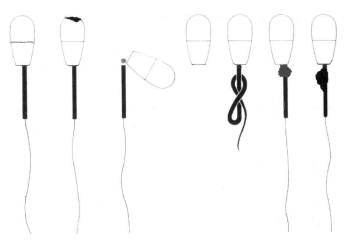

Stallion spermatozoa. From left, normal, knobbed, or folded acrosomal defect; detached head; tailless or separated head; coiled mid-piece; proximal cytoplasmic droplet; and mitochondrial midpiece defect. The normal attachment of the principal piece to the head in the stallion sperm is abaxial.

103. What is the best way to perform a sperm motility analysis in stallions?

Prerequisites include a freshly collected, warm (37° C) semen sample; an appropriate filtration of the semen to separate the gel from the gel-free portions of the ejaculate; a clean, prewarmed (37° C) microscope slide and coverslip; a good bright-field or phase-contrast microscope (preferred) that can provide either × 150 or × 200 magnification; and a draft-free area to prevent rapid cooling of the slide once it is prepared. The fresh gel-free semen should be gently mixed. A clean pipette is used to obtain a small sample to place on the prewarmed microscope slide. A clean coverslip is gently applied on top of the small drop of semen, and the slide is placed carefully on the microscope stage. The progressive motility of the raw sample should be assessed in at least 5 different fields.

It is important to make a judgment about the kind of movement that the sperm cells exhibit; not all sperm move in a progressively forward fashion. The overall number of sperm cells that move progressively forward is then estimated in each field of view. The result is a subjective estimate of progressive motility expressed as a percentage. The same technique is repeated with a sample of semen that has been diluted or extended. An appropriately prewarmed (37° C) extender should be added to the raw semen in a ratio that produces an approximate final concentration of 50×10^6 spermatozoa/ml. Most extenders are skim milk-based, with or without antimicrobials. Extended semen samples often have an improved progressive motility compared with raw (undiluted) semen samples of the same ejaculate.

104. What is the relationship between the breeding soundness examination of the stallion and fertility ?

Fertility depends on (1) libido, (2) mating ability, and (3) semen quality. The breeding soundness examination attempts to make an evaluation of all three factors and to determine the stallion's potential reproductive efficiency. However, it does not judge the stallion's fertility or sterility. The total number of progressively motile, morphologically normal sperm per ejaculate is still the best predictor of overall fertility.

105. Is there an official breeding soundness examination format to follow for stallions?

In 1992, the Society for Theriogenology and the American College of Theriogenologists modified the Stallion Breeding Soundness Examination form that was originally published in 1983. The format of the new form consists of 14 different sections: (1) stallion information, (2) owner/veterinary information, (3) history, (4) physical breeding condition, (5) external genital examination, (6) internal genital examination, (7) behavior and breeding ability, (8) other examination findings, (9) diagnostic tests, (10) semen evaluation, (11) sperm morphology, (12) longevity (viability) tests, (13) culture and sensitivity, and (14) classification.

The breeding soundness examination classifies as satisfactory a stallion that has more than 1 billion progressively motile, morphologically normal sperm in the second ejaculate collected 2 hours after the first on any given day of the year.

Society for Theriogenology, 2727 West Second Street, P.O. Box 2118, Hastings, NE 68902-2118. Office: (402) 463-0392; fax: (402) 463-5683; website: www.therio.org

American College of Theriogenologists, 2727 West Second Street, P.O. Box 2118, Hastings, NE 68902-2118. Office: (402) 463-0392; fax: (402) 463-5683; website: 128.192.20.19/ACT/ACT.HTML

106. What is the best way to determine that a stallion has ejaculated during collection with an artificial vagina?

Ejaculation can best be determined by palpating the contractions of the urethra at the base of the penis. In addition, stallions also exhibit a characteristic "flagging" of the tail during ejaculation. This sign is a less reliable indicator of ejaculation, because some stallions do not flag the tail consistently.

107. What is the significance of the Flehmen response in stallions?

The role of the Flehmen response in stallion behavior has been investigated under field and laboratory conditions. Results have indicated the following:

1. The Flehmen response is most frequently preceded by nasal rather than oral investigation of substances.

2. The stallions' rate of Flehmen response varies with the stage of the estrous cycle of the mare.

3. The rate of Flehmen response shows no variation with time of day.

4. The Flehmen response is most frequently followed by marking behavior rather than courtship behavior.

These results suggest that the Flehmen response is not an immediate component of sexual behavior (e.g., courtship) of the stallion but may be involved in the overall monitoring of the mare's estrous cycle. Therefore, the Flehmen response may contribute to the chemosensory priming of the stallion for reproduction.

108. Is gonadotropin-releasing hormone (GnRH) therapy beneficial for a stallion with low conception rate?

Although GnRH therapy is unlikely to be beneficial to most stallions suffering from fertility problems, it is not likely to be harmful. Poor fertility has been associated with hormonal imbalances in the stallion. The primary cause of this imbalance is unknown, but it may be related to abnormal secretion of gonadotropins (i.e., luteinizing hormone [LH] and follicle-stimulating hormone [FSH]). Secretion of GnRH from the hypothalamus causes the release of LH and FSH from the anterior pituitary; these gonadotropins help to maintain adequate steroid levels so that normal spermatogenesis can occur. Hypogonadotropic hypogonadism has not been documented in stallions; however, GnRH therapy has improved the fertility of a limited number of horses. Downregulation of the hypothalamic-pituitary-testicular (HPT) axis readily occurs in intact males of most other species treated with GnRH; however, the horse seems to be unusually resistant to the development of refractoriness. Complete endocrine and semen evaluations should be performed on all stallions that are considered candidates for GnRH therapy. Sequential evaluations also are necessary to monitor response to therapy.

109. What is known about inhibin activity in stallions?

The dynamic relationship of inhibin and FSH has been investigated during the annual reproductive cycle of the stallion. Plasma inhibin and FSH levels changed during the year. The inhibin profile reflected seasonal changes in testicular activity, with highest concentrations in late spring and lowest concentrations in the fall. Plasma concentrations of inhibin were positively correlated with FSH concentrations throughout the year. The testicles appear to be the source of bioactive and immunoreactive inhibin in stallions.

Roser JF, McCue PM, Hoye E: Inhibin activity in the mare and stallion. Domest Animal Endocrinol 11:87–100, 1994.

110. Does testicular size change with age or season of the year in stallions?

Yes. Seasonal and/or age-related differences in daily sperm production (DSP) and testis size were associated with significant elevations in serum concentrations of FSH, LH, and testosterone; testicular weights; numbers of elongated spermatids per Sertoli cell; and elevation of the Sertoli cell population. Testis and blood samples were obtained from 201 stallions aged 6 months to 20 years in either December–January (nonbreeding season) or June–July (breeding season) to study the effect of age and season on reproductive parameters. Seasonal differences in the Sertoli cell population of adult horses (4–20 years old) were characterized by a 36% larger number of Sertoli cells in the breeding season than in the nonbreeding season. Seasonal elevation in the Sertoli cell population was associated with an increase in testicular weight and daily sperm production per testis (DSP/testis). Concentrations of LH and testosterone in serum varied with season. Although FSH concentrations also tended to be higher in the breeding season, this trend was not statistically significant ($p > 0.05$). The number of Sertoli cells averaged over both seasons (like testicular weights) increased with age until 4–5 years of age but stabilized thereafter. This age-related difference was also associated with increased concentrations of FSH, LH, and testosterone and increased DSP/testis. The Sertoli cell population was capable of increasing in adult horses by fluctuating its size with season. The number of elongated spermatids per Sertoli cell over both seasons increased with age up to 4–5 years of age and stabilized thereafter.

Johnson L, Thompson DL Jr: Age-related and seasonal variation in the Sertoli cell population, daily sperm production and serum concentrations of follicle-stimulating hormone, luteinizing hormone and testosterone in stallions. Biol Reprod 29:777–789, 1983.

111. Can fescue grass mycotoxicity interfere with sperm production?

Despite the paucity of research in this area, at least one recent report indicates that fescue grass mycotoxicity may interfere with sperm production in stallions. To test the hypothesis that prolactin mediates the increase in seminal volume induced by sexual stimulation in stallions, semen was collected from 6 stallions every other day for 26 days. For each stallion, four treatments were randomly assigned to the first 4 of the 8 collection days and then repeated in reverse order on the last 4 collection days:

1. Control: semen was collected by normal procedures.

2. Sexual stimulation: stallions were presented to mares in a chute for 10 minutes before collection.

3. Bromocriptine (a dopamine agonist similar to the mycotoxin found in infected fescue grass) plus sexual stimulation: stallions were administered bromocriptine 10 minutes before 10 minutes of sexual stimulation prior to collection.

4. Sulpiride (dopamine antagonist): stallions were administered sulpiride 25 minutes before collection.

Prolactin concentrations in plasma were increased by sexual stimulation ($p < 0.01$) and by sulpiride ($p < 0.001$) administration and decreased ($p < 0.01$) when bromocriptine was administered before sexual stimulation. Sexual stimulation alone increased ($p < 0.01$) the volume of gel-free semen relative to control values (102 vs. 81 ml), and bromocriptine prevented this response (89 ml; $p < 0.075$ relative to sexual stimulation). Sulpiride had no effect ($p > 0.1$) on gel-free volume. Volume of gelatinous material, number of mounts, sperm concentration, motility, pH of gel-free semen, number of spermatozoa per ejaculate, and prolactin concentration in gel-free semen were not affected ($p > 0.1$) by treatment. The diminished seminal volume observed with bromocriptine treatment may indicate that stallions consuming mycotoxin(s) in fescue hay or grass are at similar risk.

Thomson CH, Thompson DL Jr, Kincaid LA, Nadal MR: Prolactin involvement with the increase in seminal volume after sexual stimulation in stallions. J Animal Sci 74:2468–2472, 1996.

112. What is the medical therapy of choice for paralysis of the equine penis (paraphimosis)?

Medical treatment is intended to contain and reverse acute problems and to obviate the need for surgery. Off-label usage of the anticholinergic drug, benztropine mesylate (Cogentin, 1 mg/ml, Merck, Sharp, & Dohme, Merck & Co., West Point, PA 19486), at a dose of 8 mg per horse by slow intravenous injection has been advocated in cases of priapism secondary to use of acepromazine or even ketamine in horses with high testosterone loading (i.e., stallions and testosterone-supplemented geldings). However, it has not always been successful. If the drug is going to work, a response usually occurs in 10–30 minutes. Control of related subcutaneous edema, both gravitational and inflammatory, is integral to a successful early resolution. Every reasonable and palliative effort must be directed at returning the penis to its normal in situ detumescent position. The passive retention of the penis in the prepuce precedes the ability to retract and retain the penis voluntarily. Judicial use of antiinflammatories and diuretics to alleviate swelling and promote urination is also indicated.

Schumacher J, Hardin DK: Surgical treatment of priapism in a stallion. Vet Surg 16:193–196, 1987.

Sharrock AG: Reversal of drug-induced priapism in a gelding by medication. Aust Vet J 58:39–40, 1982.

113. Describe the clinical findings in a stallion with evidence of seminiferous tubule degeneration.

An older (e.g., > 10 yr) stallion may be presented with a chief complaint of decreasing fertility over the past 1 or more years. The history may reveal that the stallion's cumulative conception rate (CCR) has fallen, whereas the number of services per conception (S/C) has increased. Examinations of semen quality reveal low or poor motility and poor morphology with decreasing overall sperm output. This type of historical information justifies an endocrine profile to support the clinical examination. Laboratory results may reflect that plasma LH is normal to high-normal; serum testosterone, low to normal; plasma estrogen, declining or decreased; plasma inhibin, below normal; and plasma FSH, abnormally high (3–10 times higher than expected).

114. How is a GnRH challenge test performed to evaluate stallion pituitary and testicular responsiveness?

Three small doses (5μ each) of GnRH should be given intravenously 1 hour apart. Plasma samples should be obtained every 30 minutes for a minimum of 1 hour before and 6 hours after the start of the GnRH challenge. Analyses should be performed for LH and testosterone. Compared with normal stallions, a decreased response in relation to the second and third dose of GnRH is observed in stallions with subfertility or infertility.

115. How is the human chorionic gonadotropin (hCG) challenge test different from the GnRH challenge test in stallions?

The hCG challenge test evaluates testicular responsiveness to exogenous hormonal stimulus. An injection of 10,000 IU hCG is administered intravenously. Plasma samples should be obtained every 30 minutes for a minimum of 1 hour before and 6 hours after the start of the hCG challenge. Analyses should be performed for estrogen and testosterone. Compared with normal stallions, a decreased response in testosterone and estrogen is observed in stallions with subfertility or infertility.

116. What ejaculatory disorders may be encountered in stallions?

The most common ejaculation disorders in stallions are emission and ejaculation failure and urine contamination of semen. Ejaculation is a sacrospinal reflex mediated by the pudendal nerve. In a large percentage of cases, however, ejaculation failure appears to result from either musculoskeletal or psychogenic disorder. Also encountered, although less frequently, are premature ejaculation, hemospermia, and azoospermia. Urethral obstructions are rare.

117. What is the breeding prognosis for a stallion with testicular torsion?

One case report describes a stallion that was twice referred for evaluation of scrotal swelling and signs of pain. The first admission followed a 3-year period of recurrent signs of left-sided scrotal pain and swelling. After the removal of the left testis because of testicular torsion, the stallion was returned to service. The conception rate was 82% for the next breeding season. Two years after initial surgery, the stallion again was evaluated because of acute signs of right-sided scrotal pain and swelling. Right-sided testicular torsion was detected and corrected, and the testis was sutured in place. The stallion's conception rate for the following breeding season was greater than 90%.

Threlfall WR, Carleton CL, Robertson J, et al: Recurrent torsion of the spermatic cord and scrotal testis in a stallion. J Am Vet Med Assoc 196:1641–1643, 1990.

118. What factors place the stallion at risk for developing postcastration scrotal infection?

Wound infections may be considerably reduced when castration is carried out under strictly aseptic conditions. One clinical review compared healing of the scrotal wound after castration with and without surgical closure. All castrations were performed in recumbent stallions under similar aseptic conditions and general anesthesia. The results indicated no significant difference in the prevalence of wound infections in scrotal wounds that were closed compared with those that were left completely open. Scrotal wound healing is more affected by the conditions (i.e., aseptic vs. not aspetic) under which surgery is performed than by the actual method of castration.

Homburg-van den Broek FT, Rutgers, LJ: A comparison of suturing and non-suturing of scrotal wounds following castration in stallions. Tijdschr Diergeneeskd 114:489–492, 1989 [in Dutch].

119. Can lymphoma involve the reproductive tract of stallions?

Yes. Aspermia was found in a 12-year-old Thoroughbred stallion that also had been diagnosed with generalized lymphoma. Invasion of the epididymis by neoplastic cells caused thickening and enlargement of both epididymides. The testes were not affected. Nodular ultrasonographic architecture of the epididymal areas was similar to that in previously reported cases of equine infectious epididymitis.

Held JP, McCracken MD, Toal R, Latimer F: Epididymal swelling attributable to generalized lymphosarcoma in a stallion. J Am Vet Med Assoc 201:1913–1915, 1992.

120. Can infection of the accessory sex glands be recognized by signs other than abnormal semen quality?

Yes. In one report a 5-year-old stallion was examined because of signs of abdominal pain consistent with colic. During the initial examination, signs of pain were elicited when the right seminal vesicle was palpated per rectum. Signs of pain were also elicited during sexual arousal and attempts at semen collection. The right seminal vesicle was subsequently determined to be abnormal by ultrasonographic and endoscopic examination. After the stallion was treated with trimethoprim/sulfamethoxazole for 6 weeks, the seminal vesiculitis resolved.

Freestone JF, Paccamonti DL, Eilts BE, et al: Seminal vesiculitis as a cause of signs of colic in a stallion. J Am Vet Med Assoc 203:556–557, 1993.

121. Has cryptorchidism in stallions been associated with chromosomal abnormality?

A bilaterally cryptorchid stallion with mild development of mammary glands was identified as an XX male by karyotyping. Necropsy revealed underdeveloped accessory sex glands and hypoplastic, inguinally located testes that were deficient of spermatogonia. Evaluation of routine hormonal profiles (without karyotyping) would have failed to diagnose this syndrome.

Constant SB, Larsen RE, Asbury AC, et al: XX male syndrome in a cryptorchid stallion. J Am Vet Med Assoc 205:83–85, 1994.

122. How can a cryptorchid testis be diagnosed with hormonal assays?

According to current recommendations, in horses less than 3 years old and in donkeys of any age a plasma/serum sample is taken for testosterone analysis, and then 6,000 IU of hCG are administered by intravenous injection. After 30–120 minutes, a second plasma/serum sample should be taken. Geldings have concentrations of testosterone < 40 pg/ml, whereas cryptorchids have concentrations > 100 pg/ml. The two groups may overlap, especially if the cryptorchid testis is intraabdominal. In such cases, the testosterone level rarely rises above twice the original (pre-hCG) sample.

In horses 3 years of age or older, estrone sulfate may be measured in a single blood sample. Geldings usually have concentrations less than 40 pg/ml, whereas cryptorchids usually have levels > 400 pg/ml.

Cox JE: Cryptorchid castration. In McKinnon AO, Voss JL (eds): Equine Reproduction. Philadelphia, Lea & Febiger, 1993, pp 915–920.

123. What methods help to differentiate the causes of an observed scrotal swelling in stallions?

Scrotal swelling in stallions may be attributed to disorders of either the testicle(s) or scrotum. Diagnostic tests useful in determining the cause of scrotal swelling include a thorough history, physical examination, careful palpation of the testicles and scrotum, rectal palpation of the inguinal rings, ultrasonographic evaluation, scrotal centesis, aspiration cytology, and perhaps biopsy.

124. Scrotal swelling in stallions may be caused by what conditions?

Trauma is a common cause of observed scrotal swelling in the stallion. A kick by the mare before, during, or after breeding or during teasing is the most common cause of traumatic orchitis. Other causes include ischemic insult to the testes (as may occur with testicular torsion and thrombosis of the testicular artery), inguinal hernia, varicocele, hydrocele, epididymitis, orchitis, and neoplasia of the testes and/or scrotum.

125. What neoplastic conditions have been observed to involve the reproductive tract of stallions?

Squamous cell carcinoma, papilloma, melanoma, and sarcoid may occur on the scrotum, although the penis and prepuce are much more common sites. Seminomas are the most common testicular tumors in stallions. They are usually benign but occasionally metastasize. Tumors of the pluripotential stem cells are uncommon. Such tumors contain elements of all three primary germ layers. Of the stem cell tumors, benign teratomas are most common. Teratomas usually occur in cryptorchid testes but occasionally are seen in scrotal testes. Teratocarcinoma and embryonic carcinoma are malignant stem cell neoplasms and occur rarely. Sertoli cell and Leydig cell tumors are also quite rare in stallions.

126. What infectious conditions involve the stallion's testis and epididymis?

Orchitis due to infectious or parasitic agents is relatively uncommon in stallions. The clinical presentation is similar to that of traumatic orchitis. Epididymitis may occur secondarily to orchitis. Primary epididymitis is rare in horses. Infectious orchitis is usually bilateral and most often also involves the epididymides. Infection may result from hematogenous spread or direct extension of a local wound. The most common bacterial etiologies are *Streptococcus equi* and *Streptococcus zooepidemicus*. Less common agents include *Pseudomonas mallei* (Glanders), *Salmonella abortusequi,* and *Klebsiella pneumoniae.* Viral etiologies include equine viral arteritis (EVA), equine infectious anemia (EIA), and equine influenza. Verminous orchitis may result from the migration of *Strongylus edentatus* larvae through the testicular parenchyma. Diagnosis of infectious or parasitic orchitis depends on history, physical examination, palpation of the testes and scrotum, ultrasonographic evaluation, and aspiration cytology. Semen collection and evaluation are useful if the stallion is willing to cooperate.

127. Are chlamydial infections of concern in the reproductive pathology of stallions?

Direct tests for Chlamydiae may need to be included in semen health and quality evaluation of stallion ejaculates as one of the major tasks of assisted reproduction in veterinary medicine. A recent study investigated the frequency of elementary and reticular chlamydial bodies by direct immunofluorescence tests in ejaculates collected from 52 men, 60 stallions, 42 bulls, and 66 boars. At the same time, qualitative semen tests, including ejaculate volume, sperm motility, percentage of live and dead spermatozoa and morphologic analyses, were done. Chlamydiae were demonstrated in 3.8%, 14.3%, *3.4%* ,and 9.1% of the human, bull, *stallion* and boar ejaculates, respectively. A relation between the presence of Chlamydiae and impaired functional and morphologic quality of ejaculates was found in human and bull ejaculates and in one of the two positive stallion ejaculates.

Veznik Z, Svecova D, Pospisil L, Diblikova I: Detection of chlamydiae in animal and human semen using direct immunofluorescence. Vet Med (Praha) 41:201–206, 1996 [in Czech].

BIBLIOGRAPHY

1. Allen WE, Noakes DE: Evaluation of uterine tube function in pony mares. Vet Rec 105:364–366, 1979.
2. Allen WR, Short RV: Interspecific and extraspecific pregnancies in equids: Anything goes. J Hered 88:384–392, 1997.
3. Atherton JG, Pitt TL: Types of *Pseudomonas aeruginosa* isolated from horses. Equine Vet J 14:329–332, 1982.
4. Blanchard TL, Varner DD, Schumacher J (eds): Manual of Equine Reproduction. St. Louis, Mosby, 1997.
5. Boening KJ, Leendertse IP: Review of 115 cases of colic in the pregnant mare. Equine Vet J 25:518–521, 1993.
6. Bruck I, Anderson GA, Hyland JH: Reproductive performance of thoroughbred mares on six commercial stud farms. Aust Vet J 70:299–303, 1993.
7. Constant SB, Larsen RE, Asbury AC, et al: XX male syndrome in a cryptorchid stallion. J Am Vet Med Assoc 205:83–85, 1994.
8. Cox JE: Cryptorchid castration. In McKinnon AO, Voss JL (eds): Equine Reproduction. Philadelphia, Lea & Febiger, 1993, pp 915–920.
9. Daunt DA, Steffey EP, Pascoe JR, et al: Actions of isoflurane and halothane in pregnant mares. J Am Vet Med Assoc 201:1367–1374, 1992.
10. Dybdal NO, Daels PF, Cuoto MA, et al: Investigation of the reliability of a single endometrial biopsy sample, with a note on the correlation between uterine cysts on biopsy grade. J Reprod Fertil Suppl 44:697, 1991.
11. Frazer GS, Perkins NR, Blanchard TL, et al: Prevalence of fetal maldispositions in equine referral hospital dystocias. Equine Vet J 29:111–116, 1997.
12. Freestone JF, Paccamonti DL, Eilts BE, et al: Seminal vesiculitis as a cause of signs of colic in a stallion. J Am Vet Med Assoc 203:556–557, 1993.
13. Ginther OJ: Prolonged luteal activity in mares—a semantic quagmire. Equine Vet J 22(3):152–156, 1990.
14. Held JP, McCracken MD, Toal R, Latimer F: Epididymal swelling attributable to generalized lymphosarcoma in a stallion. J Am Vet Med Assoc 201:1913–1915, 1992.
15. Hodge SL, Kreider JL, Potter GD, et al: Influence of photoperiod on the pregnant and postpartum mare. Am J Vet Res 43:1752–1755, 1982.
16. Homburg-van den Broek FT, Rutgers, LJ: A comparison of suturing and non-suturing of scrotal wounds following castration in stallions. Tijdschr Diergeneeskd 114:489–492, 1989 [in Dutch].
17. Hong CB, Donahue JM, Giles RC Jr, et al: Etiology and pathology of equine placentitis. J Vet Diagn Invest 5:56–63, 1993.
18. Honnas CM, Spensley MS, Laverty S, Blanchard PC: Hydramnios causing uterine rupture in a mare. J Am Vet Med Assoc 193:334–336,1988.
19. Johnson L, Thompson DL Jr: Age-related and seasonal variation in the Sertoli cell population, daily sperm production and serum concentrations of follicle-stimulating hormone, luteinizing hormone and testosterone in stallions. Biol Reprod 29:777–789, 1983.
20. Katila T, Celebi M, Koskine, E: Effect of timing of frozen semen insemination on pregnancy rate in mares. Acta Vet Scand 37:361–365, 1996.
21. Keiper R, Houpt K: Reproduction in feral horses: An eight-year study. Am J Vet Res 45:991–995, 1984.
22. Kikuchi N, Iguchi I, Hiramune T: Capsule types of *Klebsiella pneumoniae* isolated from the genital tract of mares with metritis, extra-genital sites of healthy mares and the genital tract of stallions. Vet Microbiol 15:219–228, 1987.
23. Ley WB, Bowen JM, Purswell BJ, et al: The sensitivity, specificity and predictive value of measuring carbon carbonate in mares' perpartum mammary secretions. Theriogenology 40:189–198, 1993.
24. MacMillan AP, Cockrem DS: Observations on the long term effects of *Brucella abortus* infection in the horse, including effects during pregnancy and lactation. Equine Vet J 18:388–390, 1986.
25. Macpherson ML, Chaffin MK, Carroll GL, et al: Three methods of oxytocin-induced parturition and their effects on foals. J Am Vet Med Assoc 210:799–803, 1997.
26. McKinnon AO, Voss JL (eds): Equine Reproduction, Philadelphia, Lea & Febiger, 1993.
27. Meyers PJ, Bowman T, Blodgett G, et al: Use of the GnRH analogue, deslorelin acetate, in a slow-release implant to accelerate ovulation in oestrous mares. Vet Rec 140:249–252, 1997.
28. Naden J, Squires EL, Nett TM: Effect of maternal treatment with altrenogest on age at puberty, hormone concentrations, pituitary response to exogenous GnRH, estrous cycle characteristics and fertility of fillies. J Reprod Fertil 88:185–195, 1990.

29. Pascoe RR: Observations on the effective length and angle of declination of the vulva and its relation to fertility in the mare. J Reprod Fertil Suppl 27:299–305, 1979.
30. Proceedings of the Annual Meeting of the Society for Theriogenology, Montreal, Quebec, Canada, September, 1997.
31. Proceedings of the Reproductive Pathology Symposium, American College of Theriogenologists and the Society for Theriogenology, Montreal, Quebec, Canada, September, 1997.
32. Proceedings of the Mare Reproduction Symposium, American College of Theriogenologists and the Society for Theriogenology, Kansas City, Missouri, August, 1996.
33. Pycock JF (ed): Self-Assessment Color Review of Equine Reproduction and Stud Medicine. Ames, IA, Iowa State University Press, 1997.
34. Pycock JF, Newcombe JR: Assessment of the effect of three treatments to remove intrauterine fluid on pregnancy rate in the mare. Vet Rec 138: 320–323, 1996.
35. Robinson, NE (ed): Current Therapy in Equine Medicine, 3rd ed., Philadelphia, W.B. Saunders, 1992.
36. Robinson, NE (ed): Current Therapy in Equine Medicine, 4th ed., Philadelphia, W.B. Saunders, 1997.
37. Roser JF, McCue PM, Hoye E: Inhibin activity in the mare and stallion. Domest Animal Endocrinol 11:87–100,1994.
38. Samper JC: The Swedish National Stud: Breeding management and stallion semen evaluation in a large scale operation. Proceedings of the Annual Meeting of the Society for Theriogenology, Toronto, Ontario, Canada, August, 1990, pp 178–186.
39. Schumacher J, Hardin DK: Surgical treatment of priapism in a stallion. Vet Surg 16:193–196, 1987.
40. Sharrock AG: Reversal of drug-induced priapism in a gelding by medication. Aust Vet J 58:39–40, 1982.
41. Smith KC, McGladdery AJ, Binns MM, Mumford, JA: Use of transabdominal ultrasound-guided amniocentesis for detection of equid herpesvirus 1-induced fetal infection in utero. Am J Vet Res 58:997–1002, 1997.
42. Smith KC, Mumford JA, Lakhani K: A comparison of equid herpesvirus-1 (EHV-1) vascular lesions in the early versus late pregnant equine uterus. J Comp Pathol 114:231–247, 1996.
43. Thomson CH, Thompson DL Jr, Kincaid LA, Nadal MR: Prolactin involvement with the increase in seminal volume after sexual stimulation in stallions. J Animal Sci 74:2468–2472, 1996.
44. Threlfall WR, Carleton CL, Robertson J, et al: Recurrent torsion of the spermatic cord and scrotal testis in a stallion. J Am Vet Med Assoc 196:1641–1643, 1990.
45. Varner DD, Schumacher J, Blanchard TL, Johnson L (eds): Diseases and Management of Breeding Stallions. Goleta, CA, American Veterinary Publications, 1991.
46. Veznik Z, Svecova D, Pospisil L, Diblikova I: Detection of chlamydiae in animal and human semen using direct immunofluorescence. Vet Med (Praha) 41:201–206, 1996 [in Czech].
47. Waelchi RO, Winder NC: Distribution of histological lesions in the equine endometrium. Vet Rec 124:274–276, 1989.
48. Youngquist RS (ed): Current Therapy in Large Animal Theriogenology. Philadelphia, W. B. Saunders, 1997.

17. ONCOLOGY

Catherine J. Savage, B.V.Sc., M.S., Ph.D., Dip. ACVIM

1. What is cancer cachexia? Does it occur in horses?

Cancer cachexia is a profound state of malnutrition and wasting despite adequate caloric intake. Evidence in other species, however, indicates that this syndrome occurs metabolically and biochemically before actual clinical manifestations of wasting are observed. Cancer cachexia occurs in horses and has the potential to decrease quality of life and possibly survival time in equine cancer patients.

Ogilvie GK: Paraneoplastic syndromes. Vet Clin North Am (Equine Pract) 14:439–450, 1998.

2. What basic mechanisms underlie cancer cachexia?

Cancer cachexia alters the metabolism of carbohydrate, lipids, and protein, essentially altering the net energy gain-to-loss ratio. The tumor experiences a net energy gain and the affected animal a net energy loss.

Glucose is the substrate preferred by tumor cells for energy production, but it is incompletely oxidized in tumor cells and yields little adenosine triphosphate (ATP). Consequently, more glucose must be utilized and metabolized to meet tumor cell demand, which prevents its use by the affected animal. The result is a shift in carbohydrate metabolism to energy requiring gluconeogenic pathways rather than the normal and efficient oxidative pathways.

Cancer cachexia is also associated with an increased degradation of the affected animal's protein store to supply the tumor cells with amino acids and to supply amino acids as substrates for hepatic gluconeogenesis, which is required because the tumor has altered carbohydrate metabolism. Because the patient affected with cancer cachexia cannot utilize the carbohydrate pathways efficiently, patient lipid stores are greatly depleted. This depletion may be the cause of most of the weight loss.

Ogilvie GK: Paraneoplastic syndromes. Vet Clin North Am (Equine Pract) 14:439–450, 1998.

3. What may cause hypercalcemia in horses?

1. Paraneoplastic hypercalcemia, sometimes termed pseudohyperparathyroidism, may be associated with cancer cachexia. It may occur in horses with lymphoma, gastric squamous cell carcinoma, other carcinomas, multiple myeloma, ameloblastoma, or parathyroid neoplasia.

2. Chronic renal failure
3. Laboratory error
4. Errors in correction of the total calcium concentration for albumin concentration
5. Consumption of vitamin D analog (the plants *Cestrum diurnum* and *Solanum malacoxylon*)
6. Iatrogenic hypervitaminosis D
7. Excessive or rapid intravenous administration of calcium solution
8. Hyperparathyroidism (uncommon)
9. Pancreatic disease, although usually hypocalcemia (uncommon)

Carlson GP: Clinical chemistry tests. In Smith BP (eds): Large Animal Internal Medicine. St. Louis, Mosby, 1990, pp 386–414.

4. Why does hypercalcemia occur in horses with paraneoplastic syndrome?

The mechanism in horses is not definitively known. A number of mechanisms may be involved, including parathyroid hormone-related peptide (PTH-rp) produced by an ectopic tumor, tumor-produced osteoclast-activating factor (OAF), and bone lysis (secondary to metastases, which are rare in horses).

Ogilvie GK: Paraneoplastic syndromes. Vet Clin North Am (Equine Pract) 14:439–450, 1998.

5. Which tumors in horses have been associated with an increased red blood cell mass?

Tumors associated with increased red blood cell mass (packed cell volume, PVC) include hepatic tumors (specifically hepatocellular carcinoma), lymphoma, and renal cell tumors. The glycoprotein hormone, erythropoietin, is produced by the equine kidney but also may be produced by some tumors. Excessive erythropoietin levels cause increased red blood cell mass.

Roby RAW, Beech J, Bloom JC, et al: Hepatocellular carcinoma associated with erythrocytosis and hypoglycemia in a yearling filly. J Am Vet Med Assoc 196:465–467, 1990.

6. What clinical signs in horses raise the suspicion of neoplasia?

The clinical signs of patients with cancer are usually nonspecific. However, if an older horse (especially > 15 years) is presented for weight loss, poor condition score, inappetance (perhaps inconsistently), intermittent fever, limb edema, chronic colic, chronic respiratory disease, chronic insidious diarrhea, or poor performance, neoplasia should be considered. Your suspicions should be made clear to the owners so that you can formulate a suitable plan.

7. What is the most commonly reported primary pulmonary tumor in horses? How may it present clinically?

The granular cell tumor (as opposed to the granulosa cell tumor of the reproductive tract of the mare) is the most commonly reported primary lung tumor, whereas lymphoma is the most commonly reported pulmonary tumor (including primary and metastatic neoplasia, which may be impossible to differentiate). The tumor is mesenchymal in origin, which makes it unique among pulmonary tumors.

Horses may have abnormal auscultatory findings (e.g., crackles and wheezes), coughing (common), tachypnea, dyspnea, weight loss, inappetance, fever, and exercise intolerance. They may appear to be clinically similar to horses with severe chronic obstructive pulmonary disease. Veterinarians have diagnosed neoplasia, with a suspicion of granular cell tumor, by performing an endoscopic examination of the trachea, corina, and secondary bronchi. In come cases, one or more masses occluding the airways have been evident. The mass lesions appear to arise in the parenchyma and protrude into the bronchi.

Misdorp W, Nauta-van Gelder HL: Granular cell myoblastoma in the horse: A report of four cases. Pathol Vet 5:385–394, 1968.

Nickels FA, Brown CM, Breeze RG: Equine granular cell tumour (myoblastoma). Mod Vet Pract 61:593–596, 1980.

Scarratt WK, Crisman MV, Sponenberg DP, et al: Pulmonary granular cell tumours in two horses. Equine Vet J 25:244–247, 1993.

8. What surfaces do mesothelial cells line? Does a mesothelioma affect only one of these mesothelial surfaces?

Mesothelial cells line the pleural, peritoneal, and pericardial cavities. Typically only one or two of the serosal surfaces are involved (e.g., peritoneum and pericardium, pleura and peritoneum). A mesothelioma usually demonstrates a benign pattern of growth and rarely undergoes metastasis by direct extension or via the hemic or lymphatic systems.

Colbourne CM, Bolton JR, Mills JN, et al: Mesothelioma in horses. Aust Vet J 69:275, 1992.

Wallace SS, Jayo MJ, Maddux JM, et al: Mesothelioma in a horse. Compend Contin Educ Pract Vet 9:210–216, 1987.

9. What are the clinical signs of a nasal passage or paranasal sinus tumor?

The clinical signs of a nasal passage or paranasal sinus tumor usually develop slowly and have a history of resistance to most forms of owner or veterinarian-initiated medical treatment. Horses may have a chronic, unilateral (occasionally bilateral) nasal discharge that is mucoid, mucopurulent, and/or sanguinous. The nasal discharge may be malodorous. Depending on the degree of occlusion of the nasal passage(s) by the mass(es) or deviation of the septum, dyspnea may be evident, especially on inspiration. Depending on the invasiveness of the tumor, facial bone distortion (usually asymmetric) may be evident. Blindness, exophthalmia, and dysphagia may occur rarely. Inappetance and weight loss may be noted in most cases eventually.

Boulton CH: Equine nasal cavity and paranasal sinus disease: A review of 85 cases. Equine Vet Sci 5:268, 1985.

Scarratt WK, Crisman MV: Neoplasia of the respiratory tract. Vet Clin North Am (Equine Pract) 14:451–474, 1998.

10. What is the most common tumor diagnosed in the equine paranasal sinuses?
Squamous cell carcinoma (SCC).

11. What diagnostic techniques should be used in the work-up of a horse with suspected neoplasia of the nasal cavity and/or paranasal sinuses? Why?

TECHNIQUE	REASON	ORDER OF PERFORMANCE
Physical examination	Assess overall condition score and weight of horse; presence of dyspnea; reduced airflow from left, right, or both nares; distortion of facial bones; character of nasal discharge; malodorous nasal discharge; and halitosis.	First
Percussion (while holding tongue in one hand for enhanced accoustics)	Ascertain whether abnormal percussion (e.g., dullness) is unilateral, bilateral, and overlying which sinuses or cavities.	Second
Endoscopic evaluation of nasal passages	Allow visualization and gross characterization of masses. Also reveals extent of masses to some degree (although radiology or CT is necessary to reveal entire extent). Allows examination of the septum until point where deformation prevents passage.	Third*
Oral examination	Useful because some tumors have capacity for aggressive local expansion and have been detected.	Fourth*
Radiographic evaluation	Determination of extent of neoplasm, tissue involvement, and destruction. Multiple views should be used to perform a complete examination, including oblique and dorsoventral views. Heavy sedation or general anesthesia is required.	Fifth*
Sinuscopy	Used to gain direct access to diseased region and to biopsy tissue.	Optional—very useful to obtain biopsy.
Computed tomography (CT)	Used to determine extent of neoplasm and tissue involvement accurately.	Optional (available only for horses at some large referral centers).
Biopsy and histopathologic evaluation	Mandatory for definitive diagnosis and important to give accurate prognosis and realistic treatment options. Histopathologic evaluation is mandatory, and culture and sensitivity techniques are desirable.	Sometimes performed with uterine biopsy forceps or other forceps using endoscopic visualization. Although biopsy instrument may be placed through biopsy instrument channel of the endoscope, this approach is not usually desirable, because biopsy sample is small and superficial.

* Depending on clinical signs, these tests may be performed in the order that the clinician believes most advisable.

12. What tumor types have the potential to metastasize to the thorax in horses?

1. Squamous cell carcinoma	7. Fibrosarcoma
2. Adenocarcinoma	8. Hepatoblastoma
3. Hemangiosarcoma	9. Chondrosarcoma
4. Renal carcinoma	10. Undifferentiated sarcoma
5. Rhabdomyosarcoma	11. Neuroendocrine tumor
6. Anaplastic malignant melanoma,	12. Undifferentiated carcinoma
dermal melanomatosis	13. Lymphoma

Scarratt WK, Crisman MV: Neoplasia of the respiratory tract. Vet Clin North Am (Equine Pract) 14:451–474, 1998.

13. Which tumors may occur in the liver of young horses?

1. Lymphoma may occur in horses of any age, including foals, and therefore poses a diagnostic challenge if only typical older horses are considered as candidates for neoplasia.

2. Hepatocellular carcinoma has been described in young horses.

Jeffcott LB: Primary liver-cell carcinoma in a young Thoroughbred horse. J Pathol 97:394–397, 1969.

Roby KA, Beech JC, Bloom JC: Hepatocellular carcinoma associated with erythrocytosis and hypoglycemia in a yearling filly. J Am Vet Med Assoc 196:465–467, 1990.

14. What is the best site to perform an ultrasonographic evaluation of a horse's spleen? What is the value of this procedure?

Transabdominal ultrasonography may be performed over the left 13th–17th intercostal spaces in a horse. This examination allows evaluation of changes that may be seen with splenic neoplasia (primary or metastatic): (1) splenic size (e.g., enlargement), (2) alterations in echogenicity, (3) homogeneity, and (4) identification of hypoechoic or hyperechoic mass(es). It is prudent also to evaluate the echogenicity of the left kidney for comparison. The left kidney should be less echogenic than the spleen.

15. What age group is typically affected by abdominal lipoma? What are the most common clinical signs?

Older horses (mean age: 16–17 years) are most typically affected with lipomas, which are benign tumors arising from mesenteric adipocytes. Because the tumors remain attached to the mesentery, typically by a stalk of variable length, they are termed pedunculated lipomas.

The most typical clinical signs are acute, severe abdominal pain, tachycardia, injected mucous membranes, and absence of borborygmi or hypomotility. In most cases, some part of the small intestine is strangulated by the stalk of the lipoma, causing physical obstruction with orad movement of small intestinal fluid into the stomach. This alkaline fluid can be retrieved by using a nasogastric tube (i.e., reflux), which is essential to avoid gastric rupture. On rectal palpation, loops of small intestine (often turgid) are usually felt. The circulation to the small intestine is severely compromised, leading to necrosis of the bowel and severe endotoxemic shock. As the bowel is compromised, abnormal peritoneal fluid (e.g., increases in protein concentration or increases in both protein concentration and nucleated cell number) is usually present.

In rare cases the lipoma may be large, causing abdominal compression and intermittent, chronic colic. Because the tumor is benign, no signs of paraneoplastic syndromes are seen.

Bilkslager AT, Bowman KF, Haven ML, et al: Pedunculated lipomas as a cause of intestinal obstruction in horses: 17 cases (1983–1990). J Am Vet Med Assoc 201:1249–1252, 1992.

Downes EE, Ragle CA, Hines MT: Pedunculated lipoma associated with recurrent colic in a horse. J Am Vet Med Assoc 204:1163–1164, 1994.

Edwards GB, Proudman CJ: An analysis of 75 cases of intestinal obstruction caused by pedunculated lipomas. Equine Vet J 26:18–21, 1994.

16. What is a pheochromocytoma? What clinical signs are associated with it? What diagnostic tests are available?

A pheochromocytoma is a tumor originating in the adrenal medulla chromaffin cells. This region is responsible for production of catecholamines (i.e., epinephrine and smaller quantities of norepinephrine and even dopamine). The tumor may be benign or malignant. Some tumors are nonfunctional (i.e., do not produce catecholamines), and some are functional, producing abnormal concentrations of catecholamines.

The clinical signs associated with pheochromocytoma are (1) tachycardia, (2) hypertension, (3) mydriasis, (4) colic, (5) inappropriate sweating, (6) muscle tremors, and (7) hemoabdomen and shock (due to tumor rupture).

The diagnostic tests for pheochromocytoma include:

1. Hyperglycemia and polycythemia (nonspecific).

2. Norepinephrine levels. One should use an ethylenediamine tetraacetic acid (EDTA) blood sample that has been separated (plasma) and chilled. Elevated levels support the existence of a pheochromocytoma. Because few equine samples are processed, it is wise also to send a control sample. The range for norepinephrine concentration in normal, resting horses (120–300 pg/ml) overlaps that of normal, excited horses (140–450 pg/ml). One should gauge the degree of excitement in the horse when the sample is taken.

3. Urinary norepinephrine, which has not been validated in horses.

4. Scintigraphic evaluation of the affected human adrenal medulla has been performed and may be used in horses with suspected pheochromocytoma.

5. Necropsy.

East LM, Savage CJ: Abdominal neoplasia (excluding urogenital tract). Vet Clin North Am (Equine Pract) 14:475–494, 1998.

Yovich JV, Ducharme NG: Ruptured pheochromocytoma in a mare with colic. J Am Vet Med Assoc 183:462–464, 1983.

Yovich JV, Horney FD, Hardee GE: Pheochromocytoma in the horse and measurement of norepinephrine levels in horses. Can Vet J 25:21–25, 1984.

17. What is the difference between lymphoma and leukemia?

Leukemias arise in the bone marrow, whereas lymphoma arises in the sarcomatous lymph tissues (i.e., lymph nodes, gut-associated lymphoid tissue [GALT], bronchus-associated lymphoid tissue [BALT], and spleen). However, some patients may pose a diagnostic challenge because lymphoma may have a leukemic phase characterized by spread from the lymphoid tissue to the blood and bone marrow.

Madewell BR, Carlson GP, MacLachlan NJ, et al: Lymphosarcoma with leukemia in a horse. Am J Vet Res 43:807–812, 1982.

Savage CJ: Lymphoproliferative and myeloproliferative disorders. Vet Clin North Am (Equine Pract) 14:563–578, 1998.

18. Why is lymphoma often termed lymphosarcoma in equine texts?

Lymphosarcoma frequently is used as a synonym for lymphoma; however, because there is no benign form of the disease, lymphoma is the correct term. The term **lymphosarcoma** was accepted parlance in the equine world because the tumors were solid and sarcomatous.

19. What are the classifications of equine lymphoma?

1. Generalized (multicentric)
2. Intestinal (alimentary)
3. Mediastinal (thoracic or thymic)
4. Cutaneous

20. What clinical signs are associated with plasma cell myeloma and multiple myeloma? How are they diagnosed?

Clinical signs suggestive of plasma cell myeloma are nonspecific. The most common are inappetance, weight loss, fever, and limb edema. Other clinical manifestations include epistaxis, pneumonia, lymphadenopathy, lameness, and ataxia. Patients with multiple myeloma may have bone pain manifested as lameness or even neurologic dysfunction, depending on location and extent of bony lesions.

Without supplemental clinicopathologic and radiographic data, immediate suspicion of plasma cell myeloma in a horse is almost impossible, although neoplasia (including plasma cell and multiple myeloma) should be on the differential diagnostic list of horses with chronic, insidious lameness. Findings on the biochemical profile, complete blood count (CBC), serum electrophoresis, and urinalysis that may assist in the diagnosis of plasma cell myeloma or even multiple myeloma include:

1. Hyperproteinemia (characterized by an hyperglobulinemia and an hypoalbuminemia)
2. Monoclonal gammopathy
3. Hypercalcemia (possible but not common)
4. Bence-Jones proteinuria
5. Anemia
6. Bicytopenia or pancytopenia (not common)
7. Systemic plasma cytosis or even circulating plasma cells (not common)
8. Bone marrow aspirate and/or biopsy (sometimes immunohistochemical staining can be used to identify plasma cell lines)
9. Radiologic evaluation of bone for cortical erosions, osteomalacia, and pathologic fractures
10. Diffuse, multifocal bone marrow involvement with actual bone destruction
11. Nuclear scintigraphy evaluation

Edwards DF, Parker JW, Wilkinson JE, et al: Plasma cell myeloma in the horse: A case report and literature review. J Vet Int Med 7:169–176, 1993.

21. What are the indications for a bone marrow aspirate?

1. Nonregenerative anemia
2. Bicytopenia (e.g., anemia and leukopenia, anemia and thrombocytopenia, or leukopenia and thrombocytopenia). Leukopenia refers to a decrease in total white cell count. It does not mean that all types of white cells have decreased numbers (e.g., the horse may be leukopenic but still have a normal number of neutrophils, eosinophils, basophils, and monocytes. The leukopenia may be characterized by a decreased number of lymphocytes (lymphopenia).
3. Pancytopenia
4. Identification of abnormal cells (e.g., immature forms in peripheral blood)
5. Hyperproteinemia or hypercalcemia suggestive of neoplasia
6. Bence-Jones proteinuria
7. Evaluation of iron store

22. At what anatomic locations can you collect a bone marrow aspirate in adult horses?

1. Sternum (routinely used)
2. Ribs (used by some clinicians)
3. Wing of ilium (used by some clinicians)
4. Proximal humerus (rarely used)
5. Proximal femur (rarely used)
6. Mandible (rarely used)
7. Vertebrae (rarely used)

23. Give one method of collecting a bone marrow aspirate in horses.

It is important to take a blood sample for concurrent evaluation. The easiest method of aspirating bone marrow in horses is to use the sternum:

1. Restrain the horse (e.g., stocks, twitch, and/or chemical sedation).
2. Clip the area of the sternum.
3. Prepare the site with betadine/chlorhexidine and alcohol (e.g., three preparations of each).
4. Select an area slightly off midline and slightly caudal to the point of the olecranon (i.e., aim to avoid the cardiac apex).
5. Infuse 1–3 ml of 2% lidocaine into the skin and subcutis, and infiltrate to the level of the periostium.
6. Prepare the site with betadine/chlorhexidine and alcohol again (e.g., three preparations of each).
7. Place sterile gloves on both hands.
8. Use a sterile, disposable spinal needle (3.5 inch, 18–20 gauge) with stylet. Some veterinarians elect to make a stab incision with a number 15 scalpel blade into the locally anesthetized area (i.e., lidocaine bleb). Insert the spinal needle either through the stab incision or directly

through the locally anesthetized area to the level of the bone. Use one hand to guide the spinal needle through the cortical bone, and use the other to guard the needle. This technique is imperative so that when the spinal needle passes through cortical bone and reaches soft cancellous bone, it is not pushed with such force that it passes through the cortical bone on the thoracic side and into the thorax and heart. Sometimes the needle stays embedded in firm osseous tissue—a marrow aspirate can still be obtained.

9. Once the spinal needle has been pushed into the cancellous bone space (i.e., resistance decreases substantially), attach the 20-ml syringe. A number of sterile syringes should be ready and precoated with EDTA so that the blood and marrow do not clot.

10. Aspirate on the syringe with considerable force to the 10–15-ml mark in an attempt to break the stromal tissue within the bone marrow so that a true representation of the cells (not just immature forms, which tend not to be firmly embedded in the stroma) can be obtained. Then allow the plunger to recoil. Bloody contents may fill the syringe; this should be avoided, if possible, by release of the syringe (i.e., release of negative pressure). In an adult horse the aim is to obtain a sample with yellowish tissue in the contents.

11. Make slides immediately for submission to the laboratory. If the laboratory is relatively close, however, you can submit the EDTA-coated syringes and slides can be made at the laboratory. Many slides should be made (regardless of who makes them), and some should be left unstained for special staining profiles if the clinical pathologists identify cells suspicious of neoplasia or other specific conditions.

12. The spinal needle can be retracted. The horse does not require suturing or antimicrobial treatment if the technique was performed aseptically.

24. From which site is it easiest to obtain a bone marrow biopsy in the standing horse restrained physically and/or chemically?

The wing of ilium.

Savage CJ, Jeffcott LB, Melsen F, Ostblom LC: Bone biopsy in the horse. I: Method using the wing of ilium. J Vet Med Assoc 38:776–783, 1991.

25. What is the most common renal tumor in horses? What are the common clinical signs?

Primary renal cell carcinoma is the most common renal tumor in horses. Clinical features seen in horses with renal cell carcinoma include weight loss, hematuria, and a palpable abdominal mass. If cystoscopy and examination of the ureteral openings are performed, hematuric fluid may be seen flowing from one or, in rare cases of bilateral involvement, both ureters. Because the right kidney cannot be palpated in normal horses, if a right-sided mass is identified, the suspicion of a mass (possibly originating from the right kidney) is confirmed.

Affected horses have an increased tendency for vascular invasion (e.g., renal vein and caudal vena cava); therefore, signs of hematuria, hemoperitoneum, and even hemothorax should be expected in advanced cases. If the owner wishes to proceed once renal cell carcinoma is suspected, the diagnostic work-up should include (1) ultrasonographic evaluation of both kidneys; (2) coagulation profile; (3) renal biopsy of the affected kidney and even the non-grossly affected kidney if the owner is interested in having a nephrectomy performed on the horse; (4) thoracic radiographs; and (5) abdominocentesis. Horses with unilateral renal cell carcinoma have survived at follow-up of 30 months after nephrectomy.

Brown PJ, Holt PE: Primary renal cell carcinoma in four horses. Equine Vet J 17:473–477, 1985.

26. Which is the most common urinary bladder tumor of horses? What is the prognosis for horses with bladder tumors?

Squamous cell carcinoma is the most common urinary bladder tumor of horses, whereas in most domestic animal species the transitional cell tumor is the most common. Squamous cell carcinomas may arise from metaplastic transformation of transitional cells of the epithelial surface into squamous epithelium or from small, isolated regions of squamous epithelium normally present in the equine bladder. Prognosis is poor because of local recurrence as well as metastasis

(1) by local spread to abdominal organs (e.g., carcinomatosis), (2) via the lymphatics (especially the internal iliac and sublumbar lymph nodes), or (3) hematogenous spread.

Traub-Dargatz JL: Urinary tract neoplasia. Vet Clin North Am (Equine Pract) 14:495–504, 1998.

27. How can ovarian tumors of the mare be classified? Give examples of tumors in each category and specify whether the tumor is benign or malignant.

Ovarian tumors may be classified according to the tissue of origin:
1. Epithelial tumors (rare). Example: cystadenoma (generally benign).
2. Germ cell tumors (rare). Examples: teratoma (benign) and dysgerminoma (potentially malignant).
3. Sex cord-stromal tumors. Example: granulosa cell tumor (most common ovarian neoplasm of mares; usually benign but may be malignant).

McCue PM: Neoplasia of the female reproductive tract. Vet Clin North Am (Equine Pract) 14:505–516, 1998.

28. Describe the typical signalment of a horse with an ovarian granulosa cell tumor.

Obviously all horses are female. All age groups reportedly have been affected (e.g., neonate, weanling foal, maiden mare, pregnant mare, foaling mare, barren mare). No breed predilection has been noted.

McCue PM: Neoplasia of the female reproductive tract. Vet Clin North Am (Equine Pract) 14:505–516, 1998.

29. How is a diagnosis of granulosa cell tumor typically made?

Diagnosis of a granulosa cell tumor in a mare is often made after alterations in behavior are observed. Techniques such as rectal palpation of the ovaries, ultrasonographic evaluation of the ovaries, and hormone analysis are commonly used. Rectal palpation usually reveals an enlarged ovary and a small, inactive contralateral ovary (although bilateral granulosa tumors and an active contralateral ovary have been reported). Ultrasonographic evaluation, using a 5-MHz, linear-array, rectal ultrasound transducer, is helpful. The most typical ultrasonographic appearance of a granulosa tumor is a "honeycombed" (multicystic) mass, although a solid ovarian mass or a single cystic lesion may be visualized in some cases. The contralateral ovary usually is small (because of feedback inhibition) and has little follicular activity; however, this finding varies.

Because granulosa cell tumors are sometimes hormonally active, hormonal profiling may be useful. Inhibin has been described as a marker hormone in mares. In one study, the inhibin concentration was elevated in over 85% of mares with granulosa cell tumors (normal: 0.1–0.7 ng/ml). Testosterone and estradiol concentrations also may be increased in some affected mares. Progesterone concentrations are invariably low; progesterone concentrations > 1.0 ng/ml are inconsistent with diagnosis of a granulosa cell tumor.

Biopsy or aspiration of the ovarian mass involves increased risk to the horse and is rarely warranted. A definitive diagnosis is made after histopathologic examination of the mass. Examination can be performed on biopsied material (rarely) or on the surgically removed mass. Sometimes a diagnosis is made incidentally at necropsy.

McCue PM: Neoplasia of the female reproductive tract. Vet Clin North Am (Equine Pract) 14:505–516, 1998.
Roser JF, McCue PM, Hoye E: Inhibin activity in the mare and stallion. Domest Animal Endocrinol 11:87, 1994.

30. Describe the most common neoplastic and nonneoplastic causes of hemoperitoneum in horses.

Neoplastic causes	Nonneoplastic causes
Pheochromocytoma	Trauma—splenic rupture
Renal cell carcinoma	Rupture of mesenteric arteries
Granulosa-thecal cell tumor	Abscessation (and vascular erosion)
Splenic hemangiosarcoma	Uterine artery rupture
Any neoplastic cause of vascular invasion and leakage	

Gatewood DM, Douglass JP, Cox JH, et al: Intra-abdominal hemorrhage associated with a granulosa-thecal cell neoplasm in a mare. J Am Vet Med Assoc 196:1827–1828, 1990.

31. How can you detect a uterine or cervical tumor in mares?

Techniques that may be of assistance in diagnosing a uterine or cervical tumor in mares include:

1. Rectal palpation
2. Ultrasonographic evaluation per rectum using a 5-MHz, linear-array transducer
3. Biopsy of the uterus using uterine biopsy forceps
4. Endoscopy of the uterus (hystoscopy) using a sterile, 1-meter endoscope. Biopsy of abnormal tissue may be performed either by using an endoscopic biopsy instrument, which takes only a small, usually superficial piece of tissue, or by carefully placing a uterine biopsy instrument in the uterus beside the endoscope so that a large specimen of the mass may be removed under direct endoscopic visualization.

32. What types of tumors affect the mare's uterus? Specify whether they are benign or malignant.

Tumors of the equine uterus are rare; however, both benign and malignant tumors have been diagnosed. Examples include:

1. Fibroma (benign)
2. Leiomyoma (benign)
3. Fibroleiomyoma (benign)
4. Leiomyosarcoma (malignant)
5. Lymphoma (malignant)
6. Rhabdomyosarcoma (malignant)
7. Adenocarcinoma (malignant)

33. Does cryptorchidism predispose stallions to any types of tumors?

Cryptorchidism is a predisposing factor for testicular seminomas in horses, dogs, and men. Teratomas may be found more commonly in cryptorchid testes than in descended (i.e., scrotal) testes in horses. Some evidence suggests that carcinoma in situ may occur in the cryptorchid testes of stallions.

Becht JL, Thacker HL, Page EH: Malignant seminoma in a stallion. J Am Vet Med Assoc 175:292–293, 1979.
Brinsko SP: Neoplasia of the male reproductive tract. Vet Clin North Am (Equine Pract) 14:517–534, 1998.
Smith BL, Morton LD, Watkins JP, et al: Malignant seminoma in a cryptorchid stallion. J Am Vet Med Assoc 195:775–776, 1989.

34. Why is the true incidence of testicular neoplasia difficult to determine?

It is difficult to determine the true incidence of testicular neoplasia because many horses are castrated at a young age before the advent of "tumor-age" (i.e., mature, older, and geriatric horses). Worldwide only a small percentage of cases are reported in the literature, and many of these reports come from equine referral centers.

Brinsko SP: Neoplasia of the male reproductive tract. Vet Clin North Am (Equine Pract) 14:517–534, 1998.

35. Which tumor may contain tissues such as bone, cartilage, teeth, hair, nervous tissue, and glandular tissue?

Testicular teratomas are more common in horses than in other domestic animal species. They are composed of many tissues foreign to testicular tissue because of their origin in pluripotent stem cells. They produce tissues from all embryonic germ layers, such as bone, cartilage, teeth, hair, nervous tissue, and epithelial glandular tissue. **Teratocarcinoma** (a highly malignant tumor) has been reported in male horses and may have tissues of both mature (as in teratomas) and juvenile germ cell tissue.

Brinsko SP: Neoplasia of the male reproductive tract. Vet Clin North Am (Equine Pract) 14:517–534, 1998.
Shaw DP, Roth JE: Testicular teratocarcinoma in a horse. Vet Pathol 23:3237–3238, 1986.

36. Summarize the clinical features of equine mandibular tumors.

1. All age groups may be affected.
2. Mandibular tumors are rare.
3. Eighty percent of reported osteosarcomas may occur in the head region.
4. Tumors vary in size but may be very large.
5. Swelling is well defined.

6. Tumors grow slowly.

7. Tumors protrude laterally, medially, or ventrally from the mandible.

8. Consistency may be hard or soft (hence tumors may be diagnostically challenging).

9. Sinus tracts are invariably absent in mandibular tumors, whereas they are common with periapical abscessation (which occurs more commonly than mandibular neoplasia).

10. If the symphysis is involved, osteogenic or odontogenic tumors should be placed higher on the differential diagnostic list.

11. Radiology is useful to differentiate neoplasm from abscessation.

12. Deep bone/mass biopsy is necessary to gain a diagnostic sample for histopathologic evaluation.

13. Tumors are difficult to excise fully; treatment may require radical resection of the mandible and/or radiotherapy.

Liversey MA, Wilkie IW: Focal and multifocal osteosarcoma in two foals. Equine Vet J 18:410–412, 1986.

Pirie RS, Dion PM: Mandibular tumors in the horse: A review of the literature and 7 case reports. Equine Vet Educ 5:287–294, 1993.

37. What signalment and signs indicate chondrosarcoma?

Usually younger horses are affected with this rare tumor. Chondrosarcomas usually form on the flatbones, including the skull, scapulae, ribs, vertebrae and pelvic bones. Long bones, including the radius, may be affected. Horses may be presented with a mass that is usually firm and nonpainful. Occasionally the mass may be slightly increased in temperature, making it imperative to rule out infective/infectious causes of inflammation. Depending on the site of the chondrosarcoma, it may cause decreased range of motion and lameness. If chondrosarcoma occurs in the long bones, its likely origin is the joint or metaphyseal physis because chondrosarcoma is composed of abnormal chondrocytes. The initial site may be the cartilage of the articular-epiphyseal cartilage complex or metaphyseal physis. Chondrosarcomas are more common in young horses, most likely because there are more cartilaginous regions in the body.

Bertone AL, Powers BE, Turner AS: Chondrosarcoma in the radius of a horse. J Am Vet Med Assoc 185:5, 1984.

38. What diagnostic plan is appropriate for a horse with a firm mass on its head?

A logical plan includes a thorough physical examination of the horse with meticulous palpation of the mass and regional lymph nodes. Radiologic examination of the mass then should be performed. Heavy sedation is usually required. If definition of the mass reveals a soft tissue component, ultrasonographic evaluation is useful; however, if it involves osseous tissue, ultrasonography is of little value. Depending on the imaging findings, the tissue may be biopsied to make a histopathologic diagnosis. If deemed necessary, a sample can be submitted for bacterial and/or fungal culture and sensitivity.

Schooley EK, Hendrickson DA: Musculoskeletal neoplasia. Vet Clin North Am (Equine Pract) 14:534–542, 1998.

39. What factors may predispose to the formation of squamous cell carcinoma of the cornea and conjunctiva?

1. Ocular pigmentation (e.g., absent or low pigmentation predisposes Paints, Pintos, and Appaloosas; Shires, Clydesdales, and Belgians frequently have nonpigmented interpalpebral conjunctiva)

2. Mature age

3. Male sex (according to some reports)

4. Genetic factors, which often may relate to lack of pigmentation; equine leukocyte antigens may be important)

5. Actinic radiation (altitude and duration of sunshine are important)

6. Chronic infection or irritation

7. Viral factors (not known)

Rebhun WC: Tumors of the eye and ocular adnexal tissues. Vet Clin North Am (Equine Pract) 14:579–606, 1998.

40. What is a dermoid? What does it look like in horses?

A dermoid is a congenital tumor that may occur on the cornea or conjunctiva (bulbar or palpebral) of foals. It is less common in foals than in other domestic species (e.g., cats, dogs, cattle). An equine dermoid may be uni- or bilateral and is flat, colored similarly to the surrounding tissues. It has projections of tiny, short hairs, which are extremely irritating to the surrounding tissues. Palpebral conjunctival dermoids tend to be the worst because they damage the cornea (e.g., ulceration). Treatment is difficult, and referral of the foal to an eye specialist should be considered.

Rebhun WC: Tumors of the eye and ocular adnexal tissues. Vet Clin North Am (Equine Pract) 14:579–606, 1998.

41. What are the most likely differential diagnoses in an 18-year-old Arabian mare with acute onset of ataxia (one grade worse in the hindlimbs than forelimbs), paresis, and proprioceptive deficits. The signs appear to be symmetric, and urinary function is normal. The manual slap test was abnormal.

The lesion appears to be located in the cervical vertebrae, and the clinical signs appear to be symmetric. It is more likely to be a compressive lesion because the hindlimbs are more severely affected than the forelimbs (i.e., the tracts for the hindlimbs are more superficially positioned in the spinal cord). The list of most likely differential diagnoses includes (1) trauma (including fracture with spinal cord compression), (2) neoplasia of the vertebral column, (3) neoplasia of the spinal cord or dura, (4) osteomyelitis, and (5) equine protozoal myeloencephalitis.

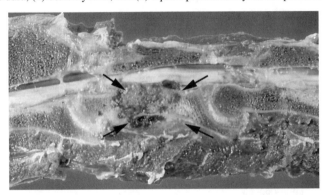

Osteosarcoma (*arrows*) of the third cervical vertebrae of an aged mare who presented with a sudden onset of severe ataxia, paresis, and proprioceptive deficits. She had an abnormal manual slap test.

42. How frequently are neoplastic cells identified when cerebrospinal fluid (CSF) is analyzed?

Neoplastic cells are identified rarely on cytologic evaluation of equine CSF. Other CSF abnormalities (e.g., elevation of protein concentration and/or elevated nucleated cell number or abnormal differential or identification of melanin granules) suggest inflammation and, in the presence of melanin granules, melanoma of the central nervous system. In two reported cases of compressive melanoma of the central nervous system, CSF from the atlantooccipital space was normal, but CSF from the lumbosacral space was abnormal. Both cases involved multiple melanomas of the central nervous system, one of which was in the region of L5–S2 (i.e., region of the lumbosacral centesis). It was believed that the tumor was aspirated directly.

Paradis MR: Tumors of the central nervous system. Vet Clin North Am (Equine Pract) 14:543–562, 1998.

Schott HC II, Major MD, Grant BD, et al: Melanoma as a cause of spinal cord compression in two horses. J Am Vet Med Assoc 196:1820–1822, 1990.

43. Horses of what color are most commonly affected with melanoma(s)?

Most horses affected with melanoma(s) are gray. In 1933 an investigator concluded that 80% of aging gray horses may develop melanocytic tumors. Usually they occur as multiple dermal tumors, primarily of the ventral tail, external genitalia, perineum, and parotid salivary glands.

McFadyean J: Equine melanomatosis. J Comp Pathol Ther 46:186–204, 1933.
Valentine BA: Equine melanocytic tumors: A retrospective study of 53 horses (1988 to 1991). J Vet Intern Med 9:291–297, 1995.

44. Describe the four forms of equine melanocytic tumors.

1. **Melanocytic nevus** may occur in younger horses of any color. It is generally a solitary and discrete superficial mass. Surgical excision is usually curative.

2. **Dermal melanoma** can be distinguished from dermal melanomatosis only by clinical impression; histopathologically the two are indistinguishable. Dermal melanomas occur as discrete masses in mature gray horses. If younger horses are affected, the form may be more aggressive.

3. **Dermal melanomatosis** usually occurs in aged (vs. mature horses affected with dermal melanoma), gray horses. Age is one of the ways to distinguish dermal melanomatosis from dermal melanoma. Dermal melanomatosis most frequently involves the external genitalia, perineum, and ventral tail. The rate of metastasis is usually high.

4. **Anaplastic malignant melanoma** has been seen in nongray horses and results in the growth of large, locally invasive tumors that metastasize within 12 months of diagnosis.

Valentine BA: Equine melanocytic tumors: A retrospective study of 53 horses (1988 to 1991). J Vet Intern Med 9:291–297, 1995.

45. A 6-year-old Thoroughbred gelding was presented with a history of bleeding from a cutaneous lesion that now appears ulcerated. What conditions are on your differential diagnostic list?

1. Cutaneous hemangiosarcoma
2. Hematoma
3. Hamartoma (tumorlike nodules that may resemble a benign neoplasm grossly and microscopically but arise from faulty tissue development). Because it is a developmental lesion, hamartoma should stop growing when the horse matures.
4. Arteriovenous fistula

46. In what tissues does hemangiosarcoma occur?

The most common primary sites of hemangiosarcoma in horses are lung, pleura, spleen, skeletal muscles, eye, and skin; some tumors are multicentric (including spleen). Hemangiosarcomas also have been detected in the pericardium, diaphragm, liver, kidney, central nervous system, sinuses, guttural pouches, vagina, and subcutaneous tissues.

Jean D, Lavoie J-P, Nunez L, et al: Cutaneous hemangiosarcoma with pulmonary metastasis in a horse. J Am Vet Med Assoc 204:776–778, 1994.
Schott HC II, Southwood LL: Disseminated hemangiosarcoma in horses. In Proceedings of the Fourteenth ACVIM 14:568, 1996.

47. Discuss the nomenclature and different forms of mast cell tumors in horses. How common are they in horses?

The nomenclature surrounding equine mast cell tumors is confusing. Many terms have been used, including mastocytoma, mast cell tumor, and cutaneous mastocytosis. The term **equine cutaneous mastocytosis** (ECM) has been endorsed recently because it is not known whether the condition is really neoplastic. However, since one of the recently described forms is malignant, it is likely that at least one form of ECM, despite its rarity, is neoplastic. There are three forms of ECM:

1. **Cutaneous nodular ECM** is the most commonly recognized form. It causes discrete, partially encapsulated, firm/fluctuant cutaneous nodules, which are usually solitary. The size varies considerably from 0.5–20 cm; the location of origin is the dermis or subcutis and, in rare cases, the muscle. The overlying skin is usually intact. Metastasis is not a feature of cutaneous nodular ECM. Tracheal, nasal, and nasopharyngeal surfaces also have been affected. It is not known whether the disease is a benign neoplasm or focal mast cell hyperplasia or dysplasia.

2. **Malignant ECM** may affect a number of different tissues, including bone. Clinical signs often include lameness and pruritus. Clinicopathologic changes may include circulating eosinophilia and hyperfibrinogenemia. Cutaneous nodular ECM and malignant ECM may be differentiated by histopathologic evaluation.

3. **Congenital ECM** is rare and affects foals at or shortly after birth. Foals have multifocal nodules that are disseminated over the body, especially along the trunk and lateral aspects of the hindlimbs. The nodules range in size from 2–3 mm to 3 cm. Bone marrow aspirates or biopsy may reveal abnormal mast cell hyperplasia.

In contrast to other domestic species, the horse is rarely affected by mast cell tumors.

Johnson PJ: Dermatologic tumors (excluding sarcoids). Vet Clin North Am (Equine Pract) 14:625–658, 1998.

Riley CB, Yovich JV, Howell JM: Malignant mast cell tumours in horses. Aust Vet J 68:346, 1991.

48. What are the categories of sarcoid? What are the most commonly affected areas of the equine body?

Sarcoids are nonmetastatic skin tumors. They are the most common tumor of equidae (specifically horses, donkeys, and mules). The four categories are based on the gross appearance: (1) flat, (2) verrucous, (3) fibroblastic, and (4) mixed verrucous and fibroblastic. The most commonly affected areas of the equine body are the head, limbs, and ventrum, although sarcoids may occur anywhere on the surface of the body.

Goodrich L, Gerber H, Marti E, et al: Sarcoids. Vet Clin North Am (Equine Pract) 14:607–624, 1998.

Ragland WL, Keown GH, Spencer GR: Equine sarcoid. Equine Vet J 2:2, 1970.

49. At what age are horses affected with sarcoids?

Most horses are between 3 and 6 years of age when sarcoids are first diagnosed, but in rare instances sarcoids have been diagnosed in yearlings.

Marti E, Lazury S, Antczak DF, et al (eds): Report of the first international workshop on the equine sarcoid. Equine Vet J 25:397, 1993.

50. What two mechanisms are believed to be important in the pathogenesis of equine sarcoids?

1. Bovine papilloma virus-like (BPV-like) DNA. Researchers have induced sarcoid-like lesions by infecting horses with BPV, but the lesions regress spontaneously and the horses develop antibodies to BPV. Naturally occurring sarcoids usually do not regress spontaneously, and antibodies to BPV have not been found in horses with sarcoids. However, BPV-like DNA has been identified in sarcoids with molecular biology techniques. Using polymerase chain reaction (PCR), 90% of sarcoids studied have contained viral sequences, the majority of which belong to BPV types 1 and 2. PCR may become important for the rapid, definitive diagnosis of sarcoid in the future.

2. Genetic influence is thought to be important in the development of sarcoids in horses. Agglomeration of sarcoid cases within particular families has occurred. The major histocompatibility complex (MHC) also appears to be important for sarcoid development within several breeds at the population level.

Goodrich L, Gerber H, Marti E, et al: Sarcoids. Vet Clin North Am (Equine Pract) 14:607–624, 1998.

Marti E, Lazury S, Antczak DF, et al (eds): Report of the first international workshop on the equine sarcoid. Equine Vet J 25:397, 1993.

51. Which H2-receptor antagonist has been proposed for treatment of melanomas in horses? What are the dose rate, route, and duration of trial treatment? What is the purported mechanism? For which clinical scenario should it be used?

H2-receptor antagonist: cimetidine (anecdotally, ranitidine does not appear to be effective).

Dose rate, route, and duration of trial treatment: 2.5 mg/kg 3 times/day orally for 2–3 months to assess response.

Proposed mechanism: unknown. One theory is that horses and other species with cancer may have an excessive number of T-suppressor (T_s) cells, which decrease the patient's ability to mount an antineoplastic response. Histamine may act as an agonist to T_s cells, further increasing the inability to mount an immunologic response against the tumor; thus an H2-receptor antagonist may decrease T_s cell activity and increase the likelihood of an antitumor response. It is not clear why other H2-receptors may not work. (**Note:** the ranitidine data are based on the response of one horse!)

Clinical scenario: melanomas should be increasing in size and appear to be assuming some characteristics of malignancy. This scenario may occur in horses that have had benign melanomas for many years.

Goetz TE, Ogilvie GK, Keegan KG, et al: Cimetidine for treatment of melanomas in three horses. J Am Vet Med Assoc 196:449–452, 1990.

52. Can chemotherapy be used for the treatment of squamous cell carcinoma (SCC) instead of surgery?

Yes. The topical use of 5-fluorouracil (5-FU) should be considered in horses with SCC as a viable alternative to radical surgical excision. 5-FU is fluorinated pyrimidine and acts as an antimetabolite (e.g., interferes with the ability of a cell to synthesize DNA), causing direct tumor cell death or increased detection by the host immunologic system. Genital SCC of male and female horses can be treated by either surgical debridement followed by topical 5-FU or topical 5-FU alone.

The procedure includes physical restraint (e.g., stocks) and chemical restraint so that the lesion can be examined and biopsied. After biopsy, tetanus toxoid should be administered to most horses. Surgical debulking of the labial region of females can be accomplished commonly in the standing position with chemical restraint. However, if the clitoral fossa is involved, and in most cases of genital SCC in males, general anesthesia should be used so that thorough debulking can take place. 5-FU may be applied as soon as the hemorrhage has ceased (usually 1–12 hours) so that it is not diluted. In females 5–FU should applied to the debulked tumor region daily (often by owners wearing latex gloves) and then checked by the veterinarian in 14 days. In males with SCC of the penis, the prepuce acts as a reservoir for 5–FU; therefore, it needs to be applied only every 2 weeks by the veterinarian. After remission of the tumor the horse should be examined every 6 months by the veterinarian to ensure no further treatments are necessary.

Fortier LA, Mac Harg MA: Topical use of 5-fluorouracil for treatment of squamous cell carcinoma of the external genitalia of horses: 11 cases (1988–1992). J Am Med Assoc 205:1183–1185, 1994.

53. Explain the treatment stages in horses after application of 5-FU to genital SCC.

Treatment stages are similar to those described in humans, although usually they are shorter in horses.

Stage 1: The initial stage is the **commencement** of an early inflammatory response 5–7 days after topical application of 5-FU.

Stage 2: The **inflammatory response** usually lasts approximately 2–4 weeks.

Stage 3: The tumor **sloughs** from 6–12 weeks. Because necrosis may be considerable during this phase, the accumulation of tissue may be malodorous.

Stage 4: **Epithelization** with little-to-no scarring occurs during the last stage of rapid healing. This stage usually lasts an additional 4–6 weeks.

Fortier LA, Mac Harg MA: Topical use of 5-fluorouracil for treatment of squamous cell carcinoma of the external genitalia of horses: 11 cases (1988–1992). J Am Med Assoc 205:1183–1185, 1994.

54. What is cis(II)-platinum diamminedichloride (cisplatin)? How does it work?

Cisplatin is a heavy metal compound that inhibits DNA synthesis by direct binding.

55. What equine tumors can be treated with intralesional cisplatin?

Tumors that can be treated with intralesional cisplatin protocols include the cutaneous forms of (1) squamous cell carcinoma, (2) papilloma, (3) sarcoid, (4) sarcomas, (5) lymphoma, and (6) melanoma. Many of these tumors also may be appropriately treated with interstitial brachytherapy.

56. What dose of cisplatin is used in horses vs. dogs?

The dose rate of cisplatin described for horses is 0.97 mg/cm^3 (i.e., approximately 1.0 mg/cm^3) of tumor every 2 weeks for approximately 4 treatments. This intralesional protocol has allowed animals with large body weights to be treated effectively as well as safely; it has obviated the need for high systemic concentrations while achieving high concentrations at the tumor level. In contrast, dogs are usually dosed systemically according to surface area, 70 mg/m^2 of surface area of the dog (not the tumor).

Theon AP: Intralesional and topical chemotherapy and immunotherapy. Vet Clin North Am (Equine Pract) 14:659–672, 1998.

Theon AP, Pascoe JR, Carlson GP, et al: Intratumoral chemotherapy with cisplatin in oily emulsion in horses. J Am Vet Med Assoc 202:261–267, 1993.

57. What is the technique for reconstitution of cisplatin?

Cisplatin should be reconstituted immediately before use; otherwise its potency may be adversely affected. Ten milligrams of cisplatin (Platinol, Bristol-Myers Squibb Co., Princeton, NJ) is first reconstituted with 1 ml of sterile water to a concentration of 10 mg/ml (saturated solution). Then it is mixed with 2 ml of medical-grade, purified sesame seed oil using a 2- or 3-way connector and Luer lock syringes for safety reasons. The suspension can be mixed by exchange of syringe contents, using two locked syringes.

Some equine veterinarians have advocated the use of aqueous preparations of cisplatin; however, this practice should be discouraged because the preparations are too dilute (1 mg/ml). Epinephrine combinations should not be used adjacent to normal tissue because of the great potential for local tissue necrosis in both normal and neoplastic tissues.

Theon AP: Intralesional and topical chemotherapy and immunotherapy. Vet Clin North Am (Equine Pract) 14:659–672, 1998.

Theon AP, Pascoe JR, Carlson GP, et al: Intratumoral chemotherapy with cisplatin in oily emulsion in horses. J Am Vet Med Assoc 202:261–267, 1993.

58. Give examples, mode of action, and side effects (known for other species) for the following groups of chemotherapeutic agents: alkylating agents, antimetabolites, antibiotics, plant alkaloids, L-asparaginase, and cisplatin.

CLASS OF CHEMOTHERAPEUTIC AGENT	EXAMPLES	MODE OF ACTION	SIDE EFFECTS
Alkylating agents	Cyclophosphamide Chlorambucil Melphalan Dacarbazine	Cause breakage of DNA and thus decrease cross-linking, replication, and transcription; *not* cell cycle-specific.	Hemorrhagic cystitis (especially cyclophosphamide) Diminished wound healing
Antimetabolites	Cytosine arabinoside Fluorouracil Methotrexate Mercaptopurine	Structural analogs of substances required for cell replication and function; S-phase specific.	Some drugs affect wound healing (especially methotrexate)
Antibiotics	Bleomycin Doxorubicin (Both are natural products derived from soil fungus.)	Damage DNA by binding to it and inhibiting replication and transcription; *not* cell cycle-specific.	Hematologic toxicity Gastrointestinal toxicity Cardiac toxicity Pulmonary fibrosis (bleomycin) Skin sloughing if injected perivascularly Diminished wound healing

Table continued on following page

CLASS OF CHEMOTHERA-PEUTIC AGENT	EXAMPLES	MODE OF ACTION	SIDE EFFECTS
Plant alkaloids	Vincristine Vinblastine	Bind microtubular protein tubulin and block mitosis by interfering with chromosomal separation in metaphase; M-phase specific.	Neural toxicity, including sensory neuropathy and paresthesia Myelosuppression Skin sloughing possible Minimal impairment to wound healing
L-asparaginase	L-asparaginase	Hydrolyses L-asparagine; G1 phase-specific.	Anaphylaxis Gastrointestinal disturbances Hepatotoxicity Pancreatitis (hemorrhagic) Coagulopathy
Cisplatin	Cis(II)-platinum diammine-dichloride	Cisplatin is a heavy metal compound that inhibits DNA synthesis by direct binding; *not* cell cycle-specific	Gastrointestinal disturbances Renal insufficiency Decreased wound healing **Note:** cisplatin is used intra-lesionally rather than systemically in horses, thereby diminishing side effects substantially.

59. What is the biologic basis of radiation therapy?

Ionizing radiation, regardless of its nature or mode of production, causes energy dissipation within the tissues. Mitotic cell death results in the failure of cells to pass through mitosis after completing one or more relatively normal mitoses. Interphase death results when more sensitive cells or cells receiving large doses of radiation degenerate during interphase and fail to reach first mitosis.

Both neoplastic and normal cells are affected (i.e., cellular DNA damage), but normal cells have greater ability to repair. This differential capability leads to the **selective effect of radiation** (i.e., tumor death with preservation of the surrounding anatomically normal tissue). However, some normal tissues are more radiosensitive (i.e., have less radiation tolerance) and may be damaged irrevocably if radiation is used. If the dose of radiation required for tumor resolution exceeds the radiation tolerance of adjacent normal tissues, radiation therapy cannot be used alone and in some cases cannot be used at all.

Theon AP: Radiation therapy. Vet Clin North Am (Equine Pract) 14:673–688, 1998.

60. What are the critical cellular target(s) of radiation therapy?

1. DNA (main target)
2. Cell membrane proteins
3. Cell membrane lipids

Blackwood L, Dobson JM: Radiotherapy in the horse. Equine Vet Educ 6:95–99, 1994.

61. Which equine tumors are radioresponsive? List them in order from most radioresponsive to least radioresponsive.

1. Squamous cell carcinoma (most radioresponsive)
2. Papilloma
3. Sarcoid
4. Soft tissue sarcomas (including neurofibrosarcoma, fibrosarcoma, hemangiosarcoma)
5. Melanoma (least radioresponsive)

Theon AP: Radiation therapy. Vet Clin North Am (Equine Pract) 14:673–688, 1998.

62. What are the three most important prognostic factors in assessing a tumor for radiation therapy?
1. Tumor type (and thus degree of radiocurability and growth rate)
2. Tumor volume
3. Tumor location
Theon AP: Radiation therapy. Vet Clin North Am (Equine Pract) 14:673–688, 1998.

63. What two types of radiation therapy are available for horses? Describe each.
1. **Teletherapy (external beam therapy).** The source is at some distance (usually approximately 1 meter) from the neoplastic site. Teletherapy is not commonly available for horses because it requires an expensive and specialized facility and owners have to agree to have the horse anesthetized a number of times. A typical treatment regimen is to give the total dose of radiation (35–45 Gy) in 6–9 dose fractions (4–5 Gy per fraction), administered 2–3 times/week over 3–4 weeks. Teletherapy is used to treat large tumors and tumors positioned deeply within tissues. It is the only type of radiation treatment that can be used to treat primary or metastatic osseous neoplasia.
2. **Brachytherapy.** The sealed radioactive source is applied directly to the neoplastic treatment area. It is a useful technique in horses because the radiation dose can be delivered precisely and safely over a short time. There are two types of brachytherapy: (1) interstitial brachytherapy (Curietherapy) and (2) plesiotherapy (surface therapy). In **interstitial brachytherapy** the radioactive sources are implanted directly into the neoplastic tissues. ^{125}Iodine and ^{192}iridium emit gamma rays. Both are available for insertion (i.e., implantation) as wires or seeds (grains). Implants may be temporary or permanent, and implantation may be performed using local anesthetic and sedation techniques or under general anesthesia. Only temporary implants are recommended because they are safer. Interstitial brachytherapy is used alone or in combination with surgery (both intraoperatively and postoperatively). The most appropriate tumors for interstitial brachytherapy are squamous cell carcinoma, sarcoids, and soft tissue sarcomas of the genitalia, head, and distal extremities. In **plesiotherapy** the radioactive sources are placed directly onto the surface of the neoplastic tissues. A strontium-90 (^{90}Sr) applicator is used commonly. ^{90}Sr decays to yttrium-90, which produces an electron beam as it decays. The depth of penetration of the electrons is small; consequently, this modality is useful only for superficial tumors (the first millimeter of tissue absorbs 60% of the electrons). The horse should have general anesthesia to ensure accuracy of and to diminish exposure of personnel. This technique is used extensively in ophthalmologic neoplasia (e.g., corneal, scleral, and conjunctival SCC and melanoma), especially intraoperatively to treat residual tumor.
Theon AP: Radiation therapy. Vet Clin North Am (Equine Pract) 14:673–688, 1998.

BIBLIOGRAPHY

1. Becht JL, Thacker HL, Page EH: Malignant seminoma in a stallion. J Am Vet Med Assoc 175:292–293, 1979.
2. Bertone AL, Powers BE, Turner AS: Chondrosarcoma in the radius of a horse. J Am Vet Med Assoc 185:5, 1984.
3. Bilkslager AT, Bowman KF, Haven ML, et al: Pedunculated lipomas as a cause of intestinal obstruction in horses: 17 cases (1983–1990). J Am Vet Med Assoc 201:1249–1252, 1992.
4. Blackwood L, Dobson JM: Radiotherapy in the horse. Equine Vet Educ 6:95–99, 1994.
5. Boulton CH: Equine nasal cavity and paranasal sinus disease: A review of 85 cases. Equine Vet Sci 5:268, 1985.
6. Brinsko SP: Neoplasia of the male reproductive tract. Vet Clin North Am (Equine Pract) 14:517–534, 1998.
7. Brown PJ, Holt PE: Primary renal cell carcinoma in four horses. Equine Vet J 17:473–477, 1985.
8. Carlson GP: Clinical chemistry tests. In Smith BP (eds): Large Animal Internal Medicine. St. Louis, Mosby, 1990, pp 386–414.
9. Colbourne CM, Bolton JR, Mills JN, et al: Mesothelioma in horses. Aust Vet J 69:275, 1992.
10. Crisman MV, Scarratt WK: See reference 38a.
11. Downes EE, Ragle CA, Hines MT: Pedunculated lipoma associated with recurrent colic in a horse. J Am Vet Med Assoc 204:1163–1164, 1994.

12. East LM, Savage CJ: Abdominal neoplasia (excluding urogenital tract). Vet Clin North Am (Equine Pract) 14:475–494, 1998.
13. Edwards DF, Parker JW, Wilkinson JE, et al: Plasma cell myeloma in the horse: A case report and literature review. J Vet Int Med 7:169–176, 1993.
14. Edwards GB, Proudman CJ: An analysis of 75 cases of intestinal obstruction caused by pedunculated lipomas. Equine Vet J 26:18–21, 1994.
15. Fortier LA, Mac Harg MA: Topical use of 5-fluorouracil for treatment of squamous cell carcinoma of the external genitalia of horses: 11 cases (1988–1992). J Am Med Assoc 205:1183–1185, 1994.
16. Gatewood DM, Douglass JF, Cox JH, et al: Intra-abdominal hemorrhage associated with a granulosa-thecal cell neoplasm in a mare. J Am Vet Med Assoc 196:1827–1828, 1990.
17. Goetz TE, Ogilvie GK, Keegan KG, et al: Cimetidine for treatment of melanomas in three horses. J Am Vet Med Assoc 196:449–452, 1990.
18. Goodrich L, Gerber H, Marti E, et al: Sarcoids. Vet Clin North Am (Equine Pract) 14:607–624, 1998.
19. Jean D, Lavoie J-P, Nunez L, et al: Cutaneous hemangiosarcoma with pulmonary metastasis in a horse. J Am Vet Med Assoc 204:776–778, 1994.
20. Jeffcott LB: Primary liver-cell carcinoma in a young Thoroughbred horse. J Pathol 97:394–397, 1969.
21. Johnson PJ: Dermatologic tumors (excluding sarcoids). Vet Clin North Am (Equine Pract) 14:625–658, 1998.
22. Liversey MA, Wilkie IW: Focal and multifocal osteosarcoma in two foals. Equine Vet J 18:410–412, 1986.
23. Madewell BR, Carlson GP, MacLachlan NJ, et al: Lymphosarcoma with leukemia in a horse. Am J Vet Res 43:807–812, 1982.
24. Marti E, Lazury S, Antczak DF, et al (eds): Report of the first international workshop on the equine sarcoid. Equine Vet J 25:397, 1993.
25. McCue PM: Neoplasia of the female reproductive tract. Vet Clin North Am (Equine Pract) 14:505–516, 1998.
26. McFadyean J: Equine melanomatosis. J Comp Pathol Ther 46:186–204, 1933.
27. Misdorp W, Nauta-van Gelder HL: Granuolar cell myoblastoma in the horse: A report of four cases. Pathol Vet 5:385–394, 1968.
28. Nickels FA, Brown CM, Breeze RG: Equine granular cell tumour (myoblastoma). Mod Vet Pract 61:593–596, 1980.
29. Ogilvie GK: Paraneoplastic syndromes. Vet Clin North Am (Equine Pract) 14:439–450, 1998.
30. Paradis MR: Tumors of the central nervous system. Vet Clin North Am (Equine Pract) 14:543–562, 1998.Pirie RS, Dion PM: Mandibular tumors in the horse: A review of the literature and 7 case reports. Equine Vet Educ 5:287–294, 1993.
31. Ragland WL, Keown GH, Spencer GR: Equine sarcoid. Equine Vet J 2:2, 1970.
32. Rebhun WC: Tumors of the eye and ocular adnexal tissues. Vet Clin North Am (Equine Pract) 14:579–606, 1998.
33. Riley CB, Yovich JV, Howell JM: Malignant mast cell tumours in horses. Aust Vet J 68:346, 1991.
34. Roby RAW, Beech J, Bloom JC, et al: Hepatocellular carcinoma associated with erythrocytosis and hypoglycemia in a yearling filly. J Am Vet Med Assoc 196:465–467, 1990.
35. Roser JF, McCue PM, Hoye E: Inhibin activity in the mare and stallion. Domest Animal Endocrinol 11:87, 1994.
36. Savage CJ: Lymphoproliferative and myeloproliferative disorders. Vet Clin North Am (Equine Pract) 14:563–578, 1998.
37. Savage CJ, Jeffcott LB, Melsen F, Ostblom LC: Bone biopsy in the horse. I: Method using the wing of ilium. J Vet Med Assoc 38:776–783, 1991.
38. Scarratt WK, Crisman MV, Sponenberg DP, et al: Pulmonary granular cell tumours in two horses. Equine Vet J 25:244–247, 1993.
38a. Scarrat WK, Crisman MV: Neoplasia of the respiratory tract. Vet Clin North Am (Equine Practice) 14:451–474, 1998.
39. Shaw DP, Roth JE: Testicular teratocarcinoma in a horse. Vet Pathol 23:3237–3238, 1986.
40. Schooley EK, Hendrickson DA: Musculoskeletal neoplasia. Vet Clin North Am (Equine Pract) 14:535–542, 1998.
41. Schott HC II, Major MD, Grant BD, et al: Melanoma as a cause of spinal cord compression in two horses. J Am Vet Med Assoc 196:1820–1822, 1990.
42. Schott HC II, Southwood LL: Disseminated hemangiosarcoma in horses. In Proceedings of the fourthteenth ACVIM 14:568, 1996.
43. Smith BL, Morton LD, Watkins JP, et al: Malignant seminoma in a cryptorchid stallion. J Am Vet Med Assoc 195:775–776, 1989.
44. Theon AP: Intralesional and topical chemotherapy and immunotherapy. Vet Clin North Am (Equine Pract) 14:659–672, 1998.

45. Theon AP: Radiation therapy. Vet Clin North Am (Equine Pract) 14:673–688, 1998.
46. Theon AP, Pascoe JR, Carlson GP, et al: Intratumoral chemotherapy with cisplatin in oily emulsion in horses. J Am Vet Med Assoc 202:261–267, 1993.
47. Traub-Dargatz JL: Urinary tract neoplasia. Vet Clin North Am (Equine Pract) 14:495–504, 1998.
48. Valentine BA: Equine melanocytic tumors: A retrospective study of 53 horses (1988 to 1991). J Vet Intern Med 9:291–297, 1995.
49. Wallace SS, Jayo MJ, Maddux JM, et al: Mesothelioma in a horse. Compend Contin Educ Pract Vet 9:210–216, 1987.
50. Yovich JV, Ducharme NG: Ruptured pheochromocytoma in a mare with colic. J Am Vet Med Assoc 183:462–464, 1983.
51. Yovich JV, Horney FD, Hardee GE: Pheochromocytoma in the horse and measurement of norepinephrine levels in horses. Can Vet J 25:21–25, 1984.

18. NUTRITION

William S. Swecker, Jr., D.V.M., Ph.D., Dip. ACVN, and
Craig D. Thatcher, D.V.M., M.S., Ph.D., Dip. ACVN

ASSESSMENT OF THE HORSE

1. Where can you obtain information about the nutrient requirements of horses?

The National Research Council prints *Nutrient Requirements of Horses*. The latest edition was printed in 1989. Categories include:

1. Maintenance horses
2. Stallions
3. Pregnant mares: 9 months, 10 months, 11 months
4. Lactating mares: foaling to 3 months, 3 months to weaning
5. Working horses: light work, moderate work, and intense work
6. Weanlings: weanling 4 months (moderate and rapid growth), weanling 6 months (moderate and rapid growth)
7. Yearlings (12 months): moderate and rapid growth
8. Long yearling (18 months): not in training, in training
9. Two years old (24 months): not in training, in training

*Nutrient Requirements of Horses**

	MAIN-TENANCE	LATE GESTATION	EARLY LACTATION	LATE LACTATION	WEANLING 6 MO	WEANLING 12 MO	MODERATE WORK[†]
Digestible energy[‡] (Mcal/lb)	0.9	1.1	1.2	1.15	1.4	1.3	1.2
Protein (%)	8	10.6	13.2	11.0	14.5	12.6	10.4
Calcium (%)	0.24	0.45	0.52	0.36	0.56	0.43	0.31
Phosphorus (%)	0.17	0.34	0.34	0.22	0.31	0.24	0.23
Copper (ppm)	10	10	10	10	10	10	10
Manganese (ppm)	40	40	40	40	40	40	40
Zinc (ppm)	40	40	40	40	40	40	40
Forage % diet	50–100	50–85	33–85	40–80	30–65	33–80	33–80
Grain % diet	0–50	15–50	15–66	20–60	35–75	20–66	20–66
Forage % body weight	1–2	1–2	1–2.5	1–2	0.5–1.8	1–2.5	1–2
Grain % body weight	0–1	0.3–1.0	0.5–2	0.5–1.5	1–3	0.5–2	0.5–2

* From Nutrient Requirements of Horses, 5th ed. Washington, DC, National Research Council, 1989.
† Examples are horses used in ranch work, jumping, etc.
‡ Assumes that hay contains 0.9 Mcal/lb and grain contains 1.5 Mcal/lb.

2. List factors that alter the nutrient requirements of the horse.

- Weight
- Type of activity (light, moderate, intense)
- Climate
- Health, condition, and temperament of horse
- Management system
- Age (growing vs. not growing)
- Pregnancy (9–11 months)
- Lactation

277

3. What scale is used to derive body condition scores for horses?

Horses are given a body condition score of 1–9 with 1 indicating extreme thinness and 9 obesity. A simpler breakdown is as follows: 1–3, thin; 4–6, moderate; and 7–9, obese. Key areas to evaluate on the horse are ribs, tuber coxae, tuber ischii, dorsal and transverse processes of the spinal column, and shoulder. In general, a horse with a condition score of 3 or less lacks subcutaneous fat and is losing muscle mass. Horses with condition scores of 4–6 are normally muscled and have increasing amounts of subcutaneous fat. Horses with condition scores of 7–9 are overconditioned. Athletes may be an exception in condition scoring with normal muscle mass and low body fat. Another equine body condition scoring system ranges from 0 (very poor) to 5 (very fat).

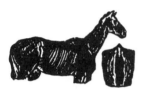

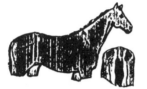

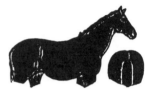

0 VERY POOR
- Very sunken rump
- Deep cavity under tail
- Skin tight over bones
- Very prominent backbone and pelvis
- Marked ewe neck

2 MODERATE
- Flat rump either side backbone
- Ribs just visible
- Narrow but firm neck
- Backbone well covered

4 FAT
- Rump well rounded
- Gutter along back
- Ribs and pelvis hard to feel
- Slight crest

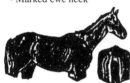

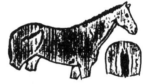

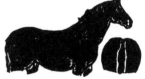

1 POOR
- Sunken rump
- Cavity under tail
- Ribs easily visible
- Prominent backbone and croup
- Ewe neck—narrow and slack

3 GOOD
- Rounded rump
- Ribs just covered but easily felt
- No crest, firm neck

5 VERY FAT
- Very bulging rump
- Deep gutter along back
- Ribs buried
- Marked crest
- Fold and lumps of fat

Equine condition score diagram. (Adapted from Huntington P, Cleland F: Horse Sense: The Australian Guide to Horse Husbandry. East Melbourne, Australia, 1992, with permission.)

4. What is a practical way to estimate a horse's body weight on the farm?

Body weight can be estimated using an equine weight tape or by measuring the girth length in inches or centimeters. The table below can be used to convert the girth length (inches) into a measure of body weight in pounds (lb).

Relationship Between Girth Measurement and Body Weight

GIRTH LENGTH (INCHES)	ESTIMATED WEIGHT (LB)	GIRTH LENGTH (INCHES)	ESTIMATED WEIGHT (LB)
40	200	68	930
45	275	70	1000
50	375	72	1070
55	500	74	1140
60	650	76	1210
62	720	78	1290
64	790	80	1370
66	860		

5. How do you assess the protein and energy status of a horse?

Decreased feed intake is reflected by decreased or low body condition scores, increased indirect (unconjugated) bilirubin concentration, and decreased serum albumin, blood urea nitrogen, and possibly serum glucose. Rarely does the serum glucose decrease in the adult horse, unless endotoxemia, septicemia, bacteremia, or hepatic disease is present. Serum nonesterified fatty acids are increased, especially in ponies, miniature horses, and azotemic adult horses.

6. Which class of horse has the highest protein requirements as a percentage of body weight?

Protein requirements are highest at birth and become progressively lower as the horse matures.

7. How do you assess the selenium, copper, and zinc status of a horse?

Blood or serum selenium can be used to assess selenium status. Liver samples are best for assessment of copper and zinc because serum levels reflect only severe deficiencies. A specific trace element tube should be used to assess zinc because blood-sampling tubes may contain zinc.

8. Contrast nutrient requirements for the equine athlete vs. the maintenance horse.

The athlete requires increased energy to meet the demands of work. Part of this increased need is met by increased intake, but the energy density of the ration also should be increased for moderate-to-heavy work or exercise. Energy density can be increased by increasing the amount of grain or by adding supplemental fat. Protein concentration of the diet does not need to be increased because of the increased intake. Electrolyte concentrations also may need to be increased to account for losses in sweat.

9. Contrast energy metabolism in the endurance horse and sprinter.

The energy requirements for endurance activity are met by the aerobic oxidation of carbohydrates, fats, or proteins. Fats are the most energy-efficient substrate for aerobic oxidation. Sprinters primarily utilize anaerobic oxidation of glycogen.

10. When do nutrient requirements increase for gestating mares?

Nutrient requirements increase above maintenance at or during the last trimester of pregnancy, primarily during the ninth, tenth, and eleventh months of gestation.

11. Contrast nutrient requirements of the lactating mare with maintenance requirements.

The mare reaches peak lactation in the second month of lactation (approximately 6 weeks), and her requirements at that time can be twice maintenance. Requirements can be met by increasing feed intake and the energy concentration of the ration through increasing the amount of alfalfa, grain, and supplemental fat.

12. What are the essential components of a good dietary history?

Record the amount offered and consumed of all forages, grains, supplements, treats, and water over a 24-hour period. In addition, document the time spent on pasture and the plants available in the pasture.

ASSESSMENT OF FEEDS

13. Water is the most important nutrient for horses and is often the most overlooked. How much water does a mature horse drink per day?

Water intake varies depending on the activity level of the horse and the temperature of the water and environment of the horse. On average, a mature horse drinks 7–15 gallons of water per day. Water intake may increase up to 25–30 gallons if the horse is working in a 100° F environment. It may be easier to calculate the amount by remembering that horses drink approximately 5–10% of their body weight at maintenance.

14. What is the first limiting amino acid for the growing horse?

Lysine is the first limiting amino acid for the growing horse. Therefore, feedstuffs high in lysine, such as soybean meal, should be used in rations for growing horses.

15. Describe the correct procedure to sample pastures, hays, and concentrates for chemical analysis.

Core samples should be obtained from 10% of the bales in the lot or a minimum of 10 bales. Square bales should be cored from the end and round bales from the side. Core samples can be mixed together and submitted for analysis. Random handfuls should be taken from grain storage bins and silos, and feedbags also can be cored. To sample a pasture, move across the pasture in a W pattern and clip samples every 25–100 yards, depending on pasture size. All samples should be placed in a plastic bag, the air removed, and the bag sealed.

16. What is recommended for a minimal database for forage analysis?

Dry matter, crude protein, fiber content, an estimate of energy content, and the macrominerals: calcium, phosphorus, potassium, and magnesium.

17. What is the fat content of most hays and grains?

Three-to-five percent on a dry matter basis.

18. How much fat can be added to an equine ration?

Horses can adapt to a ration that contains up to 15% fat, but they must be given a period of several weeks to adapt. The increase in fat should be slow and incremental.

19. Describe the importance of visual appraisal of hays.

1. The hay is identified as a legume (clover, alfalfa) or grass (e.g., timothy, orchard grass, fescue).

2. Estimate the maturity of the plant when it was harvested. Seed heads or flowers indicate a mature to overly mature plant.

3. Evaluate the ratio of leaves (highest content of nutrients) to stems (lowest content of nutrients).

4. High-quality hay should be green with a pleasant odor. Black discoloration may indicate overheating, gray discoloration may indicate the presence of mold, and brown or yellow coloration may indicate overmaturity or rain damage between cutting and harvesting.

20. Contrast grass hay, legume hay, corn, and oats in terms of protein, energy, calcium, and phosphorus content.

Legume hays contain more proteins, energy, and calcium than grass hays. Corn has a higher energy density than oats. Both corn and oats have a low calcium-to-phosphorus ratio (i.e., more phosphorus than calcium).

FEED TYPE	PROTEIN (% DM)	ENERGY (MCAL DE/LB)	CALCIUM (% DM)	PHOSPHORUS (% DM)
Grass	7–12	0.7–1	0.2–0.3	0.2–0.3
Alfalfa/clover	14–22	0.9–1.3	1.0–1.5	0.2–0.4
Corn	8–10	1.7	0.05	0.3
Oats	10–14	1.4–1.8	0.1	0.3–0.4

21. Does feeding wheat bran to horses prevent colic by serving as a laxative?

No. Bran does not have a laxative effect because it does not increase fecal water content and therefore does not soften the stool. Furthermore, no evidence based on controlled studies indicates that bran treats or prevents colic. The high phosphorus content of bran may be harmful if a sufficiently high amount (by weight, not density) is fed over a long period and not balanced with adequate calcium.

22. Why should horses not be grazed on sorghum grass pastures?

Sorghum grass (Sudan grass) pastures have been associated with cyanide and nitrate toxicosis in horses, resulting in sudden death. Posterior ataxia and cystitis also have been associated with the consumption of sorghum pasture. Cystitis occurs in horses regardless of stage of maturity or growing conditions of sorghum grasses. (See question 5 in chapter 7.)

23. Which vitamins are produced by the bacteria in horse's cecum and colon?

. Vitamin K and the B-complex vitamins.

24. What is the tolerable range of the calcium-to-phosphorus ratio for growing horses and adult horses?

Growing horses: 1–3:1; adult horses: 1–6:1.

ASSESSMENT OF FEEDING MANAGEMENT

25. Describe dry matter intake for different groups of horses by percentage of body weight.

Maintenance horses should consume 1–2% of body weight, depending on the quality of feed, which is 10–20 lb for a mature 1000-lb horse. Growing foals, working horses, and lactating mares consume up to 2–5% of body weight.

26. Many people feed by volume: coffee cans, scoops, or flakes of hay. Why is it important to know the weight of feed rather than the volume?

The weight of feed per unit volume varies widely, depending on the feedstuff (e.g., bran vs. corn), and therefore provides different energy values per volume. There is over a fourfold difference in the amount of energy provided by the same volume of bran vs. corn.

27. At what age should creep feed be supplied to nursing foals? Why?

Creep feed should be provided to the foal around 2 months of age. Milk produced by the mare is usually sufficient to meet all of the foal's nutritional needs, except for copper, for about the first 2 months of life; in the first 2 months of life the foal draws on hepatic copper reserves. After 2 months of age, the amount of milk produced by most mares no longer meets all of the foal's nutritional requirements. Creep feed also ensures that after weaning the foal is accustomed to eating a grain mix separate from what it may eat with the mare.

28. Why should fat be considered in the feeding of heavily worked equine athlete?

- Fat increases the energy density of the diet without a proportionate increase in feed intake. Therefore, one can limit the amount of grain fed, which may be beneficial in preventing colic.
- Fat decreases the amount of energy used for heat production and increases the amount available for performance.
- Fat increases glycogen if fed for 6 weeks before expected performance.
- Horses fed a high-fat diet have greater utilization of muscle glycogen.
- Fat can decrease the amount of fecal mass in the horse and thus decrease the weight that the horse must carry.

29. What is the minimal forage (hay or pasture) intake for a mature 1000-lb (450-kg) horse?

Forage intake should be at least 1% of body weight or 10 lb (4–5 kg) for a 1000-lb (450-kg) horse.

30. How often should a horse be fed hay and concentrates?

Forage (pasture or hay) should be available at all times. Stabled horses should be offered forage 3 times daily. If pasture time is available, hay can be fed once or twice daily. If the horse is on pasture all of the time, the pasture should be assessed for nutrient value and supply; otherwise, hay or concentrates may still be required. Concentrates should be fed a minimum of twice daily with no more than 5 lb (2–3 kg) of grain per feeding because of the small stomach size and normal behavior (frequent small meals) of horses. To avoid gastric ulceration, forage should always be available; however, if a horse has right dorsal colitis, a low-bulk (low-forage) diet with increased corn oil may be advocated.

31. Describe indications for enteral and parenteral alimentation of horses.

Enteral feeding should be used when gastrointestinal function and motility are present but the horse will not eat. Enteral diets may consist of a slurry of pelleted feeds or a commercial equine enteral product (e.g., Nutriprime, Kenvet, Ashland, OH 44805). Parenteral feeding is indicated when gastrointestinal function and/or motility is not present or enteral feeding is not possible.

32. Describe the maximal grain content of rations for the weanling and yearling horse.

In weanlings, grain must be less than 70% of the diet (i.e., < 70% concentrate, > 30% forage), whereas in yearlings grain must be less than 60% of the diet (i.e., < 60% concentrate, > 40% forage). These percentages reflect the minimal amount of forage; ideally it should be substantially greater (e.g., > 60% forage).

33. Describe three methods to provide milk to an orphan foal.

Allow the foal to nurse from a bottle or to drink from a pan, or place a nasogastric tube and provide milk through the tube. The optimal method is to allow the foal to drink from a pan; this low-intensity method does not run the risk of milk aspiration into the trachea.

34. How much milk should be fed to a 50-kg (110-lb) foal in a 24-hour period?

Consider 10–15% of body weight to maintain the foal and up to 22–25% body weight to provide for growth. This recommendation corresponds to 5 liters (11 pints) for maintenance and 12.5 liters (27.5 pints) for growth over a 24-hour period. In the first 3 weeks, it is optimal to divide the total volume by 12 and to feed every 2 hours. Incrementally the volume may be divided by 8 and fed every 3 hours with slow changes so that the foal at 8 weeks of age can be fed every 6 hours. Creep feed should be started.

35. Should trace-mineralized salt be provided to horses?

Trace element content of grains and forages is variable. Trace-mineralized salt provides trace elements not provided in forages and grains and should be offered as a free choice for all classes of horses. However, provision of free-choice trace-mineralized salt blocks does not ensure consumption. Sometimes trace-mineralized salt should be added directly to the concentrate. The ingestion of salt has the added benefit of increasing water consumption and putatively decreasing impaction colic in the winter months when water intake otherwise may be decreased.

NUTRITION AND DISEASE

36. Discuss the nutritional etiologies of colic.

Researchers have found that nutritional causes of colic include changes in hay and concentrate feeding; level of concentrate; certain feedstuffs such as coastal Bermuda grass, spoiled feed, young protein-rich grass, and coarse, poor-quality roughages; overfeeding; underfeeding; pelleted feeds; and inadequate water supply.

37. Which B vitamin may be supplemented in horses with poor hoof growth and integrity?

Biotin may be helpful in the repair of hoof wall defects and prevent their recurrence. Biotin improves hoof strength and decreases heel, heel-horn junction, and sidewall hoof cracks. Such hoof conditions may benefit from biotin supplementation at 15–20 mg/day for light horses and 30–40 mg/day for draft horses.

38. List the disorders of growing horses that are commonly considered developmental orthopedic diseases (DODs).

- Physitis
- Angular limb deformities
- Acquired flexor deformities
- Cervical compressive myelopathy
- Osteochondrosis (osteochondritis dissecans)
- Subchondral bone cysts

39. What is the role of nutrients in the etiology and expression of DOD?

Excessive energy intake and sudden increases in energy intake have been associated with an increase in DOD. Deficiencies of copper and imbalances in the calcium-to-phosphorus ratio also have been associated with DOD. Other nutrients that may play a role in DOD are zinc and manganese.

40. Red maple trees (*Acer rubrum*) are common throughout eastern North America and are found as far south as Florida and Texas. Describe the clinical presentation of a horse that has been poisoned by eating wilted red maple leaves or the bark of the red maple tree.

Acute hemolytic Heinz body anemia causes the horse to be weak with increased respiration and heart rate. The mucous membrane (i.e., oral and vulval) may be brown-tinged due to myoglobinemia, and there may be a red-brown discoloration to the urine (myoglobinuria and hemoglobinuria).

41. What is the cause of leukoencephalomalacia (LEM) in horses?

The primary risk factor for LEM is the feeding of mold-damaged corn. The mold responsible is *Fusarium moniliforme*. LEM (moldy corn poisoning) is a liquefactive necrosis of the white matter of the brain. The horse may present clinically with liver failure, LEM, or both. Clinical signs include ataxia, paresis, head pressing, wandering, circling, recumbency, hyperexcitability, and death.

42. Describe the toxic agents associated with fescue and the associated clinical syndromes.

Fescue toxicosis is associated with fescue pastures or hays infected with the fungus *Neotyphodium coenophialum (Acremonium coenophialum)*. Several compounds have been suspected as toxic agents, including alkaloids such as ergovaline and n-acetyl loline. Fescue toxicosis has been suspected as a cause of embryonic loss, prolonged gestation, thick placentas, and diminished lactation (agalactia). The fungal ergopeptine alkaloids inhibit prolactin secretion and therefore may be associated with decreased udder development. Weak foals have been associated with a late-gestation ration of fungus-infested fescue.

43. What nutrients and feeding strategies have been associated with exertional myopathy?

High-grain diets (high in carbohydrate and digestible energy), especially when fed while the horse is not working, have been associated with an increased occurrence of exertional myopathy. In addition, deficiencies of selenium and vitamin E may increase the risk of exertional myopathy.

44. Describe the role of nutrients and feeding systems in the etiology of laminitis.

High-grain, low-forage diets as well as a sudden change in diet and/or low water consumption have been associated with laminitis.

45. Describe the role of nutrient management in chronic obstructive pulmonary disease (COPD).

Dusty grains and hays should be avoided in the management of COPD. Strategies include adding molasses to grain mixes, feeding pelleted feeds, and soaking hay in water (for a maximum of 10 minutes) before feeding.

BIBLIOGRAPHY

1. Bridges CH, Harris ED: Experimentally induced cartilaginous fractures (osteochondrosis dissecans) in foals fed low-copper diets. J Am Vet Med Assoc 193:215, 1988.
2. Bridges CH, Moffit PG: Influence of variable content of dietary zinc on copper metabolism of weanling foals. Am J Vet Res 51:275, 1990.
3. Buechner-Maxwell VA: Enteral feeding of sick newborn foals. Compend Cont Educ Pract Vet 20:222, 1998.
4. Carroll CL, Huntington PJ: Body condition scoring and weight estimation of horses. Equine Vet J 20:41–45, 1988.
5. Cohen ND, Matejka PL, et al: Case-control study of the association between various management factors and development of colic in horses. J Am Vet Med Assoc 206:667, 1995.
6. Cohen ND, Peloso JG: Risk factors for history of previous colic and for chronic intermittent colic in a population of horses. J Am Vet Med Assoc 208:697, 1996.
7. Frape DL: Dietary requirements and athletic performance of horses. Equine Vet J 20:163, 1988.
8. Hanson RR, Pugh DG, Schumacher J: Feeding equine athletes. Compend Cont Educ Pract Vet 18:175, 1996.
9. Henneke DR, Potter GD, Krieder JL, et al: Relationship between condition score, physical measurements, and body fat percentage in mares. Equine Vet J 15:371–372, 1983.
10. King SS, Nequin LG: An artificial method to produce optimum growth in orphaned foals. Equine Vet Sci 9:319, 1989.
11. Kronfeld DS, Meacham TN, Donoghue S: Dietary aspects of orthopedic diseases in young horses. Vet Clin North Am Equine Pract 6:451, 1990.
12. Lewis LD (ed): Equine Clinical Nutrition: Feeding and Care. Baltimore, Williams & Wilkins, 1995.
13. Naylor JM, Freeman DE, Kronfield DS: Alimentation of hypophagic horses. Compend Cont Educ Pract Vet 6:S93, 1984.
14. Naylor JM, Ralston SL (eds): Large Animal Clinical Nutrition. St. Louis, Mosby, 1991.
15. Nutrient Requirements of Horses, 5th ed. Washington, DC, National Research Council, 1989.
16. Thatcher CD: Nutritional aspects of developmental orthopedic disease in growing horses. Vet Med July:743, 1991.
17. Valentine BA, Hintz HF, et al: Dietary control of exertional rhabdomyolysis in horses. J Am Vet Med Assoc 212:1588, 1998.

19. ENDOSCOPY

Susan J. Holcombe, V.M.D., M.S., Ph.D., Dip. ACVS

1. How should the horse be restrained for an endoscopic examination of the upper respiratory tract?

Minimal restraint is required for the upper respiratory tract endoscopic examination. The horse should be positioned in a set of stocks, a stanchion, or a stall. A lip twitch may be applied to the upper labia to provide additional restraint. Chemical sedation should *not* be used if upper airway function is to be assessed because sedation affects nasopharyngeal and laryngeal function. Nasopharyngeal collapse (dorsal pharyngeal collapse or dorsal displacement of the soft palate) or laryngeal paralysis may be misdiagnosed if the horse has received sedation before the examination. Chemical restraint is appropriate for endoscopic examination of the nares, guttural pouches (remnants of the eustachian tubes), and trachea.

Gaughan EM, Hackett RP, Ducharme NG, et al: Clinical evaluation of laryngeal sensation in horses. Cornell Vet 80:27–34, 1990.

2. Does the maxillary sinus communicate with the nasal passage?

Yes. The nasomaxillary opening forms the communication between the maxillary sinus and the nasal cavity and lies in the middle meatus. Purulent exudate, blood, or serous discharge draining from the middle meatus indicates sinus pathology.

Nickels FA: The nasal passage. In Traub-Dargatz JL, Brown CM (eds): Equine Endoscopy, 2nd ed. St. Louis, Mosby, 1997, p 29.

3. What are the differential diagnoses for a horse with unilateral, serosanguinous nasal discharge, reduced airflow through the nostril, and nasal stertor?

Differential diagnoses include ethmoid hematoma, fungal granuloma, nasal tumor or polyp, foreign body, paranasal sinusitis, or trauma that may have caused a nasal bone fracture. Endoscopic examination of the nasal passage confirms the presence of a mass. The biopsy instrument can be passed through the biopsy channel of the endoscope, and the mass can be biopsied to confirm its origin. Alternately, a uterine biopsy forceps can be advanced along the ventral meatus, ventral or dorsal to the endoscope, and used to obtain a biopsy. If no mass is seen within the nasal passage or ethmoid turbinate region, skull radiographs help to confirm or refute the presence of a nasal or incisive bone fracture or a mass within the conchae or sinuses.

4. Which sinuses can be examined during sinoscopy?

The dorsal conchal, frontal, caudomaxillary, and sphenopalatine sinuses can be examined during sinoscopy. The rostromaxillary and ventrocochal sinuses cannot be readily evaluated during this procedure. The rostromaxillary sinus may be visualized if the septum between it and the caudomaxillary sinus has been destroyed during the disease process.

Ruggles AJ, Ross MW, Freeman DE: Endoscopic examination of normal paranasal sinuses in horses. Vet Surg 20:418–423, 1991.

5. What are the differential diagnoses for mucopurulent discharge at the nasomaxillary opening?

Primary sinusitis and secondary sinusitis caused by a tooth root abscess, sinus cyst, or neoplasia are possible diagnoses. Skull radiographs or direct examination of the sinus via sinoscopy may be valuable diagnostic tools. Masses may be biopsied during the sinoscopy procedure, and debridement and lavage of the sinus may be therapeutic.

Ruggles AJ, Ross MW, Freeman DE: Endoscopic examination and treatment of paranasal sinus disease in 16 horses. Vet Surg 22:508–514, 1993.

6. Why can horses breathe only through the nose?

The horse is an obligate nasal breather, perhaps to allow maintenance of the olfactory senses during deglutition. The normal epiglottis is positioned dorsal to the soft palate and contacts the caudal free margin, forming a tight seal around the base of the larynx. The pillars of the soft palate form the lateral margins and converge dorsally, forming the palatal pharyngeal arch (Fig. 1, see page 292). The epiglottic-soft palate conformation necessitates nasal breathing in the horse. However, if the soft palate is displaced dorsal to the epiglottis, the rima glottis communicates with the oral pharynx, and the horse is capable of oral breathing, which occurs in some horses during episodes of dorsal displacement of the soft palate.

Niinimaa V, Cole P, Mintz S: The switching point from nasal to oronasal breathing. Respir Physiol 42:61–71, 1980.

7. What is dorsal displacement of the soft palate (DDSP)?

DDSP is a performance-limiting upper airway obstructive disease that occurs during high-intensity exercise. The caudal free margin of the soft palate displaces dorsal to the epiglottis so that the epiglottis cannot be seen in the nasopharynx (Fig. 2). The soft palate billows across the rima glottis during exhalation, creating an expiratory obstruction (Fig. 3).

Haynes PF: Dorsal displacement of the soft palate and epiglottic entrapment: Diagnosis, management, and interrelationship. Compend Cont Educ 5:S379–S388, 1983.

Rehder RS, Ducharme NG, Hackett RP, et al: Measurement of upper airway pressures in exercising horses with dorsal displacement of the soft palate. Am J Vet Res 56:269–274, 1995.

8. How is DDSP diagnosed?

There are two distinct clinical presentations of DDSP: permanent and intermittent. **Permanent DDSP** usually occurs in dysphagic horses and is caused by damage to the pharyngeal plexus of nerves, which provides motor innervation to some of the soft palate muscles (palatinus, palatopharyngeus, and levator veli palatini) and the dorsal pharyngeal constricting muscles (pterygopharyngeus, hyopharyngeus, thyropharyngeus, and cricopharyngeus). Guttural pouch empyema, abscessed retropharyngeal lymph nodes, and guttural pouch lavage with caustic solution can cause dysphasia and permanent DDSP. Permanent DDSP is easily diagnosed by endoscopic examination of the nasopharynx.

Intermittent DDSP is a dynamic condition that occurs during intense exercise. The nasopharynx may appear normal during endoscopic examination at rest. A 60-second nasal occlusion test can be performed by manually occluding the horse's nares. Breathing against the nasal obstruction crudely mimics the pressure changes that occur in the nasopharynx and trachea during intense exercise. Tracheal and nasopharyngeal inspiratory and expiratory pressures achieved during 60 seconds of nasal occlusion equal or exceed the airway pressures during intense exercise. DDSP was induced by nasal occlusion in 11% of horses examined at rest. Fifty-seven percent of these horses displaced the soft palate during incremental treadmill exercise test, whereas only 14% of horses that did not displace at rest exhibited DDSP during treadmill exercise, suggesting that DDSP during resting endoscopic examination is a strong indication of DDSP during intense exercise.

Hare WCD: Equine respiratory system. In Getty R (ed): Sisson and Grossman's The Anatomy of Domestic Animals, 5th ed. Philadelphia, W.B. Saunders, 1975, pp 504–511.

Holcombe SJ, Derksen FJ, Stick JA, et al: Effects of nasal occlusion on tracheal and pharyngeal pressures in horses. Am J Vet Res 57:1258–1260, 1996.

Parente EJ: Diagnosing upper airway obstructive disease. In Proceedings of the Sixth Symposium of the American College of Veterinary Surgeons. 1996, pp 172–173.

9. Why is it important to watch the horse swallow during the endoscopic examination of the larynx and nasopharynx?

The horse can be stimulated to swallow by spraying water into the nasopharynx through the endoscope or by tactile stimulation of the piriform recesses or epiglottis. The swallow tests the neuromuscular coordination of many muscles in the nasopharynx, including the soft palate, dorsal pharyngeal constrictor, and intrinsic laryngeal muscles. Specifically, the sphincter that forms in the nasopharynx during swallowing is formed by the dorsal pharyngeal constrictor muscles and the levator veli palatini muscles (Fig. 4). In addition, the corniculate processes of the arytenoid cartilages completely adduct (Fig. 5) during the swallow and then maximally abduct after the swallow (see Fig. 1). Therefore, if laryngeal hemiplegia is suspected, swallowing tests the adduction and maximal abduction of the corniculate processes.

10. What is pharyngitis?

Pharyngitis is inflammation of the nasopharynx and enlargement of the diffuse lymph tissue in the nasopharynx. Pharyngitis or lymphoid hyperplasia ranges from mild to severe (grades 1–4) and occurs during viral or bacterial upper respiratory tract infections or environmentally induced inflammation. Typically, young horses have grades 2–4 lymphoid hyperplasia, which does not affect performance.

Baker GJ: Diseases of the pharynx. In Robinson NE (ed): Current Therapy in Equine Medicine, 2nd ed. Philadelphia, W.B. Saunders, 1987, pp 609–610.

11. What is grade 3 laryngeal hemiplegia?

Laryngeal function has been classified by a four-tier grading scheme:

Grade 1 arytenoid function: normal function; right and left arytenoids move symmetrically; both right and left arytenoids can abduct maximally.

Grade 2 arytenoid function: normal function; right and left arytenoids move asymmetrically; both right and left arytenoids can abduct maximally.

Grade 3 arytenoid function: abnormal function; right and left arytenoids move asymmetrically; either the right or the left arytenoid (usually the left) arytenoid cannot abduct maximally but has motion (Fig. 6).

Grade 4 arytenoid function: abnormal function; right and left arytenoids move asymmetrically; either the right or the left arytenoid (usually the left) has no motion (complete paralysis) (Fig. 7).

Horses with grade 3 left laryngeal hemiplegia cannot maximally abduct the left arytenoid cartilage.

12. Is grade 3 left laryngeal hemiplegia performance-limiting? How is this determined?

Some diagnosed with grade 3 laryngeal hemiplegia collapse the left corniculate process during intense exercise, resulting in airway obstruction. Therefore, if the horse is diagnosed with grade 3 laryngeal hemiplegia, endoscopic examination of the airway during incremental treadmill exercise testing is indicated to determine whether the corniculate process collapses during intense exercise.

Rakestraw PC, Hackett RP, Ducharme NG, et al: Arytenoid cartilage movement in resting and exercising horses. Vet Surg 20:122–127, 1991.

13. What is epiglottic retroflexion?

Epiglottic retroflexion is an uncommon obstructive airway disease that occurs when the epiglottis moves during inhalation into the rima glottis, creating airway obstruction, and returns to a normal position during exhalation (Fig. 8). The cause of this syndrome is unknown.

14. Why is endoscopic examination of the guttural pouches an important part of the upper respiratory tract examination?

The guttural pouches or eustachian tube remnants are unique to the horse and may be considered the "hard drive" of the upper airway. Most of the efferent and afferent innervation of the nasopharynx and larynx courses through the guttural pouch. The glossopharyngeal and hypoglossal nerves course through the medial compartment and provide sensory innervation to the nasopharynx and tongue and motor innervation to the tongue and cranial hyoid muscles, respectively (Fig. 9). The pharyngeal branch of the vagus nerve branches from the parent nerve at the level of the sympathetic ganglion in the medial compartment and travels rostroventrally, crossing the longus capitis muscle before ramifying in the pharyngeal plexus of nerves. This nerve is intimately associated with the retropharyngeal lymph nodes, which can be seen beneath the membrane in the floor of the medial compartment. Bacterial and fungal infections also may occur in the guttural pouch. Fungal plaques may adhere to and grow in the vicinity of the internal carotid artery and, less frequently, the maxillary and external carotid arteries.

Hare WCD: Equine respiratory system. In Getty R (ed): Sisson and Grossman's The Anatomy of Domestic Animals, 5th ed. Philadelphia, W.B. Saunders, 1975, pp 504–511.

15. How is the guttural pouch examined?

Insert the endoscope through the ventral meatus to a length of approximately 25–35 cm to visualize the nasopharyngeal openings of the guttural pouches (plica salphingopharyngea). If the endoscope is in the left nasal passage, rotate the endoscope so that the left guttural pouch opening is viewed in a horizontal fashion with the slit on the topside. Then slide the endoscope biopsy instrument under the nasopharyngeal opening of the guttural pouch (keep the biopsy instrument in the mid-to-dorsolateral region to ensure that it does not get caught on the sides of the opening). Rotate the endoscope, which will abduct the opening of of the guttural pouch. At this stage, advance the endoscope (it will follow the line of the biopsy instrument) into the guttural pouch. Immediately retract the biopsy instrument into the endoscope. To enter the right guttural pouch, the guttural pouch opening may be viewed in a vertical manner. (**Note:** Different techniques may be used for the right and left pouches because of the asymmetric exit position of the biopsy instrument form the end of the endoscope.) The biopsy instrument is advanced into the right guttural pouch, and the endoscope is rotated to open the plica salphingopharyngea. Then the endoscope is advanced in the manner described above. Note that the larger compartment is the medial compartment; this distinction helps to orient the endoscope.

A Chamber's catheter may be used also to elevate the cartilaginous flap that forms the nasopharyngeal opening of the guttural pouch. It may be used as a guide and opener to advance the endoscope into the pouch; however, there is greater risk of damaging the endoscope when an external instrument is used. The endoscope should be advanced dorsally and laterally over the plica salphingopharyngea. Once the endoscope is positioned within the guttural pouch, the Chamber's catheter should be retracted gently.

16. What are the differential diagnoses for hemorrhage from the guttural pouch? How are these conditions distinguished?

Guttural pouch mycosis may result in hemorrhage from the guttural pouch. The mycotic plaque may erode through a blood vessel within the guttural pouch (most frequently the internal carotid artery, but the maxillary and external carotid arteries also may be affected), resulting in life-threatening hemorrhage. Guttural pouch hemorrhage also may be caused by avulsion of the rectus capitis and longus capitis muscles, usually as a result of trauma. Endoscopic examination of the guttural pouches, the history, and skull radiographs help to differentiate the two causes of guttural pouch hemorrhage.

Freeman DE: Guttural pouches. In Beech J (ed): Equine Respiratory Disorders. Philadelphia, Lea & Febiger, 1991, pp 305–330.

Sweeney CR, Freeman DE, Sweeney RW, et al: Hemorrhage into the guttural pouch (auditory tube diverticulum) associated with rupture of the longus capitis muscle in 3 horses. J Am Vet Med Assoc 202:1129–1131, 1993.

17. Why may a horse with strangles (*Streptococcus equi* infection) have purulent exudate draining from the guttural pouch?

The retropharyngeal lymph node chain can be seen beneath the floor of the ventromedial compartment of the guttural pouch. Abscess and rupture into the guttural pouch, especially of the median retropharyngeal lymph node, may lead to purulent drainage from the pouch (Fig. 10).

18. How can arytenoid chondritis be distinguished from left laryngeal hemiplegia?

Both diagnoses can be made by endoscopic examination. Arytenoid chondritis is similar to laryngeal hemiplegia because in both cases the arytenoid cartilage may have little-to-no movement other than passive movement. However, in arytenoid chondritis the arytenoid cartilage is deformed, the mucosa is swollen and hyperemic, and frequently a bud of granulation tissue and exudate protrude from the axial aspect of the cartilage into the rima glottis. In addition, horses with arytenoid chondritis frequently have rostral displacement of the palatopharyngeal arch (Fig. 11). In left laryngeal hemiplegia, the arytenoid cartilage has little-to-no movement other than passive movement, but the cartilage is not deformed, and no abscess or granulation tissue is present (see Fig. 7).

19. Which laryngeal cartilages can be seen during endoscopy of the upper airway?

The larynx is formed by paired arytenoid and thyroid cartilages, the cricoid cartilage, and the epiglottic cartilage. The corniculate processes of the arytenoid cartilages and the epiglottic cartilage can be seen during the endoscopic examination.

20. How are epiglottic entrapment and DDSP differentiated?

Although both syndromes can cause upper respiratory obstruction, they are very different, and the differences are clear during the endoscopic examination. DDSP occurs when the caudal free margin of the soft palate displaces dorsally to the epiglottis so that the epiglottis is no longer visible in the nasopharynx (see Fig. 2). The soft palate billows across the rima glottis during exercise and causes the obstruction. Epiglottic entrapment results from inflammation of the aryepiglottic tissue beneath the epiglottis. This tissue swells and envelops the epiglottis, forming the entrapping membrane. The redundant aryepiglottic tissue billows in the airway, causing the obstruction (Fig. 12).

21. Can other structures associated with the larynx create dynamic obstructions?

Yes. The vocal folds may collapse during intense exercise, causing inspiratory obstruction, and the aryepiglottic folds may invert axially, resulting in airway obstruction (Fig. 13). Vocal fold collapse may accompany grades 3 and 4 laryngeal hemiplegia or be the sole obstructive airway lesion.

22. Can a tracheal wash or bronchoalveolar lavage (BAL) be performed using the endoscope?

Yes. Both procedures can be performed using the endoscope. Performing a **tracheal wash** with the endoscope avoids the complications associated with percutaneous tracheal puncture. Because of contamination of the endoscope as it is passed transnasally, a guarded catheter is passed through the biopsy channel. To retrieve fluid that is valuable for culture and sensitivity techniques, the endoscope and the water bottle must be thoroughly cleaned between each use. The **BAL** can be performed using the 2–3-meter endoscope. The endoscope is advanced and wedged in a bronchus. Three hundred milliliters of saline are injected through the biopsy port and aspirated in 100-ml aliquots.

23. Why is it necessary to evaluate the trachea during endoscopic examination of the upper airway?

Tracheal deformity and intraluminal masses such as granulomas, neoplasia, and chondritis are rare but may cause airway obstruction when they occur. More common, however, is the presence in the trachea of (1) exudate, (2) blood, or (3) food-tinged fluid, which may indicate (1) inflammation and/or infection, (2) exercise-induced pulmonary hemorrhage or pulmonary abscess/neoplasia, or (3) dysphasia, respectively.

24. If upper airway conformation and function are normal during standing endoscopic examination, when is it necessary to evaluate the airway during an incremental exercise test on the treadmill?

The tendency for dynamic collapse of the unsupported structures of the upper airway is increased during intense exercise because of greater negative inspiratory pressure (from -2 cm H_2O to -40 cm H_2O) generated by thoracic expansion as peak airway flow increases from 5 L/sec at rest to 75 L/sec during intense exercise. Upper airway patency is maintained in the face of negative inspiratory pressure by upper airway muscle contraction, and neuromuscular response increases with increasing negative airway pressure. Therefore, nasopharyngeal and laryngeal dilating muscles show increased activity during intense exercise, and pathologies relating to dysfunction of this neuromuscular mechanism, such as laryngeal hemiplegia, DDSP, and aryepiglottic fold collapse, may be observed.

Lumsden JM, Derksen FJ, Stick JA, et al: Use of flow-volume loops in evaluating upper airway obstruction in exercising horses. Am J Vet Res 54:766–774, 1993.

25. What airway abnormalities can be diagnosed with endoscopic treadmill evaluation?

Dynamic obstructive airway lesions may be diagnosed during treadmill endoscopic examination. Such conditions include corniculate process collapse in a horse with grade 3 left laryngeal hemiplegia (Fig. 14), DDSP (see Fig. 3), vocal fold collapse (see Fig. 13), aryepiglottic fold collapse (Fig. 15), epiglottic retroflexion (see Fig. 8), and dorsal pharyngeal collapse (Fig. 16).

26. Why may esophagoscopy (endoscopic examination of the esophagus) be performed on a horse with esophageal obstruction (choke)?

Esophagoscopy is useful in a horse with esophageal obstruction because the obstructing mass can be identified and the position of the obstruction within the esophagus monitored (Fig. 17). After resolution of the obstruction, the esophagus can be examined and monitored (Fig. 18) for contusion, tears, and preexisting conditions such as strictures and diverticula.

27. How should the horse be prepared for gastroscopy?

The horsed should be fasted for a minimum of 12 hours, although water intake is allowed. A 3-meter endoscope is used to allow visualization of the entire stomach, including the antrum and pylorus. Chemical restraint such as xylazine hydrochloride (0.3–1 mg/kg IV) or detomidine (0.01 mg/kg IV) may be used in combination with butorphenol (0.01–0.02 mg/kg IV).

28. In performing gastroscopy, is there a safe method of passing the endoscope into the horse's esophagus to minimize the hazard that the endoscope will enter the oral cavity and be damaged by chewing?

Yes. The endoscope is advanced through the ventral meatus into the nasopharynx. The biopsy instrument is inserted into the biopsy channel of the endoscope and advanced into the nasopharynx. The biopsy instrument is advanced beneath the palatopharyngeal arch, dorsal to the larynx, and into the esophagus. The endoscope is then advanced over the biopsy instrument and into the esophagus. In essence, the biopsy instrument is used as a guidewire. Once the endoscope is within the proximal esophagus, the biopsy instrument is retracted into the endoscope. Then, using endoscopic insufflation, the esophagus is inflated so that the esophageal mucosa can be identified.

29. Why is gastroscopy performed?

The most common reason that the stomach is examined endoscopically is to confirm the presence of gastric ulcers. Most gastric ulcers occur in the nonglandular region of the stomach (i.e., squamous mucosa) along the margo plicatus, often around or below the cardia of the stomach (Fig. 19). Other reasons that gastroscopy may be performed include assessment of the stomach for gastric neoplasia, such as squamous cell carcinoma, or foreign body obstruction.

30. Can the urinary tract of the horse be examined endoscopically?

Yes. The urinary tract of both male and female horses can be examined endoscopically. The urethra, bladder, urethral openings of the accessory sex glands (male), and ureters can be evaluated. Endoscopic examination of the urinary tract is warranted in horses with abnormal urination or hemospermia. In addition, if one kidney is abnormal endoscopically or cannot be imaged or if one needs to confirm which kidney may be hemorrhaging or producing abnormal urine, both ureters can be evaluated endoscopically from within the bladder.

Vatistas NJ, Snyder JR, Johnson B: Adult stomach and duodenum. In Traub-Dargatz JL, Brown CM (eds): Equine Endoscopy, 2nd ed. St. Louis, Mosby, 1997, pp 172–186.

31. How should the horse and the endoscope be prepared for endoscopic examination of the urinary tract?

Endoscopic examination of the urinary tract is performed in the standing horse. Chemical restraint is suggested to alleviate the horse's anxiety and to allow the penis of male horses to be extended for passage of the endoscope. The endoscope should be sterilized before the examination.

32. If a horse has hematuria, how can the source of hemorrhage be determined?

The source of blood in the urine may be the urethra, accessory sex glands (male), urinary bladder, ureters, or kidneys. The sterilized endoscope is advanced proximally along the urethra. For best visualization of the urethra, air is insufflated to expand it. Evidence of inflammation, such as hyperemia or edema, should be noted, although the urethra generally looks mildly hyperemic when inflated with air. Differential diagnoses for urethral bleeding include proximal urethral defects (in entire and castrated male horses; see chapter 11), urethral viscosities, urethral masses, and urethritis (which must not be confused with the normal mildly hyperemic urethral mucosa seen after air expansion). The colliculus seminalis with paired ejaculatory orifices, bulbourethral gland openings, urethral gland openings, and prostatic ductule openings can be examined in male horses.

Once the endoscope is advanced into the bladder, the mucosal surface of the urinary bladder should be examined for evidence of cystitis or masses that may be the source of hemorrhage. Dorsally, on either side of midline, two slitlike openings can be seen. These are the openings of the ureters. A small volume of urine should be expelled from each opening approximately once per minute. Unilateral hematuria, pyuria, or anuria may be diagnosed by observing urine flow from the ureters. The ureters can be catheterized using endoscopic guidance.

33. Can the accessory sex glands of a stallion be assessed endoscopically?

The urethral openings of the accessory sex glands of the stallion, including the paired ampullae on the colliculus seminalis, prostate gland, seminal vesicles, and paired bulbourethral glands can be seen endoscopically.

Little TV, Holyoak GR: Reproductive anatomy and physiology of the stallion. In Blanchard TL, Varner DD (eds): Stallion Management. Philadelphia, W.B. Saunders, 1992, p 13.

Schott HJ, Narner DD: Urinary tract. In Traub-Dargatz JL, Brown CM (eds): Equine Endoscopy, 2nd ed. St. Louis, Mosby, 1997, pp 187–203.

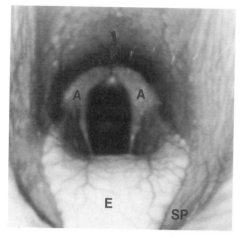

Figure 1. Endoscopic image of a normal nasopharynx and larynx of a horse. Note that the epiglottis (E) is positioned dorsal to the soft palate (SP) and the that the lateral margins of the soft palate or pillars converge dorsal to the corniculate processes of the arytenoid cartilages (A). The palatopharyngeal arch cannot be seen but is formed by the convergence of the lateral pillars of the soft palate and is positioned dorsal to the larynx *(curved arrow).*

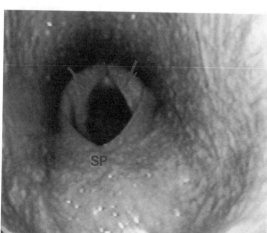

Figure 2. Endoscopic image of the larynx and nasopharynx of a horse with dorsal displacement of the soft palate (DDSP). Note that the epiglottis cannot be seen because the soft palate (SP) is positioned dorsally. The paired corniculate processes of the arytenoid cartilages *(arrows)* are seen.

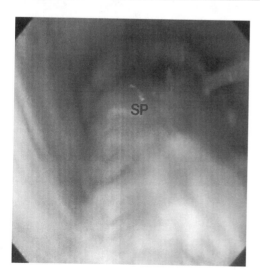

Figure 3. Endoscopic image of the nasopharynx during an episode of DDSP induced by incremental treadmill exercise test. Note that the soft palate (SP) almost completely obstructs the rima glottis during exhalation. Only a small portion of the right corniculate process *(arrow)* is seen.

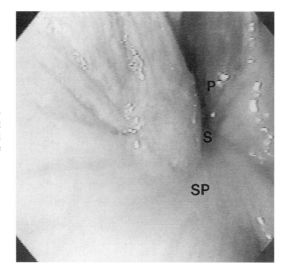

Figure 4. Endoscopic image of the nasopharynx during swallowing. Note that the sphincter (S) is formed as the distal pharynx (P) constricts and the soft palate (SP) is elevated.

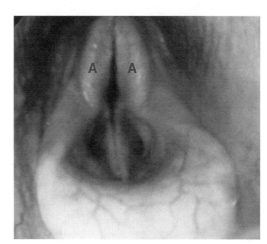

Figure 5. Endoscopic image of the larynx of a horse when the corniculate processes of the arytenoid cartilages (A) are adducted.

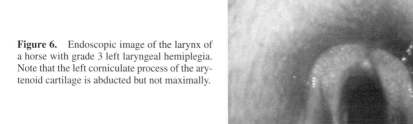

Figure 6. Endoscopic image of the larynx of a horse with grade 3 left laryngeal hemiplegia. Note that the left corniculate process of the arytenoid cartilage is abducted but not maximally.

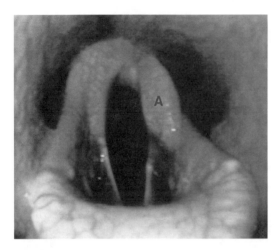

Figure 7. Endoscopic image of the larynx of a horse with grade 4 left laryngeal hemiplegia. Note that the left corniculate process of the arytenoid cartilage (A) remains in a paramedian position.

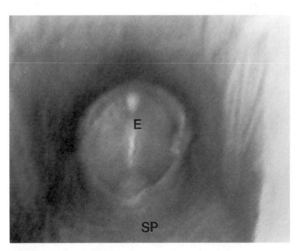

Figure 8. Endoscopic image of the larynx of a horse with epiglottic retroflexion. Note that the ventral surface of the epiglottis (E) is seen and that the caudal free margin of the soft palate (SP) is visible.

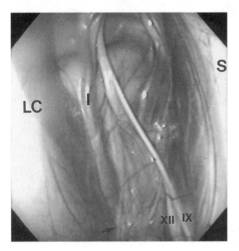

Figure 9. Endoscopic image of the medial compartment of the left guttural pouch of the horse. Note the internal carotid artery (I); glossopharyngeal and hypoglossal nerves (IX and XII) coursing together, with IX dorsal to XII; the longus capitis muscle (LC); and the pharyngeal branch of the vagus nerve (arrow) in the medial compartment. The stylohyoid bone (S) divides the guttural pouch into medial and lateral compartments.

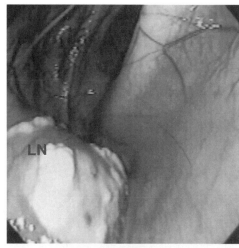

Figure 10. Endoscopic image of the guttural pouch of a horse with strangles. A retropharyngeal lymph node (LN) has ruptured into the guttural pouch. Note the purulent material within the pouch *(arrow)*.

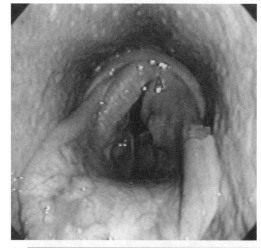

Figure 11. Endoscopic image of the larynx of horse with left arytenoid chondritis. Note the deformed left arytenoid cartilage (A), the granulation tissue *(arrow)*, and the rostral displacement of the palatopharyngeal arch *(curved arrow)*.

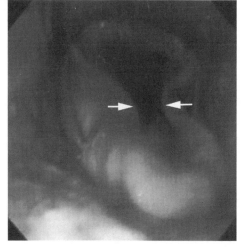

Figure 12. Endoscopic image of the larynx of a horse with collapse of the aryepiglottic folds. This upper airway obstruction was induced during an incremental treadmill examination. Note that the aryepiglottic folds are collapsed axially *(arrows)*, creating an inspiratory obstruction.

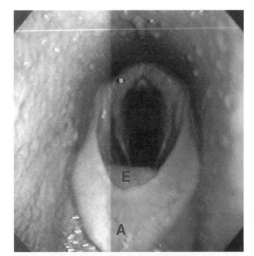

Figure 13. Endoscopic image of the larynx of a horse with epiglottic entrapment. Note the redundant aryepiglottic tissue (A) enveloping the epiglottis (E).

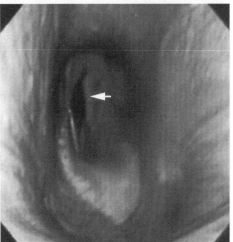

Figure 14. Endoscopic image of the larynx of a horse with grade 3 laryngeal hemiplegia during an incremental treadmill exercise test. Note the dynamic collapse of the left arytenoid cartilage *(arrow)*.

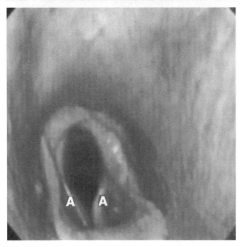

Figure 15. Endoscopic image of the larynx of a horse with vocal fold collapse. This upper airway obstruction was induced during an incremental treadmill examination. Note the vocal folds (V) collapsing axially into the rima glottis.

Figure 16. Endoscopic image of the nasopharynx and larynx of a horse with dorsal pharyngeal collapse. Note the dorsal pharynx (DP) collapsing ventrally into the nasopharynx.

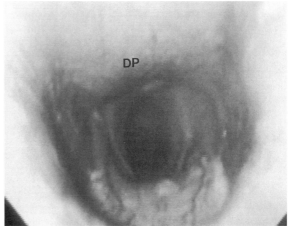

Figure 17 *(right).* Endoscopic image of the esophagus (E) of a horse with esophageal obstruction. Note the fibrous feed causing the obstructing mass (F).

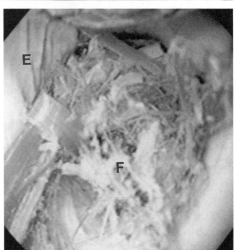

Figure 18 *(below).* Endoscopic image of the esophagus of a horse after an esophageal obstruction has been relieved. *Left,* Note the linear ulceration (U) within the esophagus (E). *Right,* Thirty days after relief, note the circumferential stricture (S) within the esophagus (E).

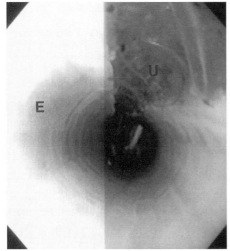

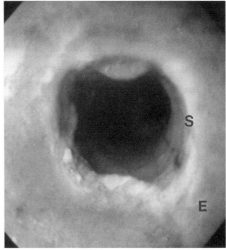

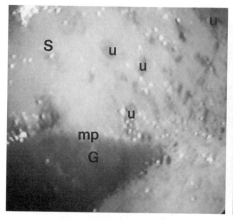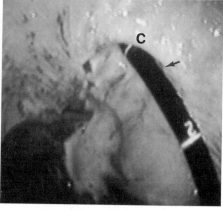

Figure 19. Endoscopic image of the stomach of a horse during gastroscopy. *Left,* Note the margo plicatus (mp), which divides the glandular (G) and squamous (S) regions of the stomach. Also note the ulcers (u) along the margo plicatus and the squamous epithelium. *Right,* Note the endoscope *(arrow)* as it is passed through the cardia (C) of the stomach. Note also the squamous ulceration of the stomach, including the cardiac region.

BIBLIOGRAPHY

1. Baker GJ: Diseases of the pharynx. In Robinson NE (ed): Current Therapy in Equine Medicine, 2nd ed. Philadelphia, W.B. Saunders, 1987, pp 609–610.
2. Freeman DE: Guttural pouches. In Beech J (ed): Equine Respiratory Disorders. Philadelphia, Lea & Febiger, 1991, pp 305–330.
3. Gaughan EM, Hackett RP, Ducharme NG, et al: Clinical evaluation of laryngeal sensation in horses. Cornell Vet 80:27–34, 1990.
4. Hare WCD: Equine respiratory system. In Getty R (ed): Sisson and Grossman's The Anatomy of Domestic Animals, 5th ed. Philadelphia, W.B. Saunders, 1975, pp 504–511.
5. Haynes PF: Dorsal displacement of the soft palate and epiglottic entrapment: Diagnosis, management, and interrelationship. Compend Cont Educ 5:S379–S388, 1983.
6. Holcombe SJ, Derksen FJ, Stick JA, et al: Effects of nasal occlusion on tracheal and pharyngeal pressures in horses. Am J Vet Res 57:1258–1260, 1996.
7. Little TV, Holyoak GR: Reproductive anatomy and physiology of the stallion. In Blanchard TL, Varner DD (eds): Stallion Management. Philadelphia, W.B. Saunders, 1992, p 13.
8. Lumsden JM, Derksen FJ, Stick JA, et al: Use of flow-volume loops in evaluating upper airway obstruction in exercising horses. Am J Vet Res 54:766–774, 1993.
9. Nickels FA: The nasal passage. In Traub-Dargatz JL, Brown CM (eds): Equine Endoscopy, 2nd ed. St. Louis, Mosby, 1997, p 29.
10. Niinimaa V, Cole P, Mintz S: The switching point from nasal to oronasal breathing. Respir Physiol 42:61–71, 1980.
11. Parente EJ: Diagnosing upper airway obstructive disease. In Proceedings of the Sixth Symposium of the American College of Veterinary Surgeons. 1996, pp 172–173.
12. Rakestraw PC, Hackett RP, Ducharme NG, et al: Arytenoid cartilage movement in resting and exercising horses. Vet Surg 20:122–127, 1991.
13. Rehder RS, Ducharme NG, Hackett RP, et al: Measurement of upper airway pressures in exercising horses with dorsal displacement of the soft palate. Am J Vet Res 56:269–274, 1995.
14. Ruggles AJ, Ross MW, Freeman DE: Endoscopic examination of normal paranasal sinuses in horses. Vet Surg 20:418–423, 1991.
15. Ruggles AJ, Ross MW, Freeman DE: Endoscopic examination and treatment of paranasal sinus disease in 16 horses. Vet Surg 22:508–514, 1993.
16. Schott HJ, Narner DD: Urinary tract. In Traub-Dargatz JL, Brown CM (eds): Equine Endoscopy, 2nd ed. St. Louis, Mosby, 1997, pp 187–203.
17. Sweeney CR, Freeman DE, Sweeney RW, et al: Hemorrhage into the guttural pouch (auditory tube diverticulum) associated with rupture of the longus capitis muscle in 3 horses. J Am Vet Med Assoc 202:1129–1131, 1993.
18. Vatistas NJ, Snyder JR, Johnson B: Adult stomach and duodenum. In Traub-Dargatz JL, Brown CM (eds): Equine Endoscopy, 2nd ed. St. Louis, Mosby, 1997, pp 172–186.

20. FLUID THERAPY

Leanne Mary Begg, B.V.Sc., Dip. VCS, M.S., MACVSc, Dip. ACVIM

1. What are the advantages of oral fluid therapy over intravenous fluid therapy?
The advantages of oral fluid therapy include (1) low expense, (2) ease of administration, (3) avoidance of complications associated with intravenous catheterization. However, the intravenous route should be used in the presence of gastric reflux (indicating ileus), other evidence of gastrointestinal dysfunction, or severe dehydration that requires rapid correction.

2. How fast can oral fluids be given?
For the average 500-kg (1100-lb) adult horse, 6–8 L may be administered every 15–20 minutes by gravity flow.

3. Which veins are used in the horse for catheter placement?
The most common veins used for catheter placement are the jugular and cephalic veins. The lateral thoracic and saphenous veins are also used.

4. What are the best methods for stabilizing catheters?
Suturing and/or Super Glue, covered with a sterile bandage.

5. What kind of fluid should you use for intravenous fluid administration?
The answer depends on (1) electrolyte status on the blood biochemistry profile and (2) knowledge of likely potential losses. If these factors are unknown, lactated Ringers' solution is probably the most logical first choice. Normal saline (0.9%) is indicated for hyperkalemia, hyponatremia, hypochloremia (e.g., foals with rupture bladder, acute renal failure), and metabolic alkalosis. The administration of 5% dextrose is appropriate for hypoglycemia and hyperkalemia.

6. What is the maintenance fluid rate for an adult 500-kg (1000-lb) horse?
70 ml/kg/24 hr (approximately 3 ml/kg/hr).

7. What is the maintenance fluid rate for a foal less than 3 weeks of age (approximate weight 50 kg)? Why is it higher than the adult maintenance fluid rate?
The maintenance fluid rate should be 90–120 ml/kg/24 hr (approximately 4 ml/kg/hr). A greater percentage of a foal's body weight is composed of extracellular fluid.

8. How fast should intravenous fluids be given?
The rate of administration of intravenous fluids depends on body size (e.g., adult horse vs. pony vs. foal), the fluid deficit calculated, and continuing losses. A practical method for patients in shock is to start at 10 times maintenance (roughly 30 ml/kg/hr) and decrease to 2–3 times maintenance when deficits have been compensated. Obviously one must be more careful of fluid rates in foals than in adults.

9. What is the ideal catheter type for long-term fluid administration?
Polyurethane catheters are the least thrombogenic and therefore the most appropriate for catheterization of the equine vein, especially if the catheter is to be maintained for longer than 24–48 hours.

10. What laboratory test abnormalities indicate dehydration?
Increased packed cell volume, increased total plasma protein concentration, and elevated serum urea nitrogen and creatinine concentration in the presence of concentrated urine (specific gravity > 1.025).

11. When do you treat an adult horse with intravenous bicarbonate?
When metabolic acidosis is severe (i.e., pH < 7.22). Moderate acidosis may respond simply to treatment of the primary disease process and restoration of the circulating fluid volume.

12. How much bicarbonate do you give?

$$HCO_3^- \text{ (mEq)} = 0.3 \times \text{body weight (kg)} \times \text{base excess (mEq/L)}$$

When bicarbonate is administered, the extracellular fluid is the principal body compartment being treated and accounts for approximately 20% of body weight; however, because some exchange occurs between cells and the extracellular fluid, 30% (0.3) is more accurate. It is safer to administer one-half of this dose and then reevaluate the patient, the blood pH, and gas values. The base excess/base deficit indicates the deviation of bicarbonate from normal (e.g., 24 mEq/L minus HCO_3^- [measured]). Bicarbonate is measured in units of mEq/L or mmol/L (equivalent units).

13. What are the possible complications of intravenous bicarbonate therapy?
- Paradoxical cerebrospinal fluid (CSF) acidosis
- Increased osmolality of the extracellular fluid and increased intravascular volume
- Overshot alkalosis
- Serum electrolyte changes due to change in pH (e.g., increased protein binding of calcium and movement of potassium intracellularly)
- Altered affinity of hemoglobin for oxygen, leading to decreased availability of oxygen at the tissue level (this complication may be associated with cardiac dysrhythmias)

14. What is paradoxical CSF acidosis?

$$HCO_3^- + H^+ = H_2O + CO_2$$

When bicarbonate is administered quickly and intravenously to an adult or immature horse with metabolic alkalosis, CO_2 is produced. CO_2 diffuses more rapidly and easily into cells and through the blood–brain barrier than the administered HCO_3^- and causes an initial intracellular acidosis that may result in altered CSF function due to acute changes in CSF pH. However, this phenomenon is rare.

15. How fast can potassium supplementation be safely given in intravenous fluids?
No faster than 1 mEq/kg/hour (to prevent cardiotoxicity). Potassium may be supplemented in intravenous fluids safely by adding 20 mEq/per liter of fluids given at a fluid rate up to 4 times maintenance.

16. How fast can calcium supplementation be safely administered in intravenous fluids?
Up to 24 mg/kg/hour has been shown to be safe in the literature. One gram of calcium borogluconate equals 4.1 mEq, which equates to roughly 0.1 mEq/kg/hour. However, equine veterinarians commonly use 20–100 ml of 23% calcium borogluconate solution diluted in a 5–6 L bag of isotonic fluids per hour (i.e., 9–46 mg calcium borogluconate/kg/hr).

17. To what solutions should calcium not be added?
Calcium should not be added to any solution containing bicarbonate because an insoluble calcium carbonate precipitate will form.

18. What is the difference between major and minor cross-matches?

A major cross-match detects recipient antibodies to donor cells (think of this as the *major* reason for which blood is given for donor cells). The minor cross-match is used to identify antibodies against recipient cells in donor serum.

19. How much blood can a horse lose before showing signs of shock?

Approximately 30% of blood volume (remember that blood volume is 7–8% of body weight).

20. After acute blood loss, how long does it take to redistribute interstitial fluid from tissue spaces into the vasculature?

Redistribution takes from 12–24 hours; therefore, hematologic changes (e.g., PCV) do not correlate with the degree of blood loss during this time. For example, in an acutely bleeding horse, the PCV may still be in the range of 20–35%.

21. What receptors are triggered during acute blood loss? What are their effects?

Arterial baroreceptors in the carotid sinus and aortic arch, together with the atrial volume receptors in the walls of the left and right cardiac atria, are triggered in patients with acute blood loss. The immediate reflex effect is to increase sympathetic tone and decrease parasympathetic tone. The atrial volume receptors also have important hormonal effects: on the hypothalamus via the pituitary to increase antidiuretic hormone (ADH) release and decrease urine production; on the hypothalamus to stimulate thirst; and on the kidney to release renin, which increases the production of angiotensin II. Angiotensin II is a potent vasopressor agent and also results in increased aldosterone production, which decreases sodium excretion and therefore increases blood volume.

22. When is a blood transfusion indicated?

A rapid decline in PCV to below 15% or massive blood loss with clinical signs of elevated heart rate, decreased pulse strength, pale mucous membranes, increased capillary refill time, poor jugular distensibility, muscular weakness, or oliguria.

23. How long do erythrocytes (red blood cells) last in the recipient after transfusion?

2–6 days.

24. How long does it take the horse to replace the erythrocyte loss if blood loss is controlled?

Bone marrow shows a proliferative response in about 3 days and begins to replace the erythrocyte loss in 5–7 days if blood loss is controlled. However, if the PCV is 15% or below, it may take 7–21 days to regain a more normal PCV.

25. What is the treatment for acute blood loss?

1. Arrest and control hemorrhage (e.g., ligation, epinephrine spray of ethmoid turbinates).

2. Commence intravenous fluid therapy. The decrease in circulating blood volume rather than a deficit of erythrocytes is responsible for the onset of shock. Therefore, the administration of isotonic fluid replacement is indicated in the immediate management of a horse with acute blood loss. Hypertonic fluid (e.g., hypertonic saline) also may be used but must be followed by isotonic fluid administration.

3. Administration of donor blood.

26. Are agglutinins more important than hemolysins in compatibility testing of horse blood?

Equine alloantibody acts more strongly as hemolysins. Unfortunately, cross-matching procedures primarily demonstrate the presence of agglutinins.

27. What is a universal donor?

The serum of universal donors lacks alloantibodies, and their erythrocytes lack alloantigens Aa and Qa. Such horses ideally should be tested negative for equine infectious anemia (i.e., Coggins test-negative).

28. If one does not have the facilities to cross-match but a blood transfusion is required, what is the safest horse to pick as a donor?

A Standardbred gelding. Naturally occurring alloantibody in horses has a low incidence and weak character. Most Standardbreds are Aa- and Qa-negative and a gelding will not have had a pregnancy to become sensitized and produce alloantibody.

29. If one does not have the facilities to cross-match, when is it safest to give a second transfusion?

Usually it requires at least 4–7 days for production of alloantibody; thus subsequent transfusions should be safe before 4 days.

30. How much blood should be administered to a horse after acute blood loss?

The following formula is used to calculate the blood volume required to restore PCV to a certain level (e.g., 30%):

$$(30 - PCV_R) (0.08 \times BW_R)/PCV_D$$

where PCV_R = PCV of the recipient, PCV_D = PCV of the donor, BW_R = body weight of the recipient, and 0.08 = 8% of body weight that is blood volume. However, if the horse has just bled, the PCV will not yet be accurate. It will not be as low as it will be after redistribution of interstitial fluid 12–24 hours later. Hence the PCV_R may not be accurate at first, and more blood may be required.

31. How much blood can be collected safely from an adult donor?

An adult horse can safely donate approximately 20% of its blood volume, i.e., 8 L from a 500-kg horse with a blood volume of approximately 40 L.

32. What reactions may be seen during administration of blood transfusion to a horse?

Anaphylactic reactions and hemolytic reactions may be seen. The transfusion should be stopped immediately if one sees restlessness, dyspnea, polypnea, tachycardia, defecation, muscle fasciculations, or sudden collapse. Then 3–5 ml of epinephrine of 1:1000 dilution should be administered intramuscularly or subcutaneously. Corticosteroid therapy (e.g., prednisolone sodium succinate, 0.25–1.0 mg/kg by slow IV infusion) also may be beneficial. Clinical signs of hemolytic reactions include fever, tachycardia, tachypnea, weakness, tremors, renal failure or collapse.

33. Does oxygen therapy help a horse with hypoxia due to acute blood loss?

No. The reduction in oxygen-carrying capacity is due to a decreased content of hemoglobin; therefore, oxygen therapy is not beneficial.

34. What is endotoxin?

Endotoxin is the lipopolysaccharide (LPS) cell wall component of gram-negative bacteria. It consists of lipid A (the common toxic moiety, which is a poor immunogen), core polysaccharide (considerable hemology exists among various gram-negative endotoxins, and it is highly antigenic), and O polysaccharides (which vary with the species and the serotype of gram-negative organism and are highly antigenic). Interaction of lipid A with tissue macrophages causes the release of several mediators, which are subsequently responsible for the pathologic changes of endotoxemia.

35. What is hyperimmune plasma? How is it made?

Horses are immunized with J5, a mutant strain of *Escherichia coli* that lacks an enzyme necessary for completion of the lipopolysaccharide core and subsequent attachment of the O polysaccharides. The incomplete core of J5 lipopolysaccharide is capable of inducing antibodies, which cross-react with a number of gram-negative organisms. Plasma is harvested from these horses and frozen.

36. How much hyperimmune plasma do you give?
4.4 mg/kg (approximately 2 L in a 450-kg horse).

37. What is the difference between fresh plasma and fresh frozen plasma?
Fresh plasma has platelets, coagulation factors (including antithrombin III), and plasma proteins. It may be stored at room temperature (25–26° C) for up to 8 hours. Fresh frozen plasma must be collected and frozen within 6 hours of collection. It provides coagulation factors (including antithrombin III) and colloid but does not provide platelets. Fresh frozen plasma may be stored at –40° C for 1 year.

38. What is the difference between fresh frozen plasma and frozen plasma?
Frozen plasma is defined as plasma collected and frozen later than 6 hours after collection. It may be used as colloid; it is not a significant source of coagulation factors or platelets. Frozen plasma may be stored at –40° C for up to 2 years.

39. How much plasma do you need to give a 500-kg (1100-lb) horse in an attempt to replace protein loss if the plasma protein of the recipient is 30 gm/L (3.0 gm/dl) and the plasma protein of the donor is 60 gm/L (6.0 gm/dl)?
The blood volume of a 500-kg horse is approximately 8% of body weight (i.e., 8/100 × 500 kg) and thus equals 40 L of blood. The plasma volume is approximately two-thirds of blood volume, which is 2/3 × 40 L = 26 L. If we aim for a plasma protein of 60 gm/L (6.0 gm/dl) for the recipient, the protein deficit = 60 – 30 gm/L = 30 gm/L × 26 L of plasma= 780 gm of protein. Therefore the plasma required is 780 gm/60 gm/L, which is approximately 13 L of plasma. Often plasma transfusions result in a lower posttransfusion total protein than expected, because low-molecular-weight proteins equilibrate with the interstitium and losses may continue as a result of the underlying disease process.

40. How much milk should you feed a sick foal that is receiving total enteral nutrition with milk?
About 20% of body weight per 24 hours divided into at least 2 hourly feedings, if the foal is a neonate.

41. What is the best way to administer milk and/or oral fluids to a foal with a poor suckle reflex?
Silicon nasogastric feeding tubes (approximately 10 French) are flexible and soft, and may be left indwelling. They allow the foal to suckle with the tube in place. One disadvantage is that they can be hard to place because they are so flexible. A stylet should be used for passage, and negative pressure on aspiration occurs only within the esophagus. Sometimes an endoscope should be used to ascertain that the tube is in the esophagus. These feeding tubes also need to be flushed with water following milk administration because they easily clog due to their small diameter.

42. If mare's milk is not available, what is the next best natural milk supplement for a foal?
Goat's milk.

43. Who is the best red blood cell donor for a foal with neonatal isoerythrolysis?
The mare, provided that the red blood cells are washed to ensure that no antibodies to the antigens Aa and Qa are administered. It is important that the donor is Aa- and Qa-negative because the foal still has circulating antibodies (i.e., from colostrum ingestion) to Aa- and Qa-positive red blood cells.

44. How much plasma should you give to a foal with failure of passive transfer?

The answer depends on the immunoglobulin level of the plasma; if the level is unknown, give 2–3 L for a 50-kg foal.

45. When can you use colostrum to treat failure of passive transfer? How much do you give?

Colostrum ideally should be used within the first 12 hours of life. If the foal is older than 24 hours, plasma should be administered intravenously. If a plentiful colostrum bank/supply exists, colostrum may still be useful after 12 hours of age for local gastrointestinal antibody administration. In general, the amount of colostrum that should be administered depends on the size of the foal, degree of failure of passive transfer, time of administration, and quality of colostrum. A minimum of 1 L of colostrum with a specific gravity of at least 1.060 to an average 50-kg foal is usually given.

46. What is the mechanism of action of hypertonic saline?

The administration of hypertonic saline (vs. isotonic 0.9% saline) leads to recruitment of extravascular fluids into the vascular compartment. Another theory proposes that a cardiovascular reflex is initiated by stimulation of pulmonary osmoreceptors.

47. What concentration of hypertonic saline is used and at what dose?

7.5% sodium chloride (saline) at 4 ml/kg (e.g., 4 ml $\times$ 500 kg = 2000 ml).

48. What are the advantages of administration of hypertonic saline?

- Small volume produces more rapid response and more marked hemodynamic effects than isotonic solutions.
- Results in increased cardiac output (CO) because of an increase in stroke volume (SV) (CO = HR $\times$ SV) due to plasma volume expansion.
- Vasodilatory effect due to release of vasoactive substances by the tissues and decrease in release of vasopressin and norepinephrine.
- Increased arterial pressure due to increased CO and plasma volume.

49. What are the disadvantages of hypertonic saline administration?

- Short duration of effect (approximately 2 hours); therefore, it must be followed by isotonic fluid administration.
- Worsening of acidosis, which is a transient effect and may be attributable to reperfusion of ischemic areas and/or an increase in anaerobic metabolism and lactate production.

50. What are the contraindications to hypertonic saline use?

- Water deprivation dehydration and sodium concentration elevation.
- May potentiate blood loss in the absence of hemostasis.

BIBLIOGRAPHY

1. Bertone JJ, Gossett KA, Shoemaker KE, et al: Effect of hypertonic vs isotonic saline solution on responses to sublethal *Escherichia coli* endotoxemia in horses. Am J Vet Res 51:999–1007, 1990.
2. Cambier C, Ratz V, Rollin F, et al: The effects of hypertonic saline in healthy and diseased animals. Vet Res Com 21:303–316, 1997.
3. Cunningham JG: Textbook of Veterinary Physiology. Philadelphia, W.B. Saunders, 1992.
4. Grubb TL, Foreman JH, Benson J, et al: Hemodynamic effects of calcium gluconate administered to conscious horses. J Vet Int Med 10:401–404, 1996.
5. Johnson PJ: Electrolyte and acid-base disturbances in the horse. Vet Clin North Am (Equine Pract) 11:491–514, 1995.
6. McGinness SG, Mansmann RA, Breuhaus BA: Nasogastric electrolyte replacement in horses. Compend Cont Educ 18:942–950, 1996.

7. Robinson NE: Current Therapy in Equine Medicine, 3rd ed. Philadelphia, W.B. Saunders, 1992.
8. Schmall LM, Muir WW, Robertson JT: Haemodynamic effects of small volume hypertonic saline in experimentally induced haemorrhagic shock. Equine Vet J 22:273–277, 1990.
9. Schmall LM, Muir WW, Robertson JT: Haematological, serum electrolyte and blood gas effects of small volume hypertonic saline in experimentally induced haemorrhagic shock. Equine Vet J 22:278–283, 1990.
10. Seahorn TL, Cornick-Seahorn J: Fluid therapy. Vet Clin North Am (Equine Pract) 10:517–525, 1994.
11. Spier SJ, Lavoie J-P, Cullor JS, et al: Protection against clinical endotoxemia in horses by using plasma containing antibody to an Rc Mutant E. coli (J5). Circ Shock 28:235–248, 1989.

21. ANTIMICROBIAL THERAPY

J. *Trenton McClure, D.V.M., M.S., Dip. ACVIM, and*
Jill J. McClure, D.V.M., M.S., Dip. ACVIM, ABVP

1. What are the sites and mechanisms of action of the various classes of antimicrobial agents? Which are bactericidal and which are bacteriostatic?

Overview of Antimicrobial Agents

CLASS	SITE OF ACTION	MECHANISM OF ACTION	BACTERI-CIDAL	BACTERIO-STATIC
Penicillin, cephalosporins (i.e., β-lactams)	Cell wall	β-lactam ring binds irreversibly with penicillin-binding proteins (enzymes) causing inhibition of cross-linking of peptidoglycan layer of cell wall. This results in structural failure of bacterial cell wall.	+	Occasionally
Vancomycin	Cell wall	Blocks transfer of pentapeptide from cytoplasm to cell membrane (i.e., inhibits cell wall micropeptide synthesis)	+	Occasionally
Polymyxin B, polymyxin C (colistin)	Cytoplasmic membrane	Bind phospholipid and disrupt cell membrane permeability.	+	
Aminoglycosides	Ribosome	Bind to 30s subunit of ribosome and therefore interfere with messenger RNA (mRNA) translation and disrupt elongation by incorporation of wrong amino acids (i.e., inhibition of attachment of mRNA); also affect transfer RNA (tRNA).	+	
Tetracyclines	Ribosome	Bind to 30s ribosomal subunit and inhibit binding of tRNA to mRNA, thereby preventing protein synthesis by bacteria.		+
Chloramphenicol	Ribosome	Binds to 50s ribosomal subunit and inhibits tRNA insertion, thus decreasing protein synthesis.	Occasionally	+
Erythromycin	Ribosome	Binds to 50s ribosomal subunit (specifically 23S ribosomal RNA molecule); inhibits mRNA translation and bacterial protein synthesis.	Occasionally	+
Rifampin	Nucleic acid synthesis	Impairs RNA and thus protein formation by binding and inhibiting DNA-dependent RNA polymerase.	+	Occasionally
Metronidazole	Nucleic acid synthesis	Damages nucleic acid structure.	+	
Quinolones	Nucleic acid synthesis	Inhibit bacterial DNA gyrase.	+	

Table continued on following page

Overview of Antimicrobial Agents (Continued)

CLASS	SITE OF ACTION	MECHANISM OF ACTION	BACTERI-CIDAL	BACTERIO-STATIC
Pyrimidines (trimethoprim, pyrimethamine)	Nucleic acid synthesis	Inhibit dihydrofolate reductase, thus inhibiting folic acid (dihydrofolic acid) conversion to folinic acid (tetrahydrofolic acid).		+
Sulfonamides	Nucleic acid synthesis	Compete with para-amino benzoic acid (PABA) for dihydropteroate syn-thetase, which is responsible for synthesis of dihydropteroate acid, the immediate precursor of folic acid; block formation of thymidine and purines		+
Trimethoprim-sulfonamides	See above	See above; synergistic effect (syner-gism promotes bactericidal effect).	+	

Beard LA: Principles of antimicrobial therapy. In Reed SM, Bayly WM (eds): Equine Internal Medicine. Philadelphia, W.B. Saunders, 1998, pp 157–187.

Hooper DC, Wolfson JS: Fluoroquinolone antimicrobial agents. N Engl J Med 324:384, 1991.

2. What is the minimal inhibitory concentration (MIC)? What is the minimal bactericidal concentration (MBC)?

The **MIC** represents the minimal concentration of a given antimicrobial that inhibits the growth of a given pathogen in vitro but will not kill it. It is usually expressed in micrograms per milliliter ($\mu g/ml$).

The **MBC** represents the minimal concentration of a given antimicrobial that kills a given pathogen in vitro. The MBC is often 2–4 times the MIC for the same isolate.

3. What determines whether an antimicrobial is considered bacteriostatic or bactericidal?

If the MIC and MBC are similar (one or two dilutions apart), a drug is considered bacterici-dal. If the MBC is several dilutions higher than the MIC, a drug is considered bacteriostatic.

4. What is the spectrum of activity of common antibacterial drugs?

	BACTERIA	MYCOPLASMA	RICKETTSIA	CHLAMYDIA	PROTOZOA
Aminoglycosides	+	+	–	–	–
Beta-lactams	+	–	–	–	–
Chloramphenicol	+	+	+	+	–
Lincosamides	+	+	–	–	+
Macrolides	+	+	–	+	–
Pleuromutilins	+	+	–	+	–
Tetracyclines	+	+	+	+	–
Quinolones	+	+	+	+	–
Sulfonamides	+	+	–	–	+
Trimethoprim	+	–	–	–	+

From Prescott JF, Baggot JD (eds): Antimicrobial Therapy in Veterinary Medicine, 2nd ed. Ames, IA, Iowa State University Press, 1993, p 4, with permission.

5. What constitutes a β-lactam antimicrobial?

An antimicrobial drug that contains a β-lactam ring structure. Examples include penicillins (e.g., procaine penicillin G, potassium penicillin, ampicillin), cephalosporins (e.g, ceftiofur, cefo-taxime), carbapenems (e.g, imipenem), and monobactams (e.g. aztreonam).

6. What are the different classifications for penicillins and their spectrum of activity?

1. **Natural penicillins.** Penicillin G is the parent drug of this family (e.g., potassium penicillin G, sodium penicillin G, procaine penicillin G, and benzathine penicillin G). The spectrum of action is primarily gram-positive aerobic and anaerobic bacteria. Natural penicillins are the drugs of choice for streptococcal infections. They are inactivated by β-lactamases. Staphylococci, enterococci, *Bacteroides fragilis*, and *Clostridium difficile* have significant and increasing resistance to penicillins. Penicillin G also has moderate activity against a few gram-negative organisms, such as *Actinobacillus* and *Pasteurella* species, although these organisms may require higher and more frequent dosing. Use against gram-negative organisms should be based on culture and sensitivity/MIC information.

2. **Broad-spectrum penicillins.** This family includes ampicillin and amoxicillin. Although broad-spectrum penicillins have slightly less activity against most gram-positive aerobes and anaerobes compared with natural penicillins, the difference in potency is rarely clinically significant. They also have an increased activity against enterococci, *Listeria* species, and gram-negative aerobic bacteria, including *Escherichia coli, Proteus mirabilis*, and *Salmonella* species. Unfortunately, because of extensive use, increasing resistance has developed among gram-negative organisms so that ampicillin's spectrum of activity is not as broad as it was originally.

3. **Extended-spectrum penicillins.** These semisynthetic drugs, derived from ampicillin, include mezlocillin and piperacillin. They have a very broad spectrum of activity, including many anaerobes, gram-positive aerobes, and gram-negative aerobes, including most Enterobacteriaceae and *Pseudomonas* species.

4. **Penicillinase-resistant penicillins.** Methicillin was the first compound in this class. Penicillinase-resistant penicillins have good activity against streptococci and staphylococci, including penicillinase-producing staphylococci. They have no activity against gram-negative bacteria. They should be used only for treating penicillinase-producing staphylococcal infections.

5. **Penicillin plus β-lactamase inhibitors.** A penicillin is combined with a β-lactamase inhibitor (clavulanic acid or sublactam). The inhibitor competes for binding β-lactamase, allowing the penicillin to remain active in the presence of β-lactamase-producing organisms, but does not change the activity of penicillin against bacteria that limit penetration into the cell wall. This combination has no activity against methicillin-resistant staphylococci.

7. What drugs belong to the different classes of penicillin?

NATURAL	BROAD-SPECTRUM	EXTENDED-SPECTRUM	PENICILLINASE-RESISTANT	PENICILLIN PLUS β-LACTAMASE INHIBITORS
Penicillin G	Ampicillin	Ticarcillin	Methicillin	Amoxicillin-clavulanic acid
Penicillin V	Amoxicillin	Carbenicillin	Oxacillin	Ampicillin-sublactam
	Hetacillin	Mezlocillin	Nafcillin	Ticaricillin-clavulanic acid
		Piperacillin	Cloxacillin	
		Azlocillin	Dicloxacillin	

8. What are the different forms of penicillin G? How do they differ?

1. **Aqueous (potassium and sodium) penicillin G** is usually administered intravenously but also can be administered intramuscularly. After administration, it achieves high serum concentrations, but because of a short half-life (30–60 minutes) it is rapidly eliminated. Therefore, frequent administration (every 4–6 hours) is required to maintain therapeutic concentrations.

2. **Procaine penicillin G** is for intramuscular injection (*never* for intravenous administration), which allows slow absorption and results in serum concentration for many hours. Thus dosage frequencies are decreased (every 12 hours). Peak serum concentrations are much lower compared with the aqueous preparation because of the slow absorption rate. However, serum concentrations are still therapeutic for most pathogens for which penicillin use is indicated.

3. **Benzathine penicillin G** is similar to procaine penicillin but allows even slower absorption, which results in a longer duration of detectable serum concentrations but, unfortunately,

much lower serum concentrations. Thus, because of the very low serum concentrations, benzathine penicillin is effective only against the most sensitive bacterial agents, specifically streptococci, and has limited therapeutic use.

9. What are the differences among first-, second-, and third-generation cephalosporins?

This classification, originally intended as a marketing tool, is used clinically to categorize the cephalosporin drugs based on their spectrum of antimicrobial activity. Unfortunately, there are significant differences in spectrums of drugs within the same generation and much overlap in antimicrobial activity among generations, especially for the second- and third-generation cephalosporins. Thus the generation classification is only a general definition with many exceptions.

10. What is the antimicrobial activity of first-, second-, and third-generation cephalosporins?

First-generation cephalosporins have a good gram-positive aerobic spectrum and a moderate spectrum of activity against gram-negative aerobic bacteria, especially *Escherichia coli, Proteus mirabilis,* and *Klebsiella* species. They have a moderate anaerobic spectrum but are inferior to the penicillins.

Compared with the first-generation cephalosporins, **second-generation cephalosporins** have less activity against streptococci and staphylococci and more activity against selected gram-negative bacteria. Some second-generation cephalosporins, specifically cefotetan and cefoxitin, have good activity against anaerobes, including *Bacteroides fragilis,* but poor activity against streptococci and staphylococci.

Third-generation cephalosporins generally have enhanced activity against gram-negative bacteria that are often multidrug-resistant. Only two third-generation cephalosporins—ceftazidime and, to a lesser extent, cefoperazone—have antipseudomonal activity. In general, third-generation cephalosporins have less potency against gram-positive aerobes than first- and second-generation drugs and no-to-moderate anaerobic activity.

11. Which cephalosporins are in which generation?

FIRST GENERATION	SECOND GENERATION	THIRD GENERATION
Cefazolin	Cefotetan	Ceftiofur
Cephalexin	Cefuroxime	Cefotaxime
Cefadroxil	Cefoxitin	Ceftizoxime
Cephapirin	Cefonicid	Ceftriaxone
Cefaclor	Cefamandole	Ceftazidime
Cephradine		Cefixime
		Cefoperazone

12. How else are cephalosporins classified?

Because the somewhat arbitrary assignment of cephalosporins to various generations has not been satisfactory, another method of classification has been used:

Parenteral group I. Examples include cephalothin, cefazolin (sometimes used in equine orthopedic patients [off-label usage]), and cephaloridine. This group has high activity against gram-positive bacteria and moderate activity against β-lactamase-producing gram-negative bacteria but no activity against *Pseudomonas* species.

Parenteral group II. Examples include ceftiofur, which is labeled for equine use (Naxcel, Pharmacea Upjohn, Kalamazoo, MI); cefotaxime, which has been used to treat equine patients with meningitis; cefotiam; cefuroxime; cefamandole; and cefmenoxime. This group has high activity against the Enterobacteriaceae.

Parenteral group III. This group has high activity against *Pseudomonas* species and related oragnisms. Examples include cefsulodin, ceftazidime, and cefoperazone.

Parenteral group IV. Drugs in this group, also termed cephamycins, have increased activity against *Bacteroides fragilis* and other *Bacteroides* species, because they are stable in the face of β-lactamase production by bacteria. Examples include cefoxitin and cefotetan.

Oral group. Drugs in this group (e.g., cephradine, cephalexin, cefaclor, cefadroxil) are absorbed from the oral route and are active in the body against gram-positive bacteria to a moderate extent. They also have a minimal amount of gram-negative activity but no activity against *Pseudomonas* species. They are not used in equine medicine.

Orsini JA, Perkons S: New beta-lactam antibiotics in critical care medicine. Compend Contin Educ Pract Vet 16:183–195, 1994.

Prescott JF, Baggott JD (eds): Antimicrobial Therapy in Veterinary Medicine, 2nd ed. Ames, IA, Iowa State University Press, 1997, pp 100–118.

13. What factors should be considered in selecting an antimicrobial drug for treatment of a bacterial infection?

1. Determine whether antimicrobial therapy is necessary. Mild infections and localized infections may not need systemic antimicrobial therapy.

2. If treatment is started before obtaining bacterial culture results, base the selection on the susceptibility pattern of the most likely organisms to be causing the disease. If culture results are available, choices should be based on the sensitivity or MIC information.

3. Use an antimicrobial with the narrowest spectrum of activity that will be effective against the known or suspected pathogen(s). This practice limits adverse effects on normal flora and acquisition of resistance.

4. Select a drug with an ability to reach therapeutic concentrations at the site of infection.

5. Consider the drug's toxicity and factors that compound it.

6. Consider the cost of therapy and ease of administration.

14. What are the indications for combination antimicrobial therapy?

• Serious life-threatening infections that are undefined
• Serious infections in hosts with impaired defenses
• Serious life-threatening infections in which the combination of antimicrobials may act synergistically against the infectious organism

15. What types of actions produce synergism between combinations of antimicrobials?

Antimicrobial combinations are frequently synergistic if they involve:

1. Inhibition of successive steps in metabolism (e.g., trimethoprim-sulfonamide)

2. Sequential inhibition of cell wall synthesis (e.g., methicillin-ampicillin)

3. Facilitation of drug entry of one antimicrobial by another (e.g., β-lactam–aminoglycoside)

4. Inhibition of inactivating enzymes (e.g., ampicillin-clavulanic acid)

5. Prevention of emergence of resistant populations (e.g, erythromycin-rifampin, streptomycin-isoniazid)

16. What types of actions generally produce antagonism between combinations of antimicrobials?

1. Combining a bacteriostatic with a bactericidal drug.

2. Antimicrobials with the same site of action (e.g., they compete for the same binding site).

3. Other cited actions of questionable clinical significance include inhibition of cell permeability mechanisms and derepression of resistance enzymes (e.g., combined β-lactam therapy).

17. How long should you wait after the onset of antimicrobial therapy before determining that a patient is not responding?

For most bacterial infections, a therapeutic response should be seen within 2 days. If an animal has been deteriorating since the onset of therapy and is at risk of dying, a change in antimicrobial therapy is justified at 24–48 hours. On the other hand, certain infections, such as equine protozoal myelitis, require weeks or months before treatment response can be appropriately evaluated.

18. What is an appropriate duration of therapy for most infections?

Treatment should continue at least 2–3 days after clinical and microbiologic resolution of the bacterial infection. For most serious infections treatment should be a minimum of 5–10 days. Infections that tend to be persistent require several weeks to months of therapy. Examples of infections that require prolonged antimicrobial therapy include internal abscesses, osteomyelitis, valvular endocarditis, septic arthritis, and equine protozoal myeloencephalitis (EPM).

19. When was penicillin discovered?

Penicillin was discovered in 1928; however, it was not until the 1940s that Florey demonstrated its effectiveness in the treatment of bacterial infections.

20. What are the two general methods for susceptibility testing? What type of results do they provide?

The dilution and agar disk-diffusion tests are the two most common susceptibility tests. The agar disk-diffusion test is qualitative (or semiquantitative), whereas the dilution test gives quantitative data.

21. What is the Kirby-Bauer antibiotic sensitivity test?

The Kirby-Bauer method is a disk-diffusion test in which pure culture of the pathogen is placed on an appropriate agar medium and individual filter paper disks impregnated with known concentrations of individual antimicrobials are placed on the pathogen-inoculated agar. The culture is incubated for 18–24 hours at 35° C. The zone of inhibition around each disk is measured, and the measurement is compared with a chart that classifies the organism into either three (sensitive, intermediate, or resistant) or four (sensitive, moderately sensitive, intermediate, or resistant) categories. Most sensitivity categories are based on drugs and pharmacokinetic data in humans. The test is relatively inexpensive.

22. How is the MIC useful clinically?

It is generally assumed that effective antimicrobial therapy requires sustained blood or tissue concentrations above MIC. Thus an organism is regarded as susceptible if it is inhibited by a concentration of drug less than that obtained in the blood of patients treated with doses normally administered for the type of infection and microorganism in question.

23. What factors may explain failure of antimicrobial susceptibility tests to predict clinical outcome?

Bacterial factors
- Improperly conducting or interpreting susceptibility criteria, such as assuming that certain concentrations of antimicrobial will be achieved in specific tissues
- Performing the sensitivity test on the wrong organisms
- Failing to recognize the organisms involved (e.g., anaerobes when only an aerobic culture was performed)
- Pathogens become resistant during the course of therapy
- Inappropriate extrapolation from bacteria cultured from an individual to an entire population
- Subinhibitory concentrations of drugs causing loss of virulence in otherwise resistant bacteria (e.g., loss of adhesive pili)

Host factors
- Degree of immunologic competence
- Inactivation of some drugs by purulent material
- Spontaneous cure of resistant bacteria by host
- Susceptible bacteria unaffected because of intracellular location
- Presence of foreign bodies or necrotic material

Drug factors
- Inadequate dosing, incorrect route of administration, or poor drug formulation
- Inactivation of drug in vivo or in vitro

• Poor drug penetration into tissues because of physiologic barriers (e.g., central nervous system and eye) or extensive necrosis

24. What is bioavailability?

Bioavailability is the fraction (F) of the drug that reaches the systemic circulation after administration by any route. For an intravenous dose, bioavailability is 100% (F= 1.0). For a drug administered extravascularly, bioavailability may be less than 100% for several reasons, such as incomplete absorption or metabolism in the gut wall or liver before entry into the systemic circulation. If only 60% of a drug reaches the systemic circulation, its bioavailability is 60% (F = 0.6). Bioavailability refers to the percentage of drug absorbed for routes other than IV but gives no indication of the rate of absorption and peak serum concentrations.

25. What is the postantibiotic effect (PAE)?

In vitro the PAE is the time before bacterial regrowth occurs after removal or inactivation of an antimicrobial from the culture environment. In vivo it is the time before bacterial regrowth occurs after antimicrobial levels fall below the MIC. Clinically, the PAE prolongs the time required between dosing intervals, because drug concentrations can be below the MIC of the organism for a period of time without significant bacterial regrowth.

26. Which antimicrobials have a PAE? How long is the PAE?

Aminoglycosides and fluoroquinolones possess PAE against most susceptible organisms. The β-lactams and bacteriostatic antimicrobials do not have a significant PAE. The one exception is penicillin, which has been shown to have a PAE against streptococcal species.

The PAE may be quite variable, lasting from 1 hour to several hours. The duration of PAE is affected by drug concentration achieved at the site of infection, duration of exposure, and bacterial strain. Because higher peak plasma concentrations are reached with longer dose interval regimens, once-daily treatment with aminoglycosides (e.g., gentamicin, amikacin) should attain a PAE of longer duration than treatment with a shorter dosing regimen (e.g., every 8 hours).

27. What is time-dependent vs. concentration-dependent killing?

The β-lactam antimicrobials, such as penicillin, have maximal killing effects at concentrations 2–4 times the MIC. When concentrations fall below MIC, bacterial growth can recommence (for most organisms). Thus the time that antimicrobial concentrations stay above MIC correlates with efficacy of therapy (time-dependent killing). Time-dependent dosing regimens exist for most antimicrobials. When dosing antimicrobials with time-dependent killing, one should use frequent dosing intervals or delayed-absorption preparations (procaine penicillin) that allow serum concentrations to remain above the MIC of the pathogen for the entire treatment duration.

A few classes of antimicrobials demonstrate concentration-dependent killing. Examples include the aminoglycosides, fluoroquinolones, and possibly metronidazole. The greater the drug concentration, the greater the bacterial killing. Therefore, dosage regimens that result in peak drug concentrations greater than 8–10 times the MIC are more effective at killing bacteria. Because aminoglycosides and fluoroquinolones also have a PAE, a large dose administered once or twice daily is efficacious, and the concerns of toxicity, cost, and owner compliance may be reduced because of the infrequent dosing intervals.

28. Why is penicillin ineffective in treating *Rhodococcus equi* infection in vivo, even though in vitro MIC data suggest that *R. equi* is highly sensitive to penicillin?

R. equi is an intracellular pathogen that infects macrophages. Penicillin does not achieve significant intracellular concentrations in vivo, resulting in treatment failure for *R. equi* pneumonia.

29. What is constitutive resistance?

The bacterium with constitutive resistance does not possess the target of the specific antimicrobial action or possesses some intrinsic protection from the specific antimicrobial.

30. How do bacteria acquire resistance to antimicrobial agents?

1. **Chromosomal mutation within the bacteria.** Chromosomal changes often result in other changes in the bacteria that make them less hardy than the nonmutated strain and less likely to survive bacterial competition without the selection pressures of antimicrobial therapy.

2. **Transduction.** Genetic material is exchanged between bacteria by plasmid DNA that is incorporated into a bacterial virus (bacteriophage), which in turn infects another bacterium.

3. **Conjugation.** In this common process of gene transfer, a donor bacterium synthesizes a sex pilus that attaches to a recipient bacterium and transfers copies of plasmid-mediated resistance genes to the recipient. The donor retains copies of the plasmid, and the recipient now becomes a potential donor. Conjugation occurs between bacterial strains of the same species, within species of the same genera, or even between species belonging to different families.

4. **Transformation.** Naked DNA passes from one cell to another. Transformation is rare compared with the other methods of resistance transfer.

The genetic elements responsible for transfer of antimicrobial resistance in transduction and transformation are the R (resistance)-plasmids or R-factors, which are extrachromosomal circular DNA. They contain regions that may code for resistance to 1–10 different antimicrobials. Transposons are short sequences of DNA that can "jump" from plasmid to plasmid, from plasmid to chromosome, or vice versa. The key property of all transposable elements is their ability to move and integrate into a foreign DNA sequence by nonhomologous recombination.

31. Which groups of bacteria acquire resistance?

Acquired resistance has been identified in virtually every pathogenic bacterial genus, although gram-positive bacteria (with the exception of staphylococci and enterococci) do not seem to acquire antimicrobial resistance readily and seem to lack the ability to acquire R-plasmids.

32. What is cross-resistance?

Cross-resistance occurs when an organism becomes resistant to one antimicrobial but also demonstrates resistance to another. The classic example is cross-resistance among aminoglycosides. Resistance to gentamicin is associated with resistance to previously released drugs, such as neomycin and kanamycin. Cross-resistance is also common among the macrolides (e.g., erythromycin, tylosin, tilmicosin).

33. What is the definition of pharmacokinetics?

Pharmacokinetics is the study of drug movement in a biologic system and is concerned with the time course of drug absorption, distribution, metabolism, and excretion.

34. What is the volume of distribution? Is it a real volume?

The volume of distribution is the apparent volume of fluid into which a drug appears to distribute in order to account for the observed plasma concentration. It accounts for all of the drug in the body and is expressed as the relationship of the amount of drug administered to the observed concentration of the drug in plasma when absorption and distribution are complete. It is neither a real value nor a real number. It is a number that represents the size of a fluid compartment required to dilute a given amount of drug in order to obtain the observed plasma concentration.

35. Why does the drug distribution differ between equine neonates and adults?

Differences in drug distribution between adults and neonates may result from crucial differences in the neonatal foal, including a larger percentage of the body weight as water, deficiencies in drug-metabolizing enzyme systems, lower glomerular filtration and renal tubular secretory mechanisms, decreased plasma protein-binding of drugs due to lower albumin levels, and impaired integrity of the blood-brain barrier. In general, kidney function of normal newborn foals is similar to that in adults within a few days of birth. Hepatic metabolizing enzymes mature over the first few months. Foals tend to have a larger volume of distribution than adults because of their high percentage of body water. The result is lower peak drug concentrations and longer elimination half-lives in foals than in adults.

36. What is the volume of distribution if the drug (1) distributes evenly throughout the body, (2) distributes into the extracellular fluid space only, and (3) widely distributes but concentrates inside cells?
(1) Approximately 1 L/kg
(2) Approximately 0.3 L/kg
(3) > 1 L/kg

37. What three factors are associated with bacterial resistance to natural penicillin?
1. Absence of a cell wall
2. Impermeable outer membrane
3. Production of β-lactamase

38. Are β-lactams and aminoglycosides antagonistic or synergistic?
The interaction of β-lactams and aminoglycosides can be synergistic because β-lactams inhibit cell wall synthesis and increase the uptake of aminoglycosides into bacteria. However, mixing β-lactams and aminoglycosides in the same syringe results in inactivation of the aminoglycoside. Inactivation also occurs in vivo as a result of high doses of penicillins; therefore, the administration of the two agents should be separated in time.

39. Erythromycin has been shown to have effects on the host as well as the bacterial parasite. Give examples.
Erythromycin is putatively an antiinflammatory or immunnosuppressive drug, may cause hyperthermia, and is a gastrointestinal prokinetic (possibly through motilin agonism).
Lakritz J: Erythromycin: Clinical uses, kinetics and mechanism of action. In Proceedings of the American College of Veterinary Internal Medicine 15. Lake Buena Vista, FL, 1997, pp 368–370.

40. What are the different formulations for oral erythromycin? Do they have any significance in terms of efficacy and safety?
Four common salts are used for oral dosing of erythromycin: base, estolate, ethylsuccinate, and stearate. Only the estolate and ethylsuccinate salts are acid-stable; thus both are available as tablet and liquid formulations. On the other hand, erythromycin base and stearate are acid-labile (sensitive) and formulated as enteric-coated tablets or delayed time-release capsules (which may contain microgranules that are individually microencapsulated or coated) so that the medication is not degraded by acid in the stomach and enters the small intestine before absorption. Acid-degraded erythromycin (anhydroerythromycin) lacks antimicrobial activity. After oral administration of crushed enteric-coated tablets of erythromycin base to foals, only approximately 20% of the parent drug is absorbed. However, after oral administration of erythromycin estolate given as a liquid suspension, approximately 60% of the erythromycin is systemically absorbed. Therefore, the acid-stable salts of erythromycin are preferred for use in horses. It is not yet known whether administration of the microencapsulated form (ERtC, Roche, Nutley, NJ, 07110; generic formulation, Faulding Pinepak Pharmaceuticals, Elizabeth, NJ 07207) has decreased absorption. It seems logical that the enteric-coated individual granules would maintain resistance to gastric acid despite removal from the outer nonprotective capsule.

41. What are the antimicrobials of choice for treatment of *R. equi* pneumonia in foals? What are the dosage recommendations?
Rifampin and erythromycin are the antimicrobials of choice for treatment of *R. equi* pneumonia in foals. Rifampin should not be used alone because resistance develops quickly. It should be administered at a dose of 5 mg/kg orally every 12 hours. Published recommendations[1,2,6,7] for the various erythromycin formulations in horses are the following:

1. Erythromycin base: 25 mg/kg orally every 6 hours
2. Erythromycin estolate: 25 mg/kg orally every 6–8 hours
3. Erythromycin stearate: 37.5 mg/kg orally every 12 hours
4. Erythromycin phosphate: 37.5 mg/kg orally every 12 hours

The stearate and phosphate doses are based on pharmacokinetic studies of adult horses fed grass hay with a grain and bran diet. Non-fasted horses fed hay diets have a gastric pH of 4.5–6.0 on average. Erythromycin base, stearate, and phosphate are inactivated by pH < 4.0. The gastric pH of foals 2 days to 12 weeks of age is below 4.0 the majority of the time. Thus, the usefulness of stearate and phosphate salts in foals based on adult horse pharmacokinetics should be interpreted with caution, especially if the enteric coating is not preserved. Also, erythromycin phosphate is a powder used for poultry, and its availability is not widespread. The esters (estolate and ethylsuccinate) are stable in low gastric pH environments.

Baker SJ, Gerring EL: Gastric pH monitoring in healthy, suckling pony foals. Am J Vet Res 54:959–964, 1993.

Ewing PJ, Burrows G, MacAllister C, Clarke C: Comparison of oral erythromycin formulations in the horse using pharmacokinetic profiles. J Vet Pharmacol Therap 17:17–23, 1994.

42. What toxicity syndromes have been associated with aminoglycosides?
1. Nephrotoxicity (primary concern in equine medicine)
2. Neuromuscular blockade
3. Ototoxicity

43. What is the mechanism of neuromuscular blockade caused by aminoglycoside antimicrobials?
Aminoglycosides result in a decrease in availability of calcium at the axonal terminal and interfere with the excitation-secretion coupling process. The postjunctional membrane has decreased sensitivity to acetylcholine because of competitive blocking of the nicotinic cholinergic receptors. Many anesthetic agents also affect calcium availability. Although the effect of either agent alone may be subclinical, effects can be additive and result in neuromusuclar blockade, particularly of respiratory muscles.

44. Which antimicrobials may cause fetal injury or abortion in pregnant mares?
Trimethoprim-sulfa may cause blood dyscrasias in the fetus if administered on a long-term basis to a pregnant mare. A case report described congenital disease in three foals born from mares that were treated during gestation for equine protozoal myeloencephalitis. The therapeutic regimen included sulfonamides, pyrimethamine, and folic acid supplementation. The foals had skin lesions, a wooly hair coat, renal failure, anemia, and leukopenia. Histologic examination revealed bone marrow aplasia, lymphoid aplasia, thin renal cortices, renal tubular nephrosis, and epidermal necrosis. The three foals and two dams that were tested had low serum folate concentrations. Although the exact cause of these congenital defects could not be documented, the authors hypothesize that the combination of folic acid inhibitors and folic acid supplements may paradoxically cause folic acid deficiency in late-term pregnant mares.

The fetus is vulnerable to many external influences at various stages of gestation; consequently, the use of drugs in the mare should be kept to a minimum because of the unpredictability of their effect on the fetus.

Toribio RE, Bain FT, Mrad DR, et al: Congenital defects in newborn foals of mares treated for equine protozoal myeloencephalopathies during pregnancy. J Am Vet Med Assoc 212:697–701, 1998.

45. How many milligrams are in a grain? How many grains are in a gram?
There are 65 mg in 1 grain. One gram contains approximately 15 grains.

46. Why are antimicrobial agents not as effective in management of infections in immunodeficient foals as in immunocompetent foals?
Inactivation of microbes is the only role played by antimicrobial drugs, whereas clinical recovery requires the patient's defense mechanisms to remove the organism and debris and to

repair and replace damaged tissue. Most infections are prevented by efficient nonspecific host defense mechanisms. Many patients recover with the aid of nonspecific and specific host mechanisms. Their importance is emphasized by the obvious failure of antimicrobials alone to protect animals adequately in the absence of inherent responses. Antimicrobials are no more or less effective in immunodeficient foals at inactivating organisms. Recovery, however, requires significant host activity, which is lacking in immunodeficient animals.

47. Which antimicrobials are well absorbed when administered orally to horses?
(1) Trimethoprim-sulfa, (2) erythromycin, (3) rifampin, (4) fluoroquinolones (e.g, enrofloxacin) (5) metronidazole, and (6) chloramphenicol.

48. Development of hyperpnea, sweating, agitation, and cutaneous wheals within 15 minutes of administration of penicillin is suggestive of what condition?
These signs are suggestive of acute anaphylaxis. Hypotension and pulmonary edema are significant findings. The severity and acuteness of onset vary. Death may occur. Onset of anaphylaxis may be delayed if the reaction is triggered by a drug metabolite rather than the parent compound.

49. What two types of reaction may occur after administration of procaine penicillin G?
1. Anaphylactic reaction.
2. Procaine reaction occurs if the procaine inadvertently enters the vascular space (e.g., entry into microvasculature after intramuscular injection; incorrect [negligent] administration intravenously). A procaine reaction may occur with the first administration of procaine penicillin G to a horse.

50. Pleuropneumonia is often caused by a mixed bacterial infection that includes anaerobic bacteria. What is a reasonable empirical choice of antimicrobials before culture and sensitivity results from tracheal lavage and thoracocentesis are available?
A combination of penicillin, gentamicin, and metronidazole provides broad-spectrum coverage for most common respiratory bacterial pathogens. For example, one may use procaine penicillin G, 20,000 IU/kg every 12 hours intramuscularly or potassium penicillin, 20,000–40,000 IU/kg every 6 hours intravenously, plus gentamicin, 6.6 mg/kg every 24 hours intramuscularly or intravenously, plus metronidazole, 15 mg/kg every 6–12 hours orally.

51. What route of administration should be used in an animal with duodenitis-proximal jejunitis (DPJ) if metronidazole is part of the antimicrobial regimen?
Most horses with DPJ (also known as proximal enteritis) produce significant amounts of reflux, because the ileus of the small intestine causes a functional obstruction. Back-up of intestinal fluid into the stomach should be relieved by indwelling nasogastric intubation and active reflux every 2–4 hours. Because a nasogastric tube will probably be in place and the small intestine will not prove reliable absorption, metronidazole should not be given orally. Instead the tablets should be crushed, added to a small volume (e.g., 20–50 ml) of water, and administered rectally by rubber tubing (e.g., 19-French). Rectal absorption of metronidazole is approximately 60% of oral absorption. Rectal metronidazole is usually administered at a dose rate of 15 mg/kg every 6 hours rather than at the oral rate of 10–15 mg/kg every 6–12 hours. Its penetration within the abdomen is excellent.

52. *Ehrlichia risticii*, the agent that causes equine monocytic ehrlichiosis (Potomac horse fever), is treated with which drug?
Oxytetracycline (6.6 mg/kg intravenous infusion every 24 hours) is effective in the treatment of ehrlichiosis. Erythromycin and rifampin also have been shown to be efficacious and have the advantage that owners can administer the drugs orally.

Palmer JE, Benson CE: Effect of treatment with erythromycin and rifampin during the acute stages of experimentally induced equine ehrlichiosis colitis in ponies. Am J Vet Res 53:2071–2076, 1992.
Palmer JE, Whitlock RH, Benson CE: Equine ehrlichial colitis: Effect of oxytetracycline treatment during the incubation period of *Ehrlichia risticii* infection in ponies. J Am Vet Med Assoc 192:343–345, 1988.

53. Which antimicrobial(s) should be used to treat a horse suffering from tetanus (*Clostridium tetani*)?

C. tetani is a gram-positive anaerobic rod, the vegetative form of which is sensitive to penicillin and tetracycline. Because the organism grows under conditions of anaerobiosis in tissues that tend to be poorly perfused, systemic administration of antimicrobials may not result in sufficiently high local levels of the drug to eliminate the organism. Thus it is important to include some form of therapy to neutralize toxins that may reach the circulation. Some veterinarians also use local antimicrobial infiltration; however, the efficacy of this approach depends on perfusion within the tissue.

54. What is the drug of choice for treating a streptococcal infection?

Considerations in selecting therapy include susceptibility, practicality, and cost. Streptococci are virtually always susceptible to penicillin, which is considered the drug of choice, but penicillins must be administered parenterally (which may mean that the horse must be hospitalized or that the owners must administer intramuscular procaine penicillin G). Streptococci are often sensitive to trimethoprim-sulfa, which is administered orally, but in many geographic regions (especially the eastern and northern states of the U.S.) more than 50% of streptococcal isolates from horses are resistant to trimethoprim-sulfa. Erythromycin, another oral alternative, has good activity against streptococci, but it can be expensive compared with the other alternatives. Erythromycin stearate and erythromycin phosphate (37.5 mg/kg every 12 hours orally) are usually cheaper than other formulations.

55. Spontaneous death (dropping dead off the needle) during a jugular vein injection is suggestive of what event?

Immediate (within seconds) reaction to an "intravenous" injection is suggestive of an inadvertent intraarterial injection (i.e., administration into the carotid artery rather than the jugular vein). An anaphylactic reaction is possible, but it requires sufficient time for the release of inflammatory mediators (e.g., minutes or longer).

56. What is the most frequent microorganism isolated from equine mastitis? Which drugs are likely to penetrate a mastitic mammary gland?

Equine mastitis is relatively rare; however, the most commonly isolated organism is *Streptococcus zooepidemicus*. Systemically administered, nonionized, nonprotein-bound, lipid-soluble agents are expected to reach the mammary gland most efficiently. When the milk is weakly acidic, antibacterial agents that are weak bases (e.g., trimethoprim, aminoglycosides, macrolides) are preferentially concentrated in the mammary gland by ion trapping. Milk from clinical mastitis may have a pH in the range of serum; thus antimicrobial agents that are weak acids (e.g., sulfonamines, penicillins, cephalosporins, rifampin) may reach effective concentrations in the milk.

57. Which drugs should be used for intraarticular injections?

Septic arthritis may result from infection with either gram-negative or gram-positive organisms. Intraarticular instillation of aminoglycosides with a gram-negative and streptococcal spectrum or cefazolin is commonly used after vigorous lavage with lactated Ringer's solution (LRS) or LRS with 5–10% dimethyl sulfoxide.

58. What antimicrobials should be used before blood culture and sensitivity results are available in patients with neonatal septicemia?

Gram-negative bacteria, most commonly *E. coli*, are predominantly isolated from cases of neonatal septicemia. Streptococci are most commonly isolated in mixed bacterial infections with gram-negative bacteria. The combination of a β-lactam antimicrobial (e.g., penicillin, ampicillin, ceftiofur, cefazolin) and an aminoglycoside (e.g., gentamicin, amikacin) usually provides good antimicrobial coverage and is indicated until blood cultures results are obtained.

59. What color is the urine from a horse treated with rifampin?

Red.

60. What is the route of excretion of penicillin and ampicillin?

Ninety percent of the dose of penicillin and ampicillin is excreted via the urinary tract in active form. Thus both drugs provide suitable coverage for treatment of urinary tract infections caused by susceptible organisms. Other antimicrobials suitable for urinary tract infections are trimethoprim-sulfa, ceftiofur, and enrofloxacin (if the bacteria are sensitive only to the latter).

61. What is the withdrawal time for procaine penicillin in a horse?

Although we seldom are concerned about the withdrawal time for antimicrobials because of potential human consumption of horse meat, some components of pharmaceuticals other than the parent compound may be detected by drug tests as forbidden substances in the body fluids of performance horses. Procaine, a local anesthetic, is a forbidden substance. It may remain in the system for more than 21 days after use of procaine penicillin.

62. Which antimicrobial provides some protection against the toxic effects of endotoxin (lipopolysaccharide) if administered before the endotoxin? How?

Polymyxin B has a detergent action on endotoxin.

63. Which antimicrobials are poorly absorbed from the gut but remain active in it?

Aminoglycosides are poorly absorbed from the gastrointestinal tract but may have an effect on intraluminal flora. They are useful for intentional efforts to sterilize the gut and may have an unintentional adverse effect on normal flora. Most β-lactams, especially penicillin and ampicillin, have poor bioavailability when administered orally to adult horses. The majority of the β-lactam remains in the intestinal tract, often adversely affecting the gastrointestinal microflora.

64. Which antimicrobial(s) should be considered for empirical treatment of respiratory bacterial infections in horses?

The most common bacteria to cause respiratory infections is *Streptococcus* species, primarily *S. zooepidemicus* and, to a lesser degree, *S. equi*. Most of the remaining isolated bacterial pathogens are gram-negative bacteria: *Actinobacillus* species, *Pasteurella* species, and *Bordetella bronchoseptica*. Gram-negative enteric organisms such as *E. coli* and *Klebsiella* species are infrequent isolates in equine bronchopneumonia but are more common in pleuropneumonia and neonatal pneumonia. Therefore, empirical treatment of equine bronchopneumonia should focus on the common organisms. Penicillin G is the drug of choice for streptococcal infections and has fair-to-good activity against *Pasteurella* and *Actinobacillus* isolates at high recommended doses (procaine penicillin G, 22,000 IU/kg twice daily intramuscularly). Ampicillin and cephalosporins (cefazolin and ceftiofur) also have good activity against streptococcal species and against many common gram-negative respiratory isolates, excluding *B. bronchoseptica*, but are more expensive than penicillin G. Trimethoprim-sulfa drugs and oxytetracycline have good activity against the common gram-negative isolates, including *B. bronchoseptica*, but their activity against streptococcal species is only fair (< 60%) in many geographic areas. Erythromycin has good activity against most of the common isolates but can be expensive to use in adult animals and, like other oral antimicrobials, has the potential to induce colic and colitis. A penicillin or cephalosporin is the most appropriate choice for empirical therapy of equine bacterial bronchopneumonia. Trimethoprim-sulfa is commonly used to treat equine bronchopneumonia because it is inexpensive and can be administered orally, but significant resistance developed by streptococcal species has reduced its effectiveness. (See chapter 11 for discussion of antimicrobials in pleuropneumonia.)

65. Aspiration pneumonia secondary to esophageal obstruction is best treated with what antimicrobial(s)?

Aspiration pneumonia is usually associated with a mixed population of bacterial agents, and broad-spectrum coverage can be assumed to be necessary. If performed, cultures often reveal a mixture of gram-positive and gram-negative organisms, both aerobes and anaerobes. Ceftiofur or a combination of penicillin and gentamicin is suitable for initial treatment. Metronidazole should be added to the therapy if a β-lactamase-producing anaerobe is isolated or if a culture is not performed.

66. Your rectal sleeve is covered with blood when you exit the rectum of a mare that you are examining for pregnancy. On repalpation you recognize a type 3 dorsal tear 12 inches cranial to the anus. In addition to other management, what antimicrobial coverage is appropriate?

Gram-negative enteric organisms and anaerobes are of primary concern. Antimicrobials with good gram-negative and anaerobic coverage are imperative. Appropriate choices are (1) gentamicin or amikacin and penicillin or (2) a cephalosporin in combination with metronidazole.

67. Three days after a mare delivered a dead foal following dystocia and suffered a retained placenta for 24 hours, she is depressed and febrile. A serosanguinous vaginal discharge is present. What type of empirical antimicrobial coverage is appropriate?

Gram-negative enteric organisms are common isolates from mares with metritis. Anaerobes are of concern with the tissue trauma associated with dystocia. Metronidazole and/or penicillin provides anaerobic coverage. An aminoglycoside, a second- or third-generation cephalosporin, or a fluoroquinolone provides gram-negative coverage. Fluoroquinolones should be used only if culture and sensitivity results reveal that other antimicrobials will not be helpful.

CONTROVERSIES

68. A yearling has swollen, painful submandibular lymph nodes, purulent nasal discharge, depression, and anorexia. Your presumptive diagnosis is "strangles." Discuss the controversy over antimicrobial treatment.

Pros: Early treatment may prevent development of full-blown strangles with lymphadenitis and overt abscessation and may reduce contamination of the premises. Systemic signs in excess of submandibular lymphadenitis, including anorexia, dysphagia, pneumonia, abdominal pain, or fever for longer than 72 hours, should be treated vigorously with antimicrobials. Little evidence suggests that metastatic strangles ("bastard strangles") is promoted by use of antimicrobials.

Cons: Treatment of *Streptococcus equi* infections with antimicrobials such as penicillin alleviates clinical signs temporarily; however, disease may recur when treatment is discontinued. Moreover, it has been proposed but not proved that treatment may predispose to occurrence of metastatic strangles with dissemination of lymphadenitis to internal lymphoid tissues.

69. Of what value are prophylactic antimicrobials for elective surgery or cases of suspected viral infections?

Pros: Prophylactic antibiotics help to prevent opportunistic bacterial organisms from establishing infection when animals are immunocompromised as a result of the stress of surgery and anesthesia or viral infections.

Cons: Administration of antimicrobials before actual surgery (e.g., the day before) has no beneficial at the time of surgery. The only beneficial effect stems from therapeutic levels at the time of surgery. The use of antimicrobials to prevent secondary bacterial infections during a viral infection should be considered an indiscriminate use that promotes resistance in bacterial populations over time, rendering the antimicrobials less effective. Such use of antimicrobials may select for multidrug-resistant secondary bacterial infections.

70. Should horses with enteric salmonellosis be treated with antibiotics?

Pros: Enteric salmonellosis may not remain limited to the intestine; septicemia may become a component of the disease. Antimicrobials may not affect the organism in the intestinal fluid or intracellularly in the enterocytes, but it may prevent severe manifestations of septicemia. Antimicrobials may protect the immunocompromised (e.g., neutropenic secondary to endotoxemia) horse from secondary bacterial infections.

Cons: Most systemic effects from salmonellosis are caused by endotoxemia, not septicemia. Furthermore, the organism is protected from most antimicrobials by virtue of its intracellular location. Antimicrobials may further alter the commensal flora of the intestine and prolong the course of *Salmonella* shedding. Resistance of *Salmonella* species to antimicrobials is highly variable, and without knowledge of the local antimicrobial sensitivity pattern, empirical selection of an appropriate antibiotic is difficult. Specific antimicrobial administration (based on culture and sensitivity) may cause an increase in endotoxemia because of death of *Salmonella* organisms and release of lipopolysaccharide.

BIBLIOGRAPHY

1. Baker SJ, Gerring EL: Gastric pH monitoring in healthy, suckling pony foals. Am J Vet Res 54:959–964, 1993.
2. Beard LA: Principles of antimicrobial therapy. In Reed SM, Bayly WM (eds): Equine Internal Medicine. Philadelphia, W.B. Saunders, 1998, pp 157–187.
3. Bertone JJ: Antimicrobial therapy for respiratory disease. Vet Clin North Am Equine Pract 13:501–518, 1997.
4. Brumbaugh GW: Rational selection of antimicrobial drugs for treatment of infections in horses. Vet Clin North Am Equine Pract 3:191–220, 1987.
5. Caprile KA, Short CR: Pharmacologic considerations in drug therapy in foals. Vet Clin North Am Equine Pract 3:123–144, 1987.
6. Ewing PJ, Burrows G, MacAllister C, Clarke C: Comparison of oral erythromycin formulations in the horse using pharmacokinetic profiles. J Vet Pharmacol Therap 17:17–23, 1994.
7. Hooper DC, Wolfson JS: Fluoroquinolone antimicrobial agents. N Engl J Med 324:384, 1991.
8. Lakritz J: Erythromycin: Clinical uses, kinetics and mechanism of action. In Proceedings of the American College of Veterinary Internal Medicine 15. Lake Buena Vista, FL, 1997, pp 368–370.
9. Orsini JA, Perkons S: New beta-lactam antibiotics in critical care medicine. Compend Contin Educ Pract Vet 16:183–195, 1994.
10. Palmer JE, Benson CE: Effect of treatment with erythromycin and rifampin during the acute stages of experimentally induced equine ehrlichiosis colitis in ponies. Am J Vet Res 53:2071–2076, 1992.
11. Palmer JE, Whitlock RH, Benson CE: Equine ehrlichial colitis: Effect of oxytetracycline treatment during the incubation period of *Ehrlichia risticii* infection in ponies. J Am Vet Med Assoc 192:343–345, 1988.
12. Plumb DC: Veterinary Drug Handbook, 2nd ed. Ames, IA, Iowa State University Press, 1995.
13. Prescott JF, Baggot JD (eds): Antimicrobial Therapy in Veterinary Medicine, 2nd ed. Ames, IA, Iowa State University Press, 1997.
14. Toribio RE, Bain FT, Mrad DR, et al: Congenital defects in newborn foals of mares treated for equine protozoal myeloencephalopathies during pregnancy. J Am Vet Med Assoc 212:697–701, 1998.

22. NONSTEROIDAL ANTIINFLAMMATORY DRUG THERAPY

Mark V. Crisman, D.V.M., M.S., Dip. ACVIM, and
Virginia Buechner-Maxwell, D.V.M., M.S., Dip. ACVIM

1. What are nonsteroidal antiinflammatory drugs?

Nonsteroidal antiinflammatory drugs (NSAIDs) are defined as substances (other than steroids) that suppress one or more components of the inflammatory cascade. The term is generally used to describe antiinflammatory agents that inhibit some component of the arachidonic acid cascade; however, the broad definition includes the flunixin meglumine-like drugs and hyaluronate, polysulfated glycosaminoglycans, and dimethyl sulfoxide. In addition to antiinflammatory properties, NSAIDs also possess analgesic and antipyretic properties. NSAIDs are among the most commonly prescribed drugs in equine medicine.

2. How are NSAIDs classified?

Chemically, NSAIDs are divided into two distinct groups based on their structural similarities; carboxylic and enolic acids. The chemical class of a particular NSAID does not predict efficacy or toxicity. Most NSAIDs are weak acids with ionization constants (pKa) between 3 and 5. At lower pHs, more drug becomes unionized and thereby increases association with the lipid bilayer of cell membrane, allowing concentration of the NSAID in areas of greater acidity (i.e., inflammation).

CARBOXYLIC ACIDS	ENOLIC ACIDS
Aspirin	Phenylbutazone
Naproxen	Dipyrone
Flunixin meglumine	Isopyrin
Meclofenamic acid	
Indomethacin	
Ketoprofen	
Carprofen	

3. What are the common clinical applications of NSAIDs in horses?

NSAIDs have been widely used in veterinary medicine for more than 30 years, primarily to treat lameness in horses. Their general antiinflammatory, analgesic, antipyretic, and antithrombotic properties make them desirable for a number of clinical situations, including musculoskeletal problems (e.g., laminitis, navicular disease, osteoarthritis) postoperative inflammation, endotoxemia, and soft tissue injuries.

4. Explain the general mechanism of action of NSAIDs.

All NSAIDs inhibit prostanoid production by inhibiting the transformation of arachidonic acid via the cyclooxygenase (COX) pathway. Inhibition of the COX pathway blocks the conversion of arachidonic acid to endoperoxides and prostaglandins G_2 (PGG_2) and H_2 (PGH_2). PGH_2 is converted to PGE_2, PGI_2 (prostacyclin), and thromboxane A_2 (TXA_2) by the enzymes endoperoxide isomerase, prostacyclin synthase, and thromboxane synthase, respectively. Endoperoxides are converted to TXA_2 in platelets and PGE_2 in inflamed tissue. The overall result of NSAID administration is a decrease in the production of prostanoids, which affect the various tissues differently. Certain NSAIDs (e.g., phenylbutazone) have a significant effect on COX inhibition, whereas others, such as the R-negative enantiomer of carprofen, are relatively weak COX inhibitors.

5. What are eicosanoids and prostanoids?

Eicosanoids are a group of compounds derived from reactions of oxygen with polyunsaturated fatty acids. The name *eicosa* derives from the Greek meaning "20" and implies that eicosanoids are derived from 20-carbon polyunsaturated fats. Eicosanoids include all of the 5-lipoxygenase products (leukotrienes) and cyclooxygenase products (prostanoids). **Prostanoids** specifically refer to the cyclooxygenase products, including prostaglandins, prostacyclin, and thromboxanes.

6. What are the important isoenzymes associated with cyclooxygenase?

1. **COX-1** is constitutively expressed in most tissues and is responsible for maintaining physiologic cellular functions such as vascular homeostasis. COX-1 is termed the "housekeeping" isoenzyme. Tissues that maintain high levels of COX-1 include vascular endothelial cells, kidney collecting tubules, platelets, and smooth muscle cells.

2. **COX-2** is the inducible enzyme and is expressed only after cellular activation (e.g., by inflammation, trauma) and the elaboration of various cytokines. Generally, COX-2 is nearly undetectable in most tissues but may increase 10–80-fold after stimulation with interleukin-1 (IL-1) or endotoxin. Glucocorticoids such as dexamethasone have little effect on COX-1, whereas they completely inhibit elaboration of COX-2.

7. Do NSAIDs uniformly inhibit both COX-1 and COX-2?

Aspirin, indomethacin, and piroxicam have been demonstrated to be more potent inhibitors of COX-1 than COX-2 and therefore affect the physiologic or homeostatic role of cyclooxygenase products. Several studies have reported that ibuprofen, naproxen, and meclofenamic acid are generally equipotent in their ability to affect the two isoenzymes. The majority of adverse effects noted with NSAID toxicosis occur with the inhibition of COX-1, whereas most of the beneficial (antiinflammatory) effects are recognized with inhibition of COX-2. An NSAID that selectively inhibits the inflammation associated with the isoenzyme COX-2, while leaving the physiologic activity of COX-1 unaffected, would greatly reduce toxicity. The presence of several forms of cyclooxygenase and the selectivity of specific NSAIDs for the different isoenzymes may account for the clinical differences observed after administration of different NSAIDs. In addition, some NSAIDs may bind irreversibly to cyclooxygenase, whereas others may not. This may explain the discrepancy between the short half-life and long duration of action that is frequently observed with NSAID administration. The discrepancy also may be due to the fact that some NSAIDs (e.g., ketoprofen, flunixin meglumine) accumulate at sites of inflammation while being cleared from the blood.

8. What are some of the important physiologic effects associated with inhibition of arachidonic acid metabolism?

1. Reduction in pain associated with arachidonic acid metabolites
2. Moderation of fever
3. Decreased platelet aggregation
4. Increased gastric acid production
5. Decreased gastric mucin production
6. Decreased renal blood flow

9. How do NSAIDs control pain?

After activation of the arachidonic acid cascade, both cyclooxygenase and 5-lipoxygenase are responsible for the subsequent elaboration of inflammatory mediators (eicosanoids). Important among these are the prostanoids, which produce pain in inflamed tissues by binding to receptors on the sensory nerve endings and lowering the threshold of nociceptors of C-fibers. In addition, prostanoids amplify the pain response associated with other mediators of inflammation, including bradykinin and histamine. By reducing local prostanoid production in tissues, NSAIDs alleviate pain in inflamed tissues. It has also been speculated that some NSAIDs, specifically flunixin meglumine, may have a central analgesic effect, as evidenced by the amelioration of abdominal pain associated with colic in horses.

10. How do NSAIDs control fever?

NSAIDs are highly effective in treating fevers of various origins in horses. Inflammation or infection stimulates the production of several cytokines, including IL-1 and tumor necrosis factor. These particular cytokines cause an increase in production of PGE_2, which acts directly on the hypothalamus to elevate the thermoregulatory set point. Administration of NSAIDs blocks the formation of PGE_2 and prevents an increase in body temperature by returning the hypothalamic regulatory set point to normal. NSAID administration is not useful in horses with hyperthermia (whether it be central hyperthermia, in which the preoptic region of the anterior hypothalamus has been damaged, postexercise hyperthermia, or erythromycin-related hyperthermia).

11. Do NSAIDs exert their effects via mechanisms other than COX inhibition?

Studies have suggested that NSAIDs demonstrate activity beyond the generally accepted hypothesis of cyclooxygenase inhibition and the subsequent elaboration of prostanoid mediators of inflammation. Reported nonprostanoid activities of NSAIDs include:

1. Inhibition of superoxide generation by neutrophils
2. Inhibition of mononuclear cell phospholipase C activity
3. Inhibition of platelet cyclooxygenase
4. Inhibition of proteoglycan synthesis by chondrocytes
5. In vitro inhibition of the lipoxygenase pathway and formation of leukotrienes

12. Give a simple, straightforward definition of pharmacokinetics and pharmacodynamics.

Pharmacokinetics refers to what the body does to the drug, whereas pharmacodynamics refers to what the drug does to the body.

13. Are there pharmacokinetic differences in NSAIDs among species?

The pharmacologic data for a particular NSAID in one species cannot be extrapolated to others. The elimination of phenylbutazone (PBZ) in horses is dose-dependent and ranges from 3.5–8 hours. Similar half-lives have been reported in dogs (6 hours). However, the elimination half live of PBZ in cattle is reported to be 40 hours, whereas in humans it is approximately 70 hours.

14. What are the differences in pharmacokinetic properties of NSAIDs commonly used in horses?

The elimination half-lives and volume of distribution for commonly used NSAIDs in adult horses are reported below. The volume of distribution of NSAIDs is quite small due to the high level of plasma protein binding of the drugs.

NSAID	ELIMINATION HALF-LIFE (T 1/2)	VOLUME OF DISTRIBUTION (L/KG)
Phenylbutazone	3.5–6 hr	0.15
Flunixin meglumine	1.6 hr	0.21
Ketoprofen	1 to 2 hr	0.16
Dipyrone	4.7 hr	0.18
Meclofenamic acid	2.5 hr	0.13
Aspirin	0.1 hr	0.08

15. What are the pharmacokinetic differences or considerations for a particular NSAID in horses?

Most NSAIDs are bound extensively (> 95%) to plasma proteins; therefore, the free or active fraction of the drug is quite small. The free or unbound fraction may increase in certain disease states, particularly those that result in hypoalbuminemia. Horses that are older, sick, or heavily parasitized may be less tolerant of the recommended dosage of a particular NSAID and therefore more susceptible to the toxic side effects. Unlike many NSAIDs, phenylbutazone demonstrates dose-dependent kinetics. A clinical dose of 4.4 mg/kg IV has a plasma half-life of about 5 hours in adult horses; at a dose of 8 mg/kg IV the plasma half-life increases to 8 hours. When administering NSAIDs to old or debilitated horses in which drug metabolism may be retarded, use of lower doses at increased intervals should be considered.

16. Do feeding schedules play any role in the pharmacokinetics of NSAIDs in horses?

The bioavailability of phenylbutazone and flunixin meglumine after oral administration results in a delay of peak serum concentrations by 6–12 hours due to binding of the drug to hay and digesta. Peak plasma concentrations are achieved more quickly in horses from which feed is withheld for a few hours before and after oral dosing compared with horses with free access to hay.

17. What importance, if any, does the age of a horse play in the pharmacokinetics of NSAIDs?

A decrease in the rate of elimination and an increase in the plasma half-life for both phenylbutazone and flunixin meglumine has been observed in older horses (> 9 yr) compared with younger horses (< 3 yr).

18. What are the special considerations in administering NSAIDs to neonatal foals?

Distinct NSAID pharmacokinetic differences exist between adult horses and neonatal foals. This difference is due primarily to a larger volume of distribution and possibly to reduced clearance mechanisms in neonatal foals. The median terminal half-life of phenylbutazone after a single 2.2 mg/kg IV dose in neonatal foals is 7.4 hours compared with 3.5 hours in adults. For flunixin meglumine, the median terminal half-life is 8.5 hours in neonates compared with 1.5–4 hours for the same 1.1 mg/kg IV dose in adult horses. In dosing neonates, comparable therapeutic effects should occur with larger doses, whereas longer dosing intervals are necessary to avoid toxicity.

19. What are the special considerations in administering NSAIDs to pregnant mares, especially late in gestation?

Phenylbutazone and probably other NSAIDs pass through placental barriers and potentially accumulate in the fetus. In one study, pregnant mares were given phenylbutazone at 2.2 mg/kg twice daily orally for 1–10 days before parturition. Sampling of their foals immediately after birth revealed an elimination half-life of phenylbutazone of 17.8 hours. It is suggested that administration of NSAIDs to pregnant mares be discontinued at least 24–48 hours before parturition to help reduce the risk of NSAID toxicosis in neonatal foals.

20. Is the plasma elimination half-life for a particular NSAID the most effective means of determining duration of action?

For many drugs, including antimicrobials, this principle may be true. NSAIDs are generally weak organic acids that tend to accumulate in inflamed tissue or inflammatory exudate. Although plasma elimination half-life (t $\frac{1}{2}$) of phenylbutazone in horses may range from 4–8 hours, the t $\frac{1}{2}$ in inflammatory exudate is 24 hours. Similar results have been reported for other NSAIDs, including flunixin meglumine, ketoprofen, and carprofen.

21. What are the manufacturers' recommended dose rates and routes of administration for NSAIDs commonly used in horses?

DRUG	ROUTE	FORMULA	DOSE
Phenylbutazone	PO, IV	Tablets, paste, injectable, Powder	Day 1: 4.4 mg/kg BID, followed by 2.2 mg/kg BID for up to 4 days
Flunixin meglumine	IV, IM*	Injectable, paste, granules	1.1 mg/kg QD for up to 5 days
Ketoprofen	IV	Injectable	2.2 mg/kg QD for up to 5 days
Aspirin	PO	Powder, tablet	25–35 mg/kg BID 5–50 mg/kg QD
Meclofenamic acid	PO	Granules	2.2 mg/kg QD for 5–7 days, then 2.2 mg/kg QOD
Naproxen	PO	Granules	10 mg/kg BID

QD = once daily, BID = twice daily, QOD = every other day
* Many clinicians elect not to administer flunixin meglumine by the intramuscular route in case of necrosis and subsequent clostridial infection.

22. How is aspirin different from other NSAIDs?

All NSAIDs potentially inhibit platelet aggregation and prolong bleeding times. Acetyl-salicylate (aspirin) differs from other NSAIDs in that it irreversibly inhibits COX. This factor is especially significant with platelets, causing them to remain ineffective for their entire lifespan of 7–12 days. Unlike aspirin, phenylbutazone and flunixin meglumine are competitive antagonists of COX; their effect depends on the continued presence of the drug in the plasma.

23. How many milligrams are in 1 grain of aspirin?

There are approximately 65 mg to 1 grain of aspirin.

24. What are the common clinical applications of aspirin in horses?

Although aspirin is the oldest (first described in 1763 to the Royal Society of London) and most widely prescribed NSAID in humans, its use in horses is limited. It is considered a poor analgesic in horses, especially for treatment of colic. Its effects on platelet function (antiaggrega-tory and decreased TXA_2) provide a clinical basis for its antithrombotic action. Aspirin has been used to treat horses with acute laminitis, navicular disease, and uveitis and to decrease further platelet aggregation in horses with thrombophlebitis.

25. What are the primary clinical applications of phenylbutazone in horses?

Phenylbutazone has been widely used in equine medicine for more than 30 years to treat lameness, especially chronic conditions such as navicular disease and osteoarthritis. In addition, phenylbutazone is often the treatment of choice for soft tissue injuries or inflammation in perfor-mance horses. Tissue injuries associated with racing or eventing, lacerations, tissue trauma, spavins, minor sprains, and muscle soreness are often treated with phenylbutazone. In a study evaluating an equine lameness model, phenylbutazone at 4.4 mg/kg IV administered once daily was effective for 24 hours, with the peak effect occurring after 8–12 hours. Phenylbutazone may be administered orally or intravenously, but because of local irritancy to tissues it must not be ad-ministered intramuscularly. When administering phenylbutazone IV, the veterinarian must ensure that none leaks perivascularly.

26. What are the important metabolites of phenylbutazone in horses?

Phenylbutazone is primarily metabolized in the liver to oxyphenbutazone and gamma-hy-droxy-phenylbutazone, which account for up to 30% of the administered dose over 24 hours. Oxyphenbutazone is the active metabolite that inhibits the metabolism and thereby increases the half-life of the parent compound, phenylbutazone.

27. What should a veterinarian do if phenylbutazone inadvertently has been administered perivascularly?

The veterinarian should inject 500–2500 ml of 0.9% saline or 0.9% saline with dimethyl sulfoxide (e.g., 50 ml and 90–99% DMSO in 1 liter of 0.9% saline) into the region of the perivascular injection. If the drug is diluted quickly, the skin may not slough.

28. Which NSAIDs have the greatest analgesic and antiinflammatory potency?

An accurate description of the potency of the various NSAIDs used in equine medicine is difficult. Both antiinflammatory and analgesic potencies of NSAIDs have been ranked in laboratory animals by their ability to inhibit cyclooxygenase activity and in the carrageenin-induced rat paw model. In horses, the *suggested* order of potency is ranked as follows: flunixin > meclofenamic acid > phenylbutazone > naproxen > salicylate.

29. What are the primary clinical applications of flunixin meglumine in horses?

Flunixin meglumine has a relatively short elimination half-life in horses compared with other species (horses: 1.6–2.5 hours; cows: 8 hours). Despite the short half-life and the relatively quick onset of action (within 2 hours) in horses, its duration of action persists up to 30 hours. A single IV dose of 1.1 mg/kg of flunixin suppresses PGE_2 production in inflammatory exudates (usually at site of NSAID accumulation) for 12–24 hours. Flunixin meglumine is considered one of the most potent analgesics and is most frequently used for the treatment of equine colic. Flunixin meglumine also has demonstrated improvement in the cardiovascular status in horses suffering from endotoxemia. Administration of low-dose flunixin meglumine (0.25 mg/kg) has been advocated for its ability to block the effects of endotoxin. These findings were based on a study of experimentally induced endotoxemia in adult horses that were *pretreated* with 0.25 mg/kg of flunixin and demonstrated a depression of thromboxane generation. Many clinicians use the dose rates of 0.25 mg/kg every 6 hours in endotoxemic horses and 0.25 mg/kg every 8–12 hours in endotoxemic horses that also have some evidence of renal compromise. Such horses should be maintained on IV fluids to minimize the effects of renal papillary necrosis.

30. What are the primary clinical applications of ketoprofen in horses?

Both clinical and research data support the use of ketoprofen as an excellent analgesic and antiinflammatory agent for musculoskeletal and gastrointestinal problems in horses. Ketoprofen was initially marketed as an inhibitor of both cyclooxygenase and 5-lipoxygenase. These claims were based on in vitro data in rat models and have as yet been unsubstantiated in horses. Several studies have evaluated the effects of ketoprofen on PGE_2 and leukotriene B_4 (LTB_4) concentrations in inflammatory exudate in horses. Results indicated that whereas PGE_2 levels were significantly suppressed, LTB_4 concentrations remained unchanged.

31. What complications are noted with NSAID administration in horses?

The toxic effects of NSAID administration, especially after high dosages for prolonged periods, have been well documented in horses. The predominant toxic side effect observed in horses is gastric ulceration.

Other adverse side effects include:

- Oral, gastric, duodenal, and colonic ulceration
- Hypoproteinemia and edema
- Anorexia, depression
- Renal papillary necrosis
- Diarrhea
- Platelet dysfunction
- Neutropenia, which is probably related to GI abnormalities and subsequent endotoxemia rather than a suppression of granulopoiesis, as originally suggested for phenylbutazone

32. Describe the general mechanism of NSAID induced gastric ulceration.

Endogenous prostanoids, particularly products of COX-1, provide a physiologic role in protection and growth of the gastrointestinal tract. Prostaglandins, particularly PGE_2, enhance mucous secretion and mucosal blood flow, decrease gastric acid and pepsin secretion, and generally stabilize cell membranes. In general, NSAIDs promote gastric acid secretion and diminished blood flow within the glandular mucosa, primarily through inhibition of PGE_2 synthesis, with resultant gastrointestinal ulceration.

33. Describe the mechanism of NSAID-induced nephrotoxicity.

Endogenous prostanoids, particularly PGE_2, maintain a cytoprotective role by modulating renal blood flow and glomerular filtration rate. The role of these prostanoids is critical during episodes of renal insults such as dehydration and hypovolemia because they primarily function in the autoregulation of renal blood flow, glomerular filtration, and modulation of renin release. Excessive NSAID administration, especially with concurrent dehydration, results in medullary ischemia with secondary renal papillary necrosis.

34. What laboratory parameters should be monitored in septic or critically ill horses on NSAID therapy?

- Hydration status (packed cell volume, serum creatinine concentration)
- Fecal occult blood
- Plasma protein and specifically albumin concentration
- Blood chemistry, specifically blood urea nitrogen, sodium, and chloride concentration
- Urinalysis, especially to evaluate enzymuria (urinary gammaglutamyl transferase [GGT] creatinine ratio) and red blood cell number/field

35. Are there differences in the ulcerogenic or nephrotoxic potential of various NSAIDs in horses?

In a recent study the toxic potentials of three NSAIDs were compared in normal adult horses in larger doses than recommended by the manufacturers. Results indicated that the ulcerogenic potential of these NSAIDs was phenylbutazone > flunixin meglumine > ketoprofen. The nephrotoxic potential of these NSAIDs was phenylbutazone > ketoprofen > flunixin meglumine.

36. What are the current recommendations for preventing NSAID toxicosis in horses?

- Administer the lowest effective dose of the NSAID.
- Limit the duration of treatment.
- Maintain adequate hydration during the course of therapy.
- Limit the viscosity of oral formulations (e.g., do not add excessive molasses) so that the oral formulation does not adhere to oral and esophageal mucosa.

37. What treatment options are available for NSAID toxicosis in horses?

Most therapies for NSAID toxicosis focus on treatment of gastrointestinal ulceration. In humans, H_2 receptor antagonists (e.g., cimetidine, ranitidine) and the proton pump inhibitor (omeprazole) are effective means of treating NSAID-induced ulcers. In addition, sulcralfate (a gastrointestinal protectant that may increase PGE_2 production) and misoprostol (a PGE_2 analog) have been used for the treatment of duodenal ulcers. Similar therapeutic regimens have been used in horses with gastric, duodenal, and colonic ulceration with mixed results.

38. What is the relationship between NSAIDs and thyroid hormones?

NSAIDs, in particular phenylbutazone, may erroneously decrease circulating thyroid hormone levels in horses, probably as a result of competitive protein binding by NSAIDs. Surprisingly, however, a recent study revealed few lower values of T3 and T4 in young horses on phenylbutazone.

39. What particular drug interactions may occur in administering NSAIDs?

All NSAIDs are acidic and highly bound to plasma proteins. An adverse drug reaction may occur if one drug displaces another from its protein binding site. Warfarin is highly bound to plasma proteins and may be removed from binding sites by phenylbutazone, leading to warfarin toxicosis. Similarly, digoxin may be displaced from protein binding sites by NSAIDs, resulting in increased plasma digoxin concentrations. The concurrent administration of aminoglycoside antimicrobials with NSAIDs may potentiate the risk of nephrotoxicity, even though the toxic effects of each drug group occur at different sites.

40. Is there a therapeutic rationale for the simultaneous administration of two different NSAIDs to the same horse?

Two different NSAIDs administered together are additive in their actions, including toxic potential. All NSAIDs function via a similar mechanism of COX inhibition; however, differences exist in their activity, toxicity, and elimination. Although clinically it may make sense to administer one NSAID that has superior antiinflammatory activity along with an NSAID that has greater antipyretic activity, it is difficult to rationalize combined usage because of the great risk of NSAID-induced toxicosis.

41. Are there any restrictions on the administration of NSAIDs, particularly to performance horses in the United States?

The use of NSAIDs in performance horses has been controversial for many years. Many racing jurisdictions in the United States as well as the American Horse Show Association permit the limited use of NSAIDs in competition. However, phenylbutazone, flunixin, and recently ketoprofen are restricted to certain concentrations in blood or urine. The question whether to allow horses to compete during treatment with analgesic drugs such as NSAIDs centers on the potential masking of pain or trauma, which may allow the horse to suffer further damage.

42. Are there differences in clinical efficacy among NSAIDs for specific conditions?

Despite the fact that the general mechanism of action of NSAIDs is similar, clinical impressions and experience over the years have led to preferences in NSAIDs for particular conditions. For example, phenylbutazone is often the treatment of choice for locomotor disorders such as navicular disease and laminitis. Flunixin meglumine or ketoprofen is often the NSAID of choice for treatment of abdominal pain or colic in horses. However, limited research suggests that flunixin meglumine may offer great pain relief for horses with osteoarthritis. There is a significant cost difference in the administration of oral phenylbutazone vs. flunixin meglumine/ketoprofen.

BIBLIOGRAPHY

1. Brooks PM, Day RO: Nonsteroidal antiinflammatory drugs—differences and similarities. N Engl J Med 324:1716–1725, 1991.
2. Kallings P: Nonsteroidal antiinflammatory drugs. Vet Clin North Am Equine Pract 9:523–541, 1993.
3. Lees P, Higgins AJ: Clinical pharmacology and therapeutic uses of non-steroidal antiinflammatory drugs in the horse. Equine Vet J 17:83–96, 1985.
4. MacAllister CG, Morgan SJ, Borne AT, et al: Comparison of adverse effects of phenylbutazone, flunixin meglumine, and ketoprofen in horses. J Am Vet Med Assoc 202:71–77, 1993.
5. May SA, Lees P: Nonsteroidal antiinflammatory drugs. In McIlwraith CW, Trotter GW (eds): Joint Disease in the Horse. Philadelphia, W.B. Saunders, 1996.
6. Semrad SD, Hardee GE, Hardee MM, et al: Low dose flunixin meglumine: Effects on eicosanoid production and clinical signs induced by experimental endotoxaemia in horses. Equine Vet J 19:201–206, 1987.

23. EPIDEMIOLOGY

David A. Dargatz, D.V.M., M.S., Ph.D., Dip. ACVIM,
and Josie L. Traub-Dargatz, D.V.M., M.S., Dip. ACVIM

DEFINITIONS

1. What is epidemiology?

Epidemiology is the study of patterns of disease in populations or groups.

2. What is the definition of molecular epidemiology?

Molecular epidemiology is the use of genetic typing techniques to determine the source and patterns of disease caused by or among specific subtypes of organisms. It may include the subtyping of disease agents or the evaluation of predisposition to disease by hosts. For example, plasmid DNA fragments can be evaluated by pulsed-field gel electrophoresis (PFGE) to determine whether the bacteria from different animals during an outbreak are the same. In addition, it can be used to determine the relatedness of organisms from diseased animals from different geographic areas.

3. What is the definition of descriptive epidemiology?

Descriptive epidemiology is the characterization of the level and distribution of disease for various subgroups in the population (e.g., age, sex, use, location, time of year).

4. What is the definition of analytic epidemiology?

Analytic epidemiology makes use of statistical techniques to draw inferences about disease occurrence and potential causal associations in populations (i.e., the study of the determinants of disease).

OUTBREAK INVESTIGATION

5. What is the definition of an outbreak?

An outbreak is the occurrence of disease at a frequency above expected levels.

6. What is outbreak investigation?

Outbreak investigation is the structured approach to data gathering that eventually leads to discovery of factors related to occurrence of disease that can be controlled. Controllable factors may then be used in intervention strategies.

7. What are five key questions in an outbreak investigation?

1. Who is affected?
2. What is the problem (case definition)?
3. When is the disease occurring?
4. Where is the disease occurring?
5. Why is the disease occurring?

8. What is a case definition?

A case definition clearly describes the attributes or characteristics of an animal that allow it to be included in the outbreak investigation (e.g., the feces are culture-positive for *Salmonella* sp.).

9. What types of measures are used to quantitate disease occurrence?

• Prevalence (e.g., proportion)
• Incidence (e.g., rate)
• Born dead:born alive in a litter (e.g., ratio)

10. What is the definition of prevalence?

Prevalence is the percentage of a group affected or diseased at any point in time (i.e., a proportion).

11. What is the definition of incidence?

Incidence is the number of new cases per unit of time (i.e., a rate).

12. What is the definition of attack rate?

The attack rate is the percentage of exposed population that develops the disease/problem.

13. What is the definition of case fatality rate?

The case fatality rate is the percentage of cases that die (see question 8 for the definition of case).

14. What is the definition of attributable rate?

(Attack rate in exposed) minus (attack rate in unexposed) = attributable rate = $[a/(a + b)]$ − $[c/(c + d)]$

	Disease	**No Disease**	
Exposed	a	b	Exposed = a + b
Unexposed	c	d	Unexposed = c + d
	Diseased = a + c	No disease = b + d	

15. How is the attributable rate useful?

The attributable rate gives an indication of how many cases of disease are attributable to the exposure and how many are related to other factors. For example, if among 100 horses exposed to a particular feed, 60 were ill and among 100 horses not exposed to the feed 10 were ill, the attributable rate would be 0.6 minus 0.1 = 0.5. From this attributable rate it is apparent that the feed is likely to be related to the illness and that it accounts for a relatively large proportion of cases.

16. What is the definition of a risk factor?

A risk factor is a factor that is associated with increased occurrence of an event, usually disease. Generally, a portion of the population is exposed and a portion is not exposed (unexposed) to this risk factor. Epidemiologists often seek to identify risk factors as the basis for developing control strategies.

DIAGNOSTIC TESTING

17. What is the definition of sensitivity?

Sensitivity = percent of true positives (diseased or infected animals) that test positive (100 − percent of false negatives). The true status (i.e., positive or negative) of a given animal is based on some best estimate of the truth relative to the disease or infection status of the animal. This best estimate of truth (i.e., the gold standard) may be based on a different laboratory test, a clinical parameter, or a postmortem finding. Depending on the choice of the standard for comparison (gold standard), the sensitivity and specificity of a test under evaluation may vary despite the assumption that they are constant. For example, if the gold standard is seroconversion to influenza and clinical signs consistent with influenza, the sensitivity of the Directogen test to detect influenza virus in nasal secretions is 45%. If the gold standard is isolation of the influenza virus, the sensitivity of the test is 83%.

18. What is the false-negative rate if the sensitivity of a test is 83%?

% false negatives = 100 − sensitivity (83%) = 17%.

19. What is the definition of specificity?

Specificity = percent of true negatives (nondiseased or noninfected animals) that test negative (100 − percent of false positive). Using the Directogen example from question 17, the specificity of the test is 98% with seroconversion and clinical signs as the gold standard and 78% with virus isolation as the gold standard.

20. What is the false-positive rate if the specificity of test is 98%?
% false positives = 100 − specificity (98%) = 2%.

21. In the chart below, define the effect of choosing each of the test result cutoff points—A, B, or C—on sensitivity and specificity.

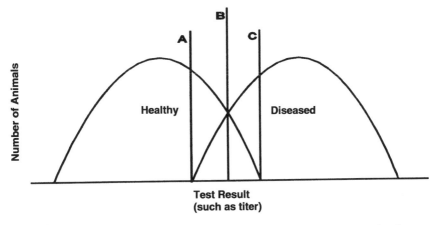

- The choice of cutoff A results in a test with 100% sensitivity, which means that there are no false-negative results, but there would be false-positive results among healthy animals.
- The choice of cufoff B results in a test with less than 100% sensitivity and specificity, which means that there would be false-negative results in some diseased animals and false-positive results in some normal animals.
- The choice of cutoff C results in a test with 100% specificity, which means that there are no false-positive results, but there would be false-negative results in the diseased population.

22. What is the definition of predictive value positive?
Predictive value positive (PVP) is the percentage of test-positive animals that are truly positive (diseased or infected) for the disease or problem for which they are tested.

23. What is the formula for calculating PVP?

$$PVP = \frac{\text{number of true-positive animals that test positive}}{\text{number of animals that test positive}}$$

24. What is the definition of PVN?
Predictive value negative (PVN) is the percentage of test-negative animals that are truly negative (nondiseased or noninfected) for the disease or problem for which they are tested.

25. What is the formula for calculating predictive value negative?

$$PVN = \frac{\text{number of true-negative animals that test negative}}{\text{number of animals that test negative}}$$

26. Can you calculate PVP and PVN based on sensitivity and specificity of a test alone?
No. You need to know the prevalence of the disease or problem in the tested population or the likelihood of disease in the tested animal. For example, the likelihood of equine protozoal myelitis (EPM) in a horse showing classic signs of EPM makes the PVP much higher than if a

neurologically normal animal is tested. When the prevalence or likelihood of a specific condition is 100%, there is no value in testing and the PVP and PVN become moot.

Formulas for Sensitivity, Specificity, PVP, and PVN

	TRUE DIAGNOSIS		
	POSITIVE	NEGATIVE	
Positive test result	a	b	a + b
Negative test result	c	d	c + d
	a + c	b + d	a + b + c + d

Sensitivity = a/(a + c)
Specificity = d/(b + d)
PVP = a/(a + b)
PVN = d/(c + d)
False positives = b
False negatives = c
Prevalence of disease in population is (a + c)

Predictive Values of Positive and Negative

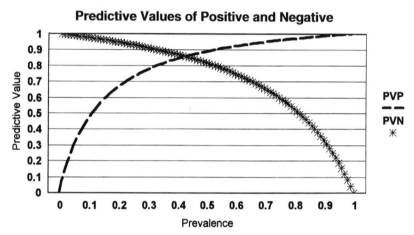

PVP increases with increasing prevalence of disease, whereas PVN decreases with increasing prevalence of disease (given a constant sensitivity and specificity for a test).

27. What is testing in parallel?

Testing in parallel is the performance of multiple tests (usually of different types) for the same disease or problem. The animal is considered diseased, infected, or abnormal if *any* test is positive. Testing in parallel uses the *or* rule: if test 1 *or* test 2 is positive, the animal is considered positive.

28. What is testing in series?

Testing in series is the performance of multiple tests for the same disease or problem. The animal is considered positive only if *both* tests or *all* tests are positive. Testing in series uses the *and* rule: if test 1 *and* test 2 are positive, the animal is considered positive.

29. What is the impact of using tests in parallel?

Parallel testing increases sensitivity of the testing process; in other words, testing in parallel results in fewer false negatives.

30. What is the impact of using tests in series?

Series testing increases the specificity of the testing process; in other words, testing in series results in fewer false positives.

31. If the consequences of a false-negative test are very high (e.g., introduction of a foreign animal disease into the U.S.), should you use parallel or series testing method?

Parallel testing minimizes the likelihood of allowing a test-negative animal with disease (i.e., false-negative animal) into the country.

32. If the consequences of a false positive test were very high (e.g., test and slaughter implications), should you use tests in parallel or series?

Series testing minimizes the likelihood of slaughtering the disease- or infection-negative animal that tested positive (i.e., false-positive animal).

33. Distinguish between accuracy and precision.

Precision is defined as the variation in values about some mean or average value (i.e., are the values tightly clustered or spread out?). Accuracy is defined as how the test result reflects the true state of nature (i.e., how well the mean value from a group of tests reflects the true mean).

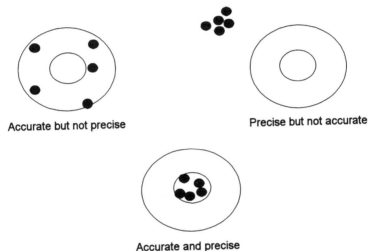

Accuracy and precision of various test results.

MEASURES OF CENTRAL TENDENCY, RISK, OR DIFFERENCES

34. What is the mean?

The mean or average is calculated by adding the values for all members of the group and dividing by the number of members in the group; for example, the mean of the packed cell volume (PCV) of 21 horses at a trainer's barn. To calculate the mean PCV, add PCV values of all 21 horses and divide by 21.

PCV values (%) of all 21 horses =

23	33	46	34	37
45	49	42	32	
38	40	36	31	
35	41	45	46	
42	45	47	48	

The mean PCV(%) = $(21 + 45 + 38 + \ldots + 37)/21 = 835/21 = 39.8$

35. What is the median?

The median is the middle value for the group if the values for the group are sorted in ascending or descending order. If there are an even number of values, the median is the value midway between the two middle values. To find the median for the PCV of 21 horses at a trainer's barn, list all 21 PCV values in ascending order. The value for the 11th horse is the median. In this example, the median PCV = 41%.

PCV (%) =	23	31	32	33	34	35	36	37	38	40	**41**
	42	42	45	45	45	46	46	47	48	49	

36. What is the geometric mean?
Take the log of each measured value (e.g., serum antibody titer), determine the mean, and then take the antilog of the mean.

37. When should you use the geometric mean?
Geometric means are usually used as a measure of central tendency among values that are nonlinear; for example, antibody titers in which the values increase by 2-fold dilutions. Serum neutralization titers for equine viral arteritis (EVA) are < 1:4, 1:4, 1:8, 1:16, and so on. Thus, extreme values can have a large effect on the mean.

38. What is an odds ratio?

	Diseased	Not Diseased	Total
Exposed	a	b	a + b
Unexposed	c	d	c + d
	a + c	b + d	n = a + b + c + d

The odds of having the disease among the exposed animals (i.e., a/b) divided by the odds of having the disease among the unexposed animals (i.e., c/d) is (a/b)/c/d), which simplifies to (ad/bc). For situations in which the disease is relatively rare (e.g., 10% or less of animals are affected), odds ratios are good approximations of relative risk.

39. What is the standard deviation?
The standard deviation is a measure of the variability in the data among individuals within a group. If the data are normally distributed (i.e., bell-shaped curve), approximately 95% of the observations fall within 2 standard deviations of the calculated mean. The standard deviation (s) is calculated as follows:

$$s = \sqrt{\frac{\Sigma(y_i - y)^2}{n - 1}}$$

where y_i = the value of the ith observation (i ranges from 1 to n, the total number of observations), y = the mean of the y_i values, and n = the number of y_i values. The standard deviation and measures of central tendency (e.g., mean and median) are calculated by many software packages, but understanding the concept of how these measures are calculated helps to understand the results.

40. What is a standard error?
The standard error is also a measure of variability in the data from a group. A confidence interval can be calculated for a population (e.g., a mean or total) using the standard error. Chances are 95% that the interval created by the estimate ± two standard errors will contain the true population value. The standard error (se) is calculated as follows:

$$se = \frac{s}{\sqrt{n}}$$

where s = the standard deviation and n = the number of observations.

41. What is the relative risk?
The relative risk (rr) is the proportion of the exposed population with the disease divided by the proportion of the unexposed population with disease.

$$(rr = [a/(a + b)] / [c/(c + d)])$$

42. What is the p-value?

The p-value is an estimate of the likelihood that the difference observed between groups may have arisen by chance alone.

43. What does p < 0.05 mean?

When two values (e.g., mean response value for two treatment groups) are compared statistically and a p-value of less than 0.05 is determined, there is less than a 5% chance that this difference arose by chance alone (i.e., not as a result of the treatment), provided there are not other biases in the ways the animals were allocated to the treatment groups. By convention, $p < 0.05$ is used to assign statistical significance; however, the use of other levels of p-value may be quite reasonable based on different circumstances.

44. What is power?

Power is the likelihood of finding a statistical difference between two groups if in fact one exists. The power for a particular study design can be calculated by making some assumptions about the magnitude of the expected differences in the outcomes of two groups. In this way the investigator can determine whether the design has sufficient power that the experiment should be undertaken or whether a new design should be considered.

EPIDEMIOLOGIC STUDY TYPE OR DESIGN

45. What is a cohort study?

In a cohort study, a group of individuals is identified for inclusion in the study based on some exposure of interest (i.e., exposed and unexposed groups). Data about the groups (exposed and unexposed) may be gathered retrospectively or prospectively.

46. What is randomization?

Randomization is the use of some method to assign individuals to groups so that each individual has a known non-zero chance to be in each group. Thus the potential for bias is minimized (e.g., random numbers table used to assign treatments to study subjects).

47. What is a cross-sectional study?

In a cross-sectional study, individuals are enrolled without regard to status of exposure to a risk factor or the presence or absence of the outcome of interest. For example, enrollment of all horses in a geographic region to look at risk factors for seropositivity to a disease agent without regard to exposure status constitutes a cross-sectional study.

48. What is an inference population?

An inference population is the larger population of individuals represented by those actually studied. For example, a study of foals on 10 randomly selected farms in Washington state revealed that if a good perinatal hygiene program was used on their dams, the risk of diarrhea in neonatal foals was reduced. If one applies this finding to all neonatal foals in the U.S., all neonatal foals in the U.S. are the inference population.

49. What is a clinical or field trial?

A clinical or field trial is a planned comparison of the outcome for groups or individuals receiving different treatments (e.g., vaccine vs. no vaccine).

50. What is a case control study?

In a case control study, a group of individuals with the disease of interest (i.e., animals meeting the case definition) is enrolled and a comparison group without the disease (i.e., controls) is also selected for study. The analysis usually focuses on the different exposures between the two groups that may account for their outcome status (i.e., cases or controls).

DATA TYPES

51. What are ordinal data?

Variables or factors with an ordered level in which differences between categories cannot necessarily be considered equal (e.g., coding severity of lameness as grade 0 [not lame] to grade 4 [non–weight-bearing]). Although grade 2 lameness is worse than grade 1 lameness, the difference between grades 1 and 2 cannot easily be equated with the difference between grades 2 and 3.

52. What are continuous data?

Variables or factors with any numerical potential outcome within a certain range (e.g., age).

53. What are interval data?

Variables or factors that are numerical with consistent distance between values, but zero is an arbitrary point.

54. What are nominal data?

Factors that are not numerical and have no logical order or named categories (e.g., breed of animal or yes/no outcome; yes = presence of cancer, no = absence of cancer).

BIBLIOGRAPHY

1. Chambers TM, Shortridge PH, Powell DG, Watkins KL: Rapid diagnosis of equine influenza by the Directogen Flu-A enzyme immunoassay. Vet Rec 135:275–279, 1994.
2. Dargatz DA, Salman MD: Application of epidemiologic principles and methods to investigating and controlling equine infectious diseases. Update on infectious diseases. Vet Clin North Am 9:247–257, 1993.
3. Martin SW, Meek AH, Willeberg P: Veterinary Epidemiology: Principles and Methods. Ames, IA, Iowa State Press, 1987.
4. Morely PS, Bogdan JR, Townsend HGG, Hanes DM: Evaluation of Directogen Flu-A assay for detection of influenza antigen in nasal secretion of horses. Equine Vet J 27:131–134, 1995.
5. Norman GR, Steiner DL: Biostatistics: The Bare Essentials. St. Louis, Mosby, 1994.
6. Rothman KJ: Modern Epidemiology. Boston, Little, Brown, 1986.
7. Smith RD: Veterinary Clinical Epidemiology: A Problem-Oriented Approach. Stoneham, MA, Butterworth-Heinemann, 1991.
8. Traub-Dargatz JL, Dargatz DA: Clinical epidemiology: Application to laboratory data. Clinical Pathology. Vet Clin North Am 11:515–524, 1995.

INDEX

Page numbers in **boldface type** indicate complete chapters.